DENTAL COCKTAIL

The Ultimate Treasure for MDS Entrance Examinations

DENTAL COCKTAIL

The Ultimate Treasure for MDS Entrance Examinations

SECOND EDITION

Thoroughly Revised and Updated

- AIIMS Dental (Nov 2014)
- AIIMS Medical (Nov 2014)
- AIIMS SRship Questions 2014 Set A
- AIIMS SR Papers 2014 Set B
- AIIMS Unreleased SR Papers
- AIIMS Endodontics Question Bank
- AIIMS Perio Question Bank
- E-Course MCQs
- COHEN's MCQs
- High-yield Facts
- Numerical Corner
- AIIMS Anesthesia Question Bank
- AIIMS Physiology SR Papers
- Trauma MCQs Set A
- Trauma MCQs Set B
- Perio Innovations
- OMFS SR Paper (Jan 2015)
- Orthodontics SR Paper (Jan 2015)
- Prosthodontics SR Paper (Jan 2015)
- AIIMS SRship Paper (July 2014)
- Some Important High-yield Facts from OP Kharbanda
- Endodontics SR Questions
- Additional Questions of Periodontics SRship (July 2014)
- Medical AIIMS (May 2015)
- AIPG 2015
- AIIMS Dental (May 2015)
- Prosthodontics SR Papers (July 2015)
- Oral Surgery SR Papers (July 2015)

Manikandan GR
Junior Resident
Department of Periodontics
Government Dental College
Thiruvananthapuram, Kerala, India

Forewords
Sivakumar Nuvvula
S Gowri Sankar
Presanthila Janam

JAYPEE *The Health Sciences Publisher*
New Delhi | London | Panama | Philadelphia

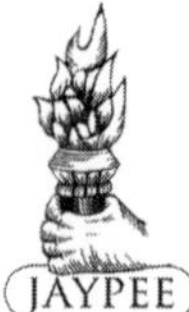

Jaypee Brothers Medical Publishers (P) Ltd

Headquarters

Jaypee Brothers Medical Publishers (P) Ltd.
4838/24, Ansari Road, Daryaganj
New Delhi 110 002, India
Phone: +91-11-43574357
Fax: +91-11-43574314
Email: jaypee@jaypeebrothers.com

Overseas Offices

J.P. Medical Ltd.
83, Victoria Street, London
SW1H 0HW (UK)
Phone: +44-20 3170 8910
Fax: +44-(0)20 3008 6180
Email: info@jpmedpub.com

JP Medical Inc.
325 Chestnut Street, Ste 412
Philadelphia, PA 19106
Phone: + 1-267-519-9789
Email: support@jpmedus.com

Jaypee Brothers Medical Publishers (P) Ltd.
Bhotahity, Kathmandu, Nepal
Phone: +977-9741283608
Email: kathmandu@jaypeebrothers.com

Jaypee-Highlights Medical Publishers Inc.
City of Knowledge, Bld. 237, Clayton
Panama City, Panama
Phone: +1 507-301-0496
Fax: +1 507-301-0499
Email: cservice@jphmedical.com

Jaypee Brothers Medical Publishers (P) Ltd.
17/1-B, Babar Road, Block-B, Shaymali
Mohammadpur, Dhaka-1207, Bangladesh
Mobile: +08801912003485
Email: jaypeedhaka@gmail.com

Website: www.jaypeebrothers.com
Website: www.jaypeedigital.com

Dental Cocktail

First Edition: 2015
(Published by author)

***Second Edition:* 2016**

ISBN: 978-93-5250-055-0

Printed at Gopsons Papers Ltd

Dedicated to

My Saviour Lord Ganesha
The God of Wisdom

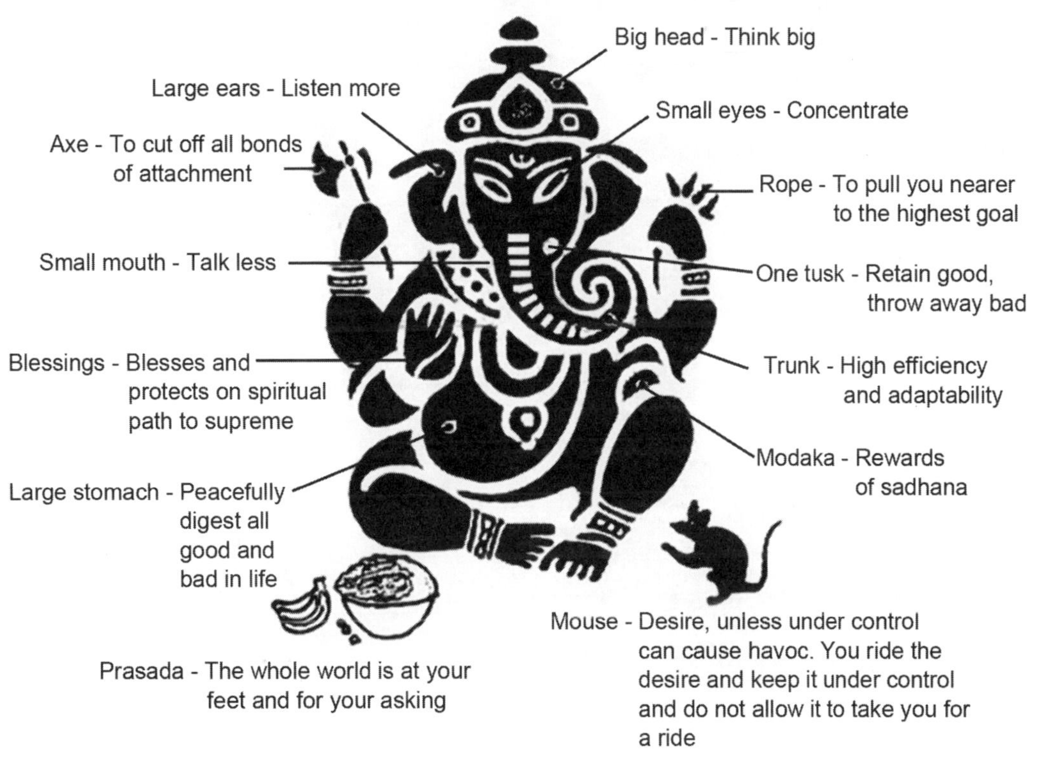

Foreword to the Second Edition

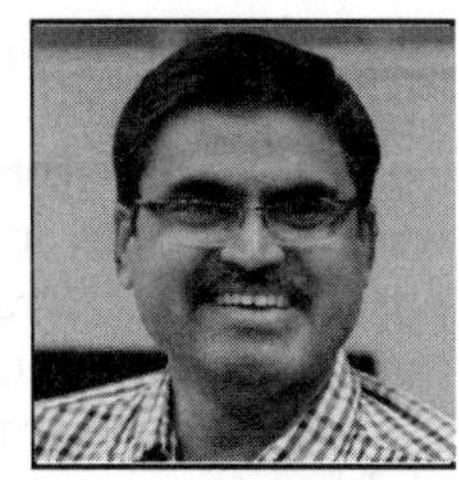

I am happy to write a foreword to this book 'Dental Cocktail' by Dr Manikandan GR, whom I know for the past few years. I knew him as an enthusiastic undergraduate student of dentistry, an aspirant of postgraduation in dentistry, who not only achieved his goal, but also helped many other aspirants achieve their goals. I remember his discussions during the preparation for PG entrance examinations on various Facebook and Whatsapp groups with many faculties across India as well as the fellow aspirants. With that experience, he has compiled many books for PG aspirants at the State and National level. He had presented some papers on oral and dental health at various platforms of State and National level and also published numerous articles and papers in various magazines and journals.

I have learnt that the second edition has a compilation of recent AIPG and AIIMS PG entrance papers, AIIMS SR papers, high-yielding facts from various standard textbooks as well as MCQs on various topics of medicine and dentistry to name a few. I am confident that this new edition will surely help the aspirants of various PG entrance examinations, and I wish Dr Manikandan GR all the success in this endeavor.

Sivakumar Nuvvula
MDS FICD
Professor and Head
Department of Pedodontics
Former Principal
Narayana Dental College and Hospital
Nellore, Andhra Pradesh, India

Foreword to the Second Edition

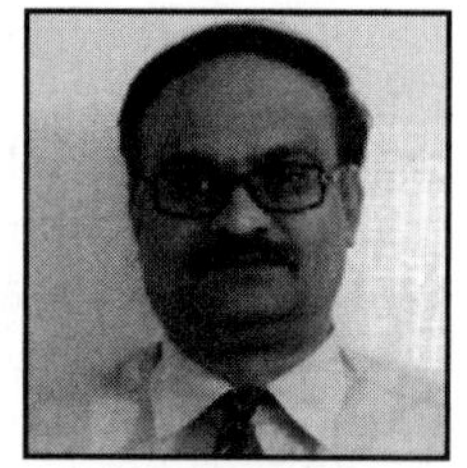

I am very much delighted to write a foreword to this small piece of great work by Manikandan. I have more than one reason to cherish. First of all, he is known to have a penchant for this type of literary work. I have seen him as a studious aspirant preparing for the MDS entrance, who transmuted into a person who inspires and guides the students for the preparation of postgraduate examinations in a proper channel. His zeal is highly infectious, especially to the young aspirants and has been very active on social media. His contribution to the field of patient's education and academic dental works in National and International works is highly commendable. He is selected into the PG course by AIPG. No doubt, anybody can guess without much anticipation the kind of smart work he can engender. The chapters are well written with brief points of importance that are very comprehensive to the core. This book will definitely be a valuable asset to those who are footing for the All India PG preparation and other state entrances. I wish Manikandan all the best in his future endeavors!.

S. Gowri Sankar

S Gowri Sankar
Professor
Department of Orthodontics
Narayana Dental College
Nellore, Andhra Pradesh, India

Foreword to the First Edition

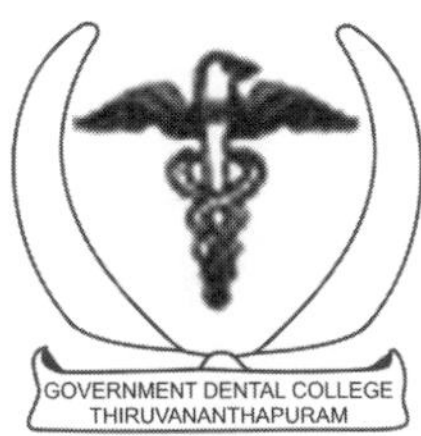

Dr Presanthila Janam, MDS
Principal

Government Dental College
Thiruvanathapuram–695011,
Kerala, India
Tel: (91)(471)2444092–40
Fax: 2444092–666
Mobile: 09387803891
Email: pjanamperio@gmail.com

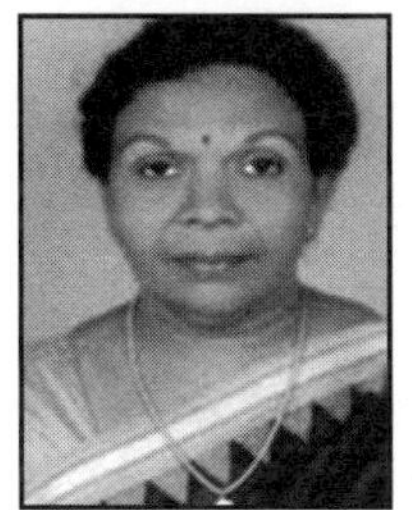

It is my great privilege to write a few words about the book Dental Cocktail, which is a great effort by Dr Manikandan GR. He is a very good student of mine, doing postgraduation in my department. He has won so many awards for various International, National and State scientific presentations within this period. The hallmark of this book is that it contains fully solved papers needed for the national-level examinations, like AIIMS and AIPG, in a simple and lucid manner. I am confident that this book will give a glance to all the related high-yield topics and will be informative and interesting for the MDS aspirants in dentistry. He deserves a hearty congratulations for all the efforts and hard work and I am sure this book will be of great help to the undergraduates gaining insight into the subjects.

Wishing this endeavour a grand success!!

Dr Presanthila Janam

Preface to the Second Edition

With warmth and happiness, I am scribbling the lines for the preface to the second edition of this book. I am happy with the overwhelming response to its first edition. I am indeed delighted to make out the second edition with the publishing tycoons, Jaypee Brothers Medical Publishers (P) Ltd. Let this effort kindle the fire of passion to seek knowledge in the proper direction in pursuit of clearing the MDS Entrance Examinations.

Wishing all my readers all the success in the name of Almighty!

When we share laughter, we share double the fun and when we share knowledge, we surpass what we had done.

Manikandan GR
e-mail: bellrings4u@gmail.com

Preface to the First Edition

"Two roads diverged in a wood, and I,
I took the one less travelled by,
And that has made all the difference."

Dreams are not which we see in the night only, real dreams are innovations with a heartfelt desire. The everlasting saga of knowledge and medical facts are such a treasure to cherish. I am happy to present before all my dear readers my sincere attempt to bring this book in a easy lucid and student friendly manner. It is indeed an amalgamation of my dreams and my efforts to make that dream come true. I hope my attempt will satisfy your thirst for a book of this manner, first ever in the history of MDS and filling the gap for a kind of book every aspirant was longing for. I hope this ray of light that I had lightened will kindle your souls with passion for reaching knowledge and go for this manner of academic endeavours. As in the poem by Robert Frost "The Road not taken" quoted above be ready to take the paths least travelled by and try to make a difference in your field rather than being idle.

Wishing all my readers prayers and success

Manikandan GR
e-mail: bellrings4u@gmail.com

Acknowledgments

First and foremost, I want to bend my head before the Almighty Lord Ganesha for helping me achieve this goal. I want to express my thanks to my mother, father, family and my dear friends who have always supported me. I would like to place a thanks note to my dear teachers right from my pre-primary till MDS, who had guided me, scolded me when it was needed and led me to the right path and supported me the most in each of my ventures. I would like to express my heartfelt thanks to my teacher Sister Fatima, who was my class teacher in the 4th standard and is now in her heavenly abode. She always inspired me to write. I am also thankful to my Teacher Usha, who filled in me a passion for literary works during my high-school classes.

I want to sincerely appreciate and thank my dear teacher and my Head of the Department Dr Presanthila Janam, who was kind enough to write a foreword to the first edition of this book and for being a constant source of inspiration for all my academic ventures. I am thankful to my dear friend Sarath SS, Junior Resident, OMFS Department, Government Dental College, Thiruvananthapuram, Kerala, India, who was always there during my MDS entrance preparation and provided me a lot of study material, which also were useful in expanding my level of knowledge.

I also want to acknowledge one of my teachers and a veteran dentist Dr C Venugopal, Civil Surgeon, General Hospital, Thiruvananthapuram; Mr Deepu and Ms Gopika, PROs, General Hospital, Thiruvananthapuram and my DEIC and dental department senior-house surgeons at General Hospital, Thiruvananthapuram, where I was working previously. They have always been so inspiring and motivating as far as my writing skills are concerned.

I also want to acknowledge one of my friends Anjana Ravindran (Junior Resident, PMS College of Dental Science & Research, Thiruvananthapuram), who had first inspired me to come up with my scientific publication.

I want to express my gratitude to the following gentlemen in dental entrance coaching for their love and support—Dr OP Kharbanda, Director, Dental Wing, Centre for Dental Education & Research, AIIMS, New Delhi; Dr Sivakumar Nuvvula, Professor and Head, Department of Pedodontics, Narayana Dental College, Nellore, Andhra Pradesh; Dr Jitendra Sharan, Research Scholar, Department of Orthodontics, AIIMS, New Delhi; Dr S Gowri Sankar, Professor, Department of Orthodontics, Narayana Dental College, Nellore, Andhra Pradesh; and Dr Sourabh Madaan, Director, Rx Dentistry.

I want to thank all my 'Dental Cocktail' Facebook and Whatsapp study-group members, who always encourage and inspire me to come up with ventures like this in a stipulated period of time.

I convey my sincere thanks to Jaypee Brothers Medical Publishers (P) Ltd, New Delhi, India for their efforts and suggestions, especially Shri Jitendar P Vij (Group Chairman), Mr Ankit Vij (Group President), Ms Chetna Vohra (Associate Director), and Ms Payal Bharti (Project Manager) for helping me through my idea. I am also grateful to Mr Venugopal, Head, Cochin Division, Kerala, Mr Arun and Mr Anoop, Thiruvananthapuram Division for helping me in the project.

Testimonials

I went through the content of this amazing book 'Dental Cocktail' written by my colleague Dr Manikandan GR, who is hardworking and always ready to bring out new things and ideas into practice. I really want to appreciate him for bringing out this much-needed book in a nice manner at the right time with well-explained keys and additional points which are high-yielding for the coming AIIMS and AIPG examinations. I am happy to see that he has included all high-yield areas and numericals as well as authentic SR Papers of AIIMS and various AIIMS Question Banks, which are crucial in getting the seat. I recommend this book to every MDS aspirant and wish this endeavor a grand success.

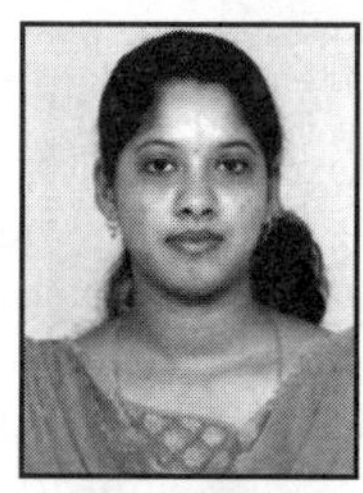

Dr Mary Diana (Rank 2)
AIIMS, November 2013

* * *

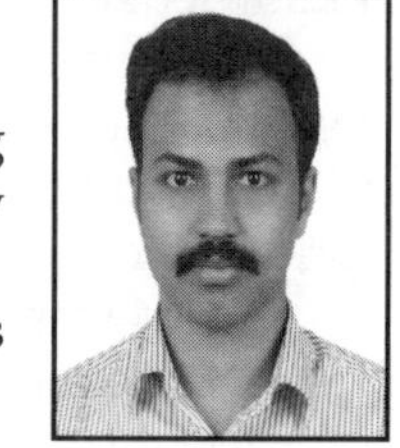

Dr Sajith Xavier (Rank 69)
AIPG 2016

'Dental Cocktail' is an essential ingredient towards the final preparation, which provides the recent AIIMS SR papers and AIIMS question banks. I am very thankful to Dr Manikandan Sir for this book.

* * *

I really want to appreciate the hard work of Dr Manikandan GR for bringing such a nice book 'Dental Cocktail' with authentic questions and explanatory answers from standard textbooks.
This book is very much useful for changing the question pattern of AIPGDEE. I recommend this book to every MDS aspirant and wishing all a great success.

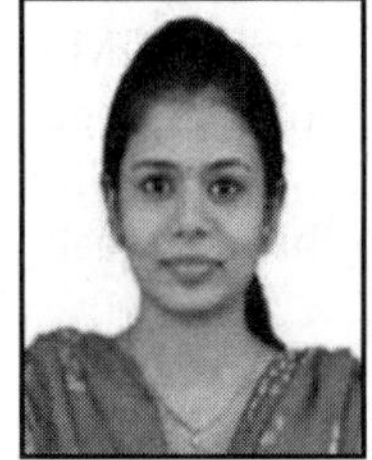

Dr Arun (Rank 76)
AIPG 2016

* * *

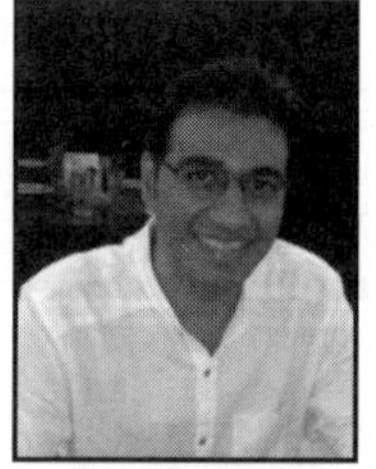

Dr Junia Devassy (Rank 148)
AIPG 2016

First of all, I want to congratulate my mentor Dr Manikandan GR on the publication of the second edition of his book 'Dental Cocktail'. It was illuminating to have the experience as a student under his guidance through his fabulous classes and Whatsapp study groups. This will indeed be a comprehensive book to guide the MDS aspirants with all the high-yield topics. I trust that the information will be of great assistance. Don't forget to grab one!!!

* * *

When the almighty is with you, you can achieve whatsoever you desire. So 'dream big! If it offends someone, so what?....dream bigger!'
And to fulfill the same, Dental Cocktail has played a major role and I sincerely want to thank Dr Manikandan for putting in best of his efforts to help the future aspirants reach their goal.
'To err is human.'

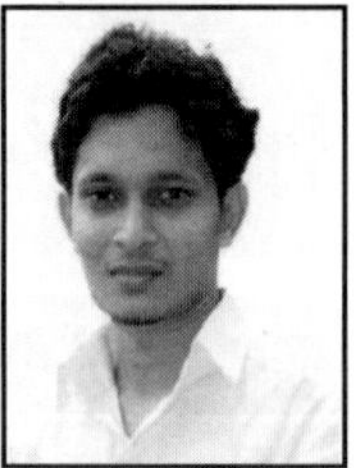

Lohit Arora
AIPG Dec 2015 (Rank 59)
PGI Nov 2015 (Rank 14)

* * *

Mohammed Fawaz (Rank 8)
AIPG 2015

Guys, never judge a book by the number of mistakes it has. You will never find a book without a single mistake. Instead, you should appreciate the hard work the author has put in to serve the best content. And, do always remember – 'Hard work beats the talent when the talent doesn't work hard'.

* * *

The most important task for the MDS aspirants is to collect the right matter for preparation; and your books undoubtedly stand among the top in this criteria for proper guidance.

* * *

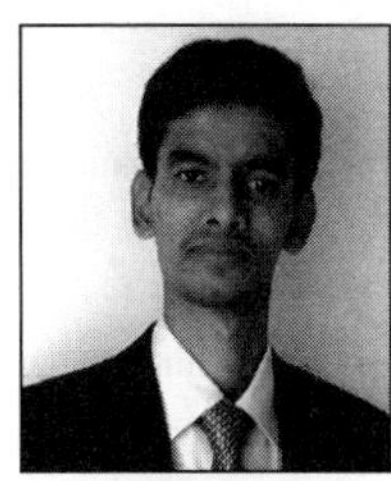
Muhammad Abdul Rahman TV (Rank 18) AIPG 2015

Right guidance and hard work are key to success. It is impossible to read all the books which are available in the market. But there are some books without which our dreams will not have been fulfilled. Thanks to Dr Manikandan GR for bringing out such books. I hope this book also will help the PG aspirants in achieving their goals.

* * *

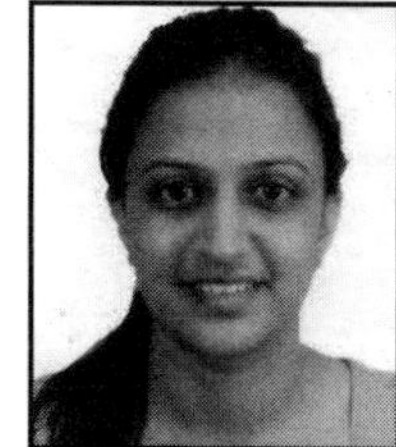
Bhagyashree (Rank 68) AIPG 2016

Getting a rank in AIPG Dental Entrance Examination as per the changed scenario requires hard work done in the correct direction.

This blend was provided to me by Dr Manikandan's sincere efforts in his DENTAL COCKTAIL BOOK SERIES AND GROUP DISCUSSIONS, which provided me with authentic papers and explanations to the points, which give it an extra edge. Keep up the great work for the benefit of the students.

* * *

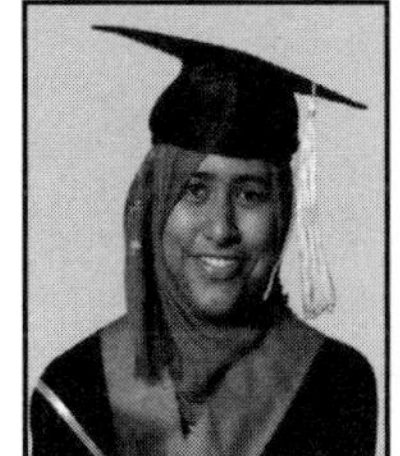
Nadira Rahman (Rank 5) AIPG 2015

Thank you Manikandan Sir for such a wonderful book and also for your inspiring 'Anybody Can Do' sessions!! The questions given in Dental Cocktail have proved to be very helpful for my examinations. Solving the SR papers has definitely reinforced my knowledge by cracking difficult questions. I strongly recommend it, especially for all the AIIMS and AIPGE aspirants. Thank you 'Dental Cocktail' and wishing you all the best for a very bright future!!

* * *

Contents

AIIMS Dental (Nov 2014)

1. **False about Phenotype is:**
   a. It is modified with passage of time
   b. It is influenced by genotype
   c. It is the genetic sequence of an individual
   d. Associated with morphological appearance
   Ans. c

Ref: Dictionary of Genetics Straight pick from AIIMS SR Ship

2. **TEN Scan be explained on the basis of:**
   a. Referred pain
   b. Allodynia
   c. Central Pain Inhibition Theory
   d. Gate Control Theory
   Ans. d

Ref: Peterson 2/e p956

3. **Platelet adhesion to collagen occurs through:**
   a. Factor IX
   b. Factor VIII
   c. Fibrinogen
   d. VWF
   Ans. d

Ref: Robbin's 8/e p116-118

4. **Auriculotemporal nerve is encircled by:**
   a. Superficial temporal vein
   b. Middle Meningeal Artery
   c. Superficial Temporal Artery
   d. Anterior Tympanic Artery
   Ans. B

Ref: BD Chourasia 4/e vol 3 p155

5. **All of the following are used as disinfectants except:**
   a. 5% chloroxylenol
   b. 1–2% cetrimide
   c. 100% alcohol
   d. 2% Lysol
   Ans. c

Ref: Ananthanarayan 7/e p30

6. **Antirabies vaccine is not given in case of:**
   a. Rat bite
   b. Cat bite
   c. Dog bite
   d. Monkey bite
   Ans. a

Ref: Harrison 18/e p1611-1616, Direct pick from AIIMS SR July 2014

7. **DPT Vaccine is not given in A/E:**
   a. Drug Reaction
   b. Severely immunocompromised state
   c. Previous allergic reaction
   d. Degenerating severe neurologic disease

   Ans. b

   Ref: CDC Recommendations regarding vaccines and immunisation

8. **False about Hemophilus Influenzae is:**
   a. Capsular polypeptide protein plays an important role in pathogenicity
   b. Needs Factor X and V for growth in culture media
   c. Most common invasive manifestation is meningitis
   d. Rare cause of meningitis in the first two months of life

   Ans. a

   Ref: Ananthanarayan 7/e p329-331

9. **The virological marker indicating active multiplication of Hepatitis B is:**
   a. Anti HbS
   b. HbeAb
   c. IgM AntiHbc
   d. HbsAg

   Ans. b

   Ref: Ananthanarayan 7/e p555

10. **All are true about Vibrio cholera except:**
    a. It is a gram positive bacteria
    b. It activates adenyl cyclase
    c. The toxin is named as cholera toxin
    d. Loss of water and Sodium ions happens in diarrhea

    Ans. a

    Ref: Ananthanarayan 7/e p305

11. **The element playing the role of a second messenger is:**
    a. Iron
    b. Magnesium
    c. Sodium
    d. Calcium

    Ans. d

    Ref: Gurkeerat Singh 2/e p222

12. **The structure that develops from second branchial arch is:**
    a. Condyle
    b. Mandible
    c. Muscles of mastication
    d. Muscles of facial expression

    Ans. d

    Ref: Langman's Embryology 10/e p367-68

13. **Which element is vital for wound healing?**
    a. Copper
    b. Ruthenium
    c. Silver
    d. Lithium

    Ans. a

    Ref: Vasudevanand Sreekumari Biochemistry 4/e p312

14. All are components of posterior triangle of neck except:
   a. EJV
   b. Phrenic Nerve
   c. Subclavian vein
   d. Hypoglossal nerve
   Ans. d

Ref: BD Chaurasia 4/e Vol 3 p72

15. When phagosome combines with lysosomes, phagolysosome forms which helps to kill intracellular bacteria by:
   a. NADPH oxidase
   b. Catalase
   c. Superoxide dismutase
   d. Peroxidase
   Ans. a

Ref: Robbin's 7/e p60, 16

16. All are part of megaloblastic anemia except:
   a. Mild to moderate splenomegaly
   b. Nucleated erythrocytes
   c. Raised bilirubin
   d. Rise in reticulocyte count
   Ans. d

Ref: Harrison 18/e ch105

17. Nausea and Vomiting is caused due to A/E:
   a. Ingested blood
   b. Acetaminophen
   c. Nitrous oxide
   d. Opiod
   Ans. b

Ref: Peterson 2/e p100

18. DOC for acute bacterial meningitis is:
   a. Cefoperazone
   b. Ceftriaxone
   c. Vancomycin
   d. Spectinomycin
   Ans. b

Ref: KD Tripathi 6/e p435

19. A 45-year-old female patient who is on insulin was brought to casualty in loss of consciousness, first line of management will be:
   a. IV Dextrose
   b. IV Corticosteroids
   c. OGTT
   d. Parenteral Insulin Administration
   Ans. d

Ref: Bailey and Love 24/e p1132

20. A patient who is refractory to multiple platelet transfusions can be dealt with:
   a. Platelet irradiation
   b. Random platelet transfusion
   c. Single donor transfusion
   d. HLA Matched platelet
   Ans. d

Ref: Harrison 18/e chap 54 p 3107

21. A lady with an age of 29 years with a pregnancy of 17 weeks and has a 10 year old boy with Down's syndrome. She does not want another Down syndrome. The best advice to her is:
   a. No test is required now as her age is below 35 years
   b. Ultrasound at this point of time will definitely tell her that next baby will be Down syndromic or not
   c. Amniotic fluid samples plus chromosomal analysis will definitely tell her that next baby will be Down syndromic or not
   d. Blood screening at this point of time will clear the exact picture
   Ans. c

Ref: Fernando Arios, High risk pregnancy p 45

22. All of the following are part of delayed transfusion reaction except:
   a. Positive DAT test
   b. Hemoglobinuria
   c. Reduced Hb
   d. Spherocytes positive
   Ans. d

Ref: Bailey and Love 25/e p21

23. Which statement about Carbamazepine is true:
   a. It is a nephrotoxic drug
   b. Serum level is more than 40 mg/ml to be fatal
   c. Serum level and rate of convulsions are unrelated
   d. It is used in the prophylaxis of migraine
   Ans. c

Ref: KD Tripathi 6/e p406

24. When Local anaesthetic is applied along with adrenaline into vessel then:
   a. Hypertension with tachycardia
   b. Hypotension with bradycardia
   c. Hypotension with tachycardia
   d. Hypertension with bradycardia
   Ans. a

Ref: Applied pharmacology by Stan. K. Bardal p337

25. All acts by competitive inhibition except:
   a. Simvastatin
   b. Sulfadiazine
   c. DFP
   d. Methotrexate
   Ans. c

Ref: KD Tripathi 6/e p614, 39

26. Office personal who are at high-risk of Nitrous oxidetoxicity, to prevent them the most sensitive test for Nitrous oxide detection is:
   a. Dosimeter
   b. Infrared spectrophotometer
   c. High Suction speed
   d. Laminar flow
   Ans. b

Ref: McDonald 8/e p296

27. Patient with prosthetic valves is planned for surgery. True statement is:
   a. Antibiotic prophylaxis is not mandatory
   b. Antibiotic prophylaxis is mandatory
   c. No specific precautions are required
   d. Oral bacteria and systemic disease are not correlated
   Ans. b

Ref: Peterson 2/e p23

28. Least shelf life is shown by:

a. Polyether
b. Addition silicon
c. Condensation silicon
d. Polysulphides

Ans. c

Ref: Philips 11/e p213

29. The second amalgam war was associated with:

a. Alfred Stock
b. Charles Bell
c. Green Black
d. Huggins

Ans. a

Ref: Sherwood Essentials of Operative Dentistry p332

30. Tooth size is affected in which stage of development?

a. Initiation
b. Histodifferentiation
c. Morphodifferentiation
d. Apposition

Ans. c

Ref: McDonald's Pediatric Dentistry 8/e p53

31. Common fact with respect to porcelain and amalgam is:

a. Decreased compressive strength and raised tensile strength
b. Raised compressive strength and reduced tensile strength
c. Decreased working and setting time
d. Increased working and setting time

Ans. b

Ref: Philips 11/e p512

32. In biopsy true about formalin as fixative is all except:

a. To prevent autolysis
b. To make tissue rigid
c. To kill micro organisms
d. 2 % formalin is used

Ans. d

Ref: Shafer's 6/e p922

33. HOX gene mutations are responsible for:

a. Polysyndactyly
b. Goltz syndrome
c. Gorlin syndrome
d. Holoprosencephaly

Ans. a

Ref: Robbins 7/e p475

34. Polymerisation shrinkage is:

a. Density changes from 0.94 gm/cm3 to 1.19 gm/cm3 and volume shrinkage is 21%
b. Density changes from 1.19 gm/cm3 to 0.94 gm/cm3 and volume shrinkage is 21%
c. Density changes from 0.94 gm/cm3 to 1.19 gm/cm3 and volume shrinkage is 7%
d. Density changes from 1.19 gm/cm3 to 0.94 gm/cm3 and volume shrinkage is 7 %

Ans. a

Ref: Philips 11/e p739

35. All of the following are animal tests for biocompatibility except:
   a. Ames Test
   b. LD50
   c. Buehler Test
   d. Implantation
   Ans. a

Ref: Philps 11/e p188

36. Most mucostatic impression material is:
   a. Alginate
   b. Plaster of Paris
   c. ZOE
   d. Impression Compound
   Ans. b

Ref: Philips 11/e p201

37. All are true about impression compound except:
   a. ADA specification No is 1
   b. Kneading in water bath make its property to get changed
   c. It can be softened in flame also
   d. It is available in various forms
   Ans. a

Ref: Craig Restorative Dental materials 13/e p248

38. Maximum biocompatibility is seen with:
   a. Polysulphide
   b. Polyether
   c. Condensation silicon
   d. Addition silicon
   Ans. a

Ref: Philips 11/e p229

39. The gelation temperature for hydrocolloid impression materials is:
   a. 37-38
   b. 25-35
   c. 18-30
   d. 35-37
   Ans. a

Ref: Philips 11/e p235

40. Back pressure porosity causes due to:
   a. Improper venting
   b. Large and long sprue
   c. Incomplete removal of wax
   d. Improper pattern build up
   Ans. a

Ref: Philips 11/e p346

41. True for beta hemihydrate is:
   a. Presence of air bubbles
   b. Absence of air bubbles
   c. Calcinations done by boiling in 3% $CaCl2$
   d. Closed vessel is used under steam
   Ans. a

Ref: Philips 11/e p257

42. Which among the following is NOT present in periodontal ligament?

a. Myelinated nerve fibers
b. Angioblast and undifferentiated cells
c. Fibronectin
d. Mature Elastic Fibers

Ans. d

Ref: Carranza 11/e p893 Straight pick from AIIMS SR Ship

43. Which of the following has least modulus of elasticity?

a. NiTi
b. Co-Cr-Ni
c. Beta Titanium
d. Stainless Steel

Ans. a

Ref: Profitt 4/e p442

44. Arrange the elastomeric materials in their increasing order of permanent deformation:

a. Addition silicone, Condensation silicone, polyether, polysulphide
b. Polyether, Addition silicone, polysulfide, Condensation silicone
c. Additional silicon, Condensation Siliconpolysulfide, polyether
d. Polyether, polysulphide, additional silicone, condensation silcone

Ans. a

Ref: Philips 11/e p227

45. Most effective method of plaque control on exposed root concavity:

a. Tooth pick
b. Tufted Floss
c. Dental Brush
d. Interdental Brush

Ans. d

Ref: Carranza 9/e p663 Straight pick from JULY AIIMS SR 2014

46. Dolichocephalic refers to:

a. Long and narrow dental arch
b. Short and narrow dental arches
c. Long and wide dental arches
d. Short and wide dental arches

Ans. a

Ref: McDonald 8/e p614

47. Most advanced technique to find out the bone density in present era is:

a. Probing
b. RVG
c. Thermography
d. Cone Beam CT

Ans. d

Ref: Carranza 9/e p951

48. Child with ankylosis of the TMJ for surgery is best intubated with:

a. Tracheostomy
b. Cricothyroidotomy
c. LA with sedation
d. Awake fibreoptic intubation

Ans. d

Ref: Neelima Malik 2/e p185

49. Throat pack is not used for:
a. Awake patient
b. After LMA
c. After surgery
d. None
Ans. a

Ref: Ajay Yadav Anaesthesia p89

50. During Lefort 1 osteotomy with midpalatine split, the free segment undergoes displacement in which direction?
a. Horizontal
b. Transverse
c. Vertical
d. Superior
Ans. b

Ref: Profitt 4/e p699-701

51. True about nasal intubation is:
a. Can be done in case of basilar skull fracture
b. Keeps surgical field free during surgery
c. Can be used to perform cleft palate surgery
d. Keeps patient intubated in postoperative period
Ans. b

Ref: Peterson's Oral and Maxillofacial Surgery 2/e p1143

52. Throat pack is done in:
a. Endotracheal tube without cuff
b. In all oral surgical intubations
c. Endotracheal tube with cuff
d. After LMA intubation
Ans. b

Ref: Peterson Oral and Maxillofaxial surgery 2/e p477

53. Microorganism found in ANUG is:
a. Eikenella corrodens
b. Tannerella forsythia
c. Fusobacterium nucleatum
d. Prevotella intermedia
Ans. c

Ref: Carranza Periodontology 11/e Vol.2

54. In a normal growing child the expected increase in weight on the first birthday as compared to birth weight is:
a. 50
b. 100
c. 200
d. 300
Ans. c

Ref: OP Ghai 7/e p6

55. Bacteria associated with rapidly progressive periodontitis:
a. P. intermedia and P. gingivalis
b. P. intermedia and F. nucleatum
c. P. gingivalis and A. comitans
d. T. forsythia and A. comitans
Ans. c

Ref: Carranza 9/e p410

56. Ocular fibrous histiocytoma most commonly occurs in:
a. Eyelid
b. Epibulbar surface
c. Intraocular surface
d. Orbit
Ans. d

Ref: Ocular Pathology by Myron Yanoff 2/e p443

57. TNM stands for:
a. Tumor, necrosis, metastasis
b. Tumor nevus, metastasis
c. Tumor, node, morphology
d. Tumor, node, metastasis
Ans. D

Ref: Peterson 2/e p623

58. Most common variant of soft tissue sarcoma is:
a. Liposarcoma
b. Synovial sarcoma
c. Malignant fibrous histiocytoma
d. Rhabdomyosarcoma
Ans. a

Ref: Shafer 6/e p160

59. School based Dental Health Care for whole country was adopted in:
a. Australia
b. Denmark
c. Myanmar
d. New Zealand
Ans. d

Ref: Soben Peter 6/e p545-553

60. Calculation of infant mortality rate does not includes:
a. Postneonatal deaths
b. Early neonatal deaths
c. Late neonatal deaths
d. Stillbirth
Ans. d

Ref: Park 22/e p521

61. Not true about incubation period is:
a. For differentiating co-primary and secondary cases
b. To find out time for quarantine
c. To prevent infection to contacts of infected person
d. To find out time for isolation
Ans. d

Ref: Park 21/e p111, 94

62. The pattern of change of disease trends of mortality and morbidity where the pandemics of infection are replaced by degenerative and manmade disorders as the main cause of morbidity and mortality is known as:
a. Parodoxical transition
b. Epidemiological transition
c. Reversal of Transition
d. Demographic transition
Ans. b

Ref: Park 21/e p337

63. In chronic gingivitis all cells are involved except:
a. Plasma cells
b. Lymphocyte
c. Neutrophils
d. Macrophages
Ans. c

Ref: Carranza Periodontology 11/e p765

64. Reed Sternberg cells in Hodgkin's lymphoma is:
a. T cell
b. B cell
c. Natural killer cell
d. Mast cell
Ans. b

Ref: Yanoff and Duker 3/e ch 8.4 and 12.12

65. Patient is treated for H.pylori can be accurately diagnosed and monitored by using:
a. Stool bacteria culture
b. Sodium chloride test
c. Urea breath test
d. Gastric acid test
Ans. c

Ref: Harrison 18/e ch293

66. Basal cell carcinoma shows hallmark feature of:
a. Nuclear/epithelial palisading
b. Foam cells
c. Psammoma bodies
d. Keratin pearls
Ans. a

Ref: Neville 2/e p374

67. Height of study model with mounted base and trimmed is:
a. 55 mm
b. 70 mm
c. 85 mm
d. 95 mm
Ans. b

Ref: Gurkeerat Singh 2/e p80

68. Which of the following is not included in IOTN?
a. Cleft lip and palate
b. Dental health
c. Aesthetics
d. Bimaxillary protrusion
Ans. d

Ref: Profitt 4/e p18

69. The agents used in day care surgery are:
a. Pethidine, isoflurane, propofol
b. Propofol, sevoflurane, halothane
c. Isoflurane, fentanyl, propofol
d. Halothane, thiopentone, haloperidol
Ans. c

Ref: Ajay Yadav Anaesthesia p75 and 83

70. **Which of the following is the most radiosensitive cell in the body?**
    a. RBC
    b. Muscle
    c. Lymphoid tissue
    d. Basal layer
    Ans. d

Ref: White and Pharaoh 5/e p30

71. **In a 10-year-old patient midline shift in central incisor can be best diagnosed by:**
    a. Lower lip stretched and by seeing the lower frenum and midline
    b. Upper lip stretched and by seeing the upper frenum and midline
    c. Comparing midline of incisors with nasal septum midline
    d. PA Cephalogram view
    Ans. d

Ref: OP Kharbanda 1/e p71

72. **Oral hygiene instructions are being given at a special school; which IQ level group find it difficult to repeat the instructions?**
    a. 36-51
    b. 55-68
    c. 71-92
    d. 95-120
    Ans. a

Ref: McDonald 8/e p40

73. **A 10-year-old growing child has unusually small mandible which of the following is correct?**
    a. Patient may develop snoring and sleep apnea
    b. Condyle fracture
    c. Growth catches up during pubertal growth spurt
    d. Treatment is needed after puberty
    Ans. a

Ref: OP Kharbanda 1/e p543

74. **When the incisal edge of the anterior teeth are placed in end to end contact, the condyle of mandible moves?**
    a. Backward
    b. Forward
    c. Downward and forward
    d. Downward
    Ans. a

Ref: A manual of Occlusion in Clinical Practice 3/e p 81

75. **Lingual placement of posterior teeth will cause all except:**
    a. Gagging
    b. Excessive force on residual ridge
    c. Tongue movement reduction
    d. Speech difficulties
    Ans. c

Ref: Nallaswamy Textbook of Prosthodontics 1/e p700

76. **In the case of a thick labial frenum which muscle entrapment happens?**
    a. Orbicularis oris
    b. Buccinator
    c. Masseter
    d. Platysma
    Ans. a

Ref: Snell's Clinical Anatomy 9/e p1136

77. The technique which cuts only mineralised tissue and not nerves and vessels is based on the principle of:
a. Electrosurgery
b. Piezoelectricity
c. Osteotome
d. Cryosurgery
Ans. b

Ref: Carranza 11/e p1797

78. If you are going to restore lower molar with amalgam which is having cavity with proximal box wide buccolingually the wedge indicated is:
a. Piggy back wedging
b. Double wedging
c. Wedge wedging
d. Triple wedging
Ans. b

Ref: Sturdevant's 4/e p723

79. In a case of 10-year-old boy with Class II division 1 an overjet of 5 mm true statement is:
a. Recurrent throat infections
b. Mandibular teeth are at high fracture risk
c. Patient may develop tongue thrusting
d. Maxillary anterior teeth are prone for fracture
Ans. d

Ref: Gurkeerat Singh 2/e p623

80. A patient aged 11 years comes for the extraction of right maxillary central incisor, after administering local anaesthetic has complained about burning sensation and pain in the right eye can be attributed to:
a. The alternative course of middle superior alveolar nerve *Ref: Monheim's Local Anaesthesia 7/e p347*
b. The reaction to the preservative used in the solution
c. Improper entry of solution through the infraorbital pathway
d. Normal occurrence and will be subsided by itself
Ans. b

Ref: Monheim's Local Anaesthesia 7/e p347 Straight pick from AIIMS SRSHIP

81. A young male present with loose motions and intermittent abdominal pain over the past 1 year. Wet mount specimen showed the presence of multiple ova which are more than 100 microns in diameter. The causative organisms for the disease includes all except:
a. Ophistorchis viverani
b. Gastrodiscoides hominis
c. Fasciola gigantica
d. Echinostema ileocaanum
Ans. a

Ref: Oxford Textbook of Medicine Vol 1 4/e p837

82. Cleft lip and Palate is:
a. Monogenic
b. Polygenic
c. Multifactorial
d. Bifactorial
Ans. c

Ref: McDonald 8/e p91-92

83. False about difference in primary and permanent teeth:
a. Size is more in permanent teeth
b. The mesiodistal length compared to the cervico incisal length is more in primary teeth
c. Cervical ridge is not prominent in primary when compared to the permanent
d. The primary teeth is more white in color
Ans. c

Ref: McDonald 8/e p66

84. A 12-year-old child with flat base skull and copious nasal discharge thick lips, large tongue and enlarged head liver and spleen was found to be normal at birth is suffering from:
   a. Proteus syndrome
   b. Lipoid proteinosis
   c. Hurler's syndrome
   d. Beckwith Wiedman syndrome

   Ans. c

Ref: Shafer 7/e p630-31

85. Immediate bacteria which are responsible for pellicle formation or initial colonisers are:
   a. Gram + aerobes
   b. Gram – anaerobes
   c. Gram + facultative
   d. Gram + anaerobe

   Ans. c

Ref: Carranza 10/e p143

86. In a national water supply and sanitation programme a problem village is defined as all except:
   a. Water is exposed to the risk of cholera
   b. Water source has excess of iron and heavy metals
   c. Water infested with guinea worm
   d. Distance of safe water greater than 1.6 km

   Ans. c

Ref: Park 20/e p391

87. All of the following are parts of NRHM except:
   a. Institutional deliveries under JSY
   b. Health and Family welfare societies
   c. State and District Health Mission
   d. Appoint ASHA

   Ans. b

Ref: Park 20/e p379-380

88. Which of the following has problem in recall bias?
   a. Case control study
   b. Randomized controlled trial
   c. Cohort study
   d. Cross sectional study

   Ans. a

Ref: Park 20/e p69

89. In a study in the UK, an association was found between sale of antiarrythmic drug and an increase in deaths due to asthma. This is an example of:
   a. Cweohort study
   b. Case control study
   c. Experimental study
   d. Ecological study

   Ans. d

Ref: Park 21/e p59

90. A 12-year-old child complained of recurrent pain over the right maxillary posterior tooth, cold and fever spells but clinically no caries was evident. The line of management is:
   a. Supportive therapy
   b. No intervention needed
   c. Refer to a physician for ruling out sinusitis
   d. Wait and watch for two weeks

   Ans. c

Ref: OP Ghai Essential Pediatrics 8/e p543

AIIMS Medical (Nov 2014)

1. **Color plate of foramen ovale was given. Which of the following structures doesn't pass through the area marked in the diagram:**
   a. Lesser petrosal nerve
   b. Maxillary nerve
   c. Motor root of trigeminal nerve
   d. Sensory branch of mandibular nerve
   Ans. b

Ref: Gray's Anatomy 40/e p528-529

2. **'Turkish Saddle' refers to:**
   a. Hypothalamus
   b. Pituitary gland
   c. Amygdaloid body
   d. Uncus
   Ans. b

Ref: Gray's Anatomy 40/e p424

3. **During pronation of foot, the axes of which two joints become parallel?**
   a. Talocrural and subtalar
   b. Talonavicular and calcaneocuboid
   c. Talonavicular and subtalar
   d. Midtarsal and tarsometatarsal
   Ans. b

Ref: www.vaslimedical.com/pdf/VasyliMedical%20Pronation.pdf

4. **Most common site of mucosa associated lymphoid tissue:**
   a. Duodenum
   b. Jejenum
   c. Ileum
   d. Stomach
   Ans. c

Ref: Gray's Anatomy 40/e p74

This is a tricky question MALT is the most commonly present in the ileum (as peyer's patcyhes), though MALT omas most commonly arise from stomach

5. **All are true about sphincter urethrae except:**
   a. Voluntary
   b. Supplied by pudendal nerve
   c. Originates from the ischiopubic rami
   d. Located at the baldder neck
   Ans. d

Ref: BD Chaurasia Human Anatomy Vol 2 6/e p356

6. **Dense regular collagen is found in all except:**
   a. Ligament
   b. Periosteum
   c. Aponeurosis
   d. Tendon
   Ans. b

Ref: http://en.wikipedia.org/wiki/Dense_regular_connective _tissue

7. Panniculus adiposus is seen in:
a. Scrotum
b. Orbit
c. Eyelid
d. Penis
Ans. b

Ref: Cunningham's Textbook of Anatomy 3/e p364

8. Membrana tectoria is derived from:
a. Anterior atlanto occipital membrane
b. Posterior atlanto ccipital membrane
c. Anterior longitudinal ligament
d. Posterior longitudinal ligament
Ans. d

Ref: BD Chaurasia Human Anatomy Vol 3 6/e p173

9. All of the following are true about cavernous sinus thrombosis except:
a. Loss of jaw jerk
b. Infection can spread to cavernous sinus from danger area of face via inferior ophthalmic vein
c. Most common cause in ethmoidal sinusitis
d. Loss of sensation around the eye
Ans. a

Ref: Gray's Anatomy 40/e p430

10. Which of the following is not carried by dorsal column:
a. Pain
b. Proprioception
c. Vibration
d. Touch
Ans. a

Ref: Gray's Anatomy 40/e p262

11. Which cranial nerve nucleus underlies the facial colliculus:
a. Sixth
b. Seventh
c. Eighth
d. Fifth
Ans. a

Ref: Gray's Anatomy 40/e p240

12. Which of the following techniques is used to study the current flow across a single ion channel:
a. Voltage clamp technique
b. Patch clamp technique
c. Iontophoresis
d. Galvanometry
Ans. b

Ref: Ganong's Review of Medical Physiology 24/e p49

13. K complexes and sleep spindles are seen in which stage of sleep:
a. REM
b. Stage 1 NREM
c. Stage 2 NREM
d. Stage 3 NREM
Ans. c

Ref: Ganong's Review of Medical Physiology 24/e p273

14. **Free nerve endings causing nociceptive fibers are seen in which of the following:**
    a. Intestine
    b. Mesentery
    c. Spleen
    d. Liver
    Ans. b

Ref: Physiology of Gastrointestinal Tract by Kim E Barrett, Fayez K Ghishan, Juanita L Merchant, Hamid M Said, Jackie D Wood p 690

15. **Attention and concentration are functions of which of the following brain areas:**
    a. Frontal lobe
    b. Parietal lobe
    c. Hypothalamus
    d. Basal Ganglia
    Ans. a

Ref: Ganong's Review of Medical Physiology 24/e p294

16. **You are testing knee jerk reflex in a patient. The afferents in deep tendon reflexes are carried by:**
    a. Nuclear bag and chain fibers
    b. Golgi tendon organ
    c. Nuclear bag and static chain fibers
    d. Dynamic intrafusal fibers
    Ans. d

Ref: Ganong's Review of Medical Physiology 24/e p229

17. **Which of the following is not a component of counter current mechanism:**
    a. Thick ascending limb of Henle
    b. Collecting duct
    c. Descending limb of Henle
    d. Vasa recta
    Ans. b

Ref: Ganong's Review of Medical Physiology 24/e p687

18. **The triad of bradycardia, hypertension and irregular respiration are called as:**
    a. Cushing's reflex
    b. Bezold Jarisch reflex
    c. Bainbridge reflex
    d. Herring's reflex
    Ans. a

Ref: Ganong's Review of Medical Physiology 24/e p607

19. **A short duration high frequency stimulation with 5Hz of perforant pathway in hippocampus leads to:**
    a. Long-term potentiation
    b. Habituation
    c. Long-term depression
    d. Post tetanic potentiation
    Ans. a

Ref: Ganong's Review of Medical Physiology 24/e p286

20. **In traumatic brain injury, changes in the brain metabolism are seen. All are true except:**
    a. There is shut down of pyruvate dehydrogenase activity
    b. There is accumulation of lactate in brain
    c. There is increased lactate uptake from circulation
    d. Increased CSF lactate is associated with good prognosis
    Ans. d

Ref: http://www.ncbi.nlm.nih.gov/pubmed/19561963

21. Which technique is used to study the structure of molecules?
   a. X-ray crystallography
   b. Electron microscopy
   c. Ion exchange chromatography
   d. Agarose gel electrophoresis
   Ans. a

Ref: Harper's Illustarted Biochemistry 28/e p37

22. A child suffered from a viral illness for which she took aspirin. 3 Days later the child presented to the emergency with altered sensorium and icterus. What is the underlying biochemical defect?
   a. Beta oxidation of fatty acids
   b. Glucose-6-phosphatase deficiency
   c. Pyruvate dehydrogenase deficiency
   d. Urea cycle defect
   Ans. a

Ref: Ghai Essential Pediatrics 8/e p570

23. All of the following amino acids are components of collagen except:
   a. Glycinc
   b. Proline
   c. Lysine
   d. Desmosine
   Ans. d

Ref: Harper's Illustarted Biochemistry 28/e p527, 530

24. Identify the disease shown in the karyotype (Color Plate was given):
   a. Bloom syndrome
   b. Cri du chat syndrome
   c. Pradeer willi syndrome
   d. Down's syndrome
   Ans. b

Ref: Harrison's Principle of Internal Medicine 18/e p517 Langman Medical Embryology 11/e p21

25. A 17-year-old female underwent a fine needle aspiration cytology for a lump in the breast which was well defined, non tender and mobile. The diagnosis of a benign lesion can be considered by which of the following pathogenic features?
   a. Dyscohesuve ductal epithelium without cellular fragments
   b. Tightly arranged ductal epithelial cells with dyscohesive bare nuclei
   c. Stromal predominance with hyperplasia of spindle cells
   d. Polymorphism with single or arranged ductal epithelial cells
   Ans. b

Ref: Winfred Gray's Diagnostic Histopathology 2/e p279-80

26. Which of the following is seen in Schwannoma?
   a. Storiform pattern
   b. Spindle cells
   c. Antoni A and B
   d. Target cells
   Ans. c

Ref: Robbins and Cotran's Pathological Basis of Disease 8/e p1340

27. A 27-year-old female with right sided thyroid nodule was operated. A 2×2 cm thyroid nodule was resected and the following histology was found. What is your diagnosis?
   a. Papillary carcinoma thyroid
   b. Adenomatous goiter
   c. Follicular adenoma
   d. Grave's disease
   Ans. a

Ref: Robbins and Cotran's Pathological Basis of Disease 8/e p1121-22

28. A patient with a history of recurrent ureteric stones presented with fever. Right sided nephrectomy was done. Diagnosis is:

a. Adult polycystic kidney disease
b. Renal cell carcinoma
c. Cystic dysplastic kidney
d. Hydronephrosis with chronic pyelonephritis

Ans. d

Ref: Robbins and Cotran's Pathological Basis of Disease 8/e p943, 961

29. Which of the following induces apoptosis in a cell:

a. Oleic acid
b. Glucocorticoids
c. Isoprenoids
d. Myristic acid

Ans. b

Ref: Underwood Pathology 5/e p78

30. A 65-year-old chronic smoker presented with a central lung mass with distal bronchiectasis and recurrent pneumonia. A greyish white tumor was resected. Which of the following histopathological finding is most likely to be seen?

a. Small cells with scant cytoplasm, ill defined cell borders and hyperchromatic nuclei with nuclear palisading
b. Derivatives of all three germ layers are seen
c. Tall columnar cells with cytoplasmic and intraalveolar mucin
d. Palisading or rosette like arrangements of cells separated by abundant fibrovascular stroma

Ans. a

Ref: Robbins and Cotran's Pathological Basis of Disease 8/e p721-727

31. About GIST all are true except:

a. Most common site is stomach
b. Originates from interstitial cells of Cajal
c. Size plays a role in prognosis
d. ALK mutation is seen in most cases

Ans. d

Ref: Robbins and Cotran's Pathological Basis of Disease 8/e p789-90

32. Which of the following changes is commonly seen in cancers:

a. Hypomethylation of oncogenes
b. Hypermethylation of tumor suppressor genes
c. Loss of heterozygosity
d. Mutation of introns

Ans. b

Ref: Harrison's Principle of Internal Medicine 18/e p677-78

33. Molecular classification of breast cancer is based on:

a. Gene expression profiling
b. Expression of hormone receptors(er/pr)
c. Serum hormone levels
d. In vitro response to chemotherapeutic agents

Ans. a

Ref: Robbins and Cotran's Pathologic Basis of Disease 8/e p1084

34. An Afroamerican boy of 6 years age presented with abdominal pain, chronic hemolysis and abnormal RBC shape on peripheral smear. Most likely disorder responsible for this condition:

a. Trinucleotide repeat
b. Point mutation

c. Antibodies against RBC membrane
d. Genetic imprinting
Ans. b

Ref: Robbins and Cotrans Pathological Basis of Disease 8/e p646

35. Which of the following is incorrect regarding tumor markers?
a. Desmin-carcinoma
b. Cytokeratin-carcinoma
c. S100-Melanoma
d. Common leukocyte antigen-lymphoma
Ans. a

Ref: Robbins and Cotrans Pathological Basis of Disease 8/e p35

36. Epigenetics deals with genetic modifications that do not alter the sequence of DNA. All of the following can detect epigenetic modification except:
a. CHIP on CHIP
b. Bisulphite method
c. HPLC
d. Methylation specific PCR
Ans. c

Ref: Robbins and Cotrans Pathological Basis of Disease 8/e p180-181

37. In a 70 years old man who was working in asbestos factory for 10-15 years. On routine X-ray a mass was seen in right apical region of the lung. Biopsy was taken from the mass. Which of the following is seen on electron microscopic examination:
a. Numerous long, slender microvilli
b. Melanosomes
c. Desmosomes
d. Neurosecretory granules in the cytoplasm
Ans. a

Ref: Robbins and Cotrans Pathological Basis of Disease 8/e p734

38. A patient is on treatment with penicillin developed pallor, there was no shortness of breath, urticarial or wheezing. On investigation antibodies against penicillin were found in blood. What type of hypersensitivity has occurred in this patient?
a. I
b. II
c. III
d. IV
Ans. b

Ref: Robbins and Cotrans Pathological Basis of Disease 8/e p653, 202

39. Dexmedetomidine is a:
a. Centrally acting alpha 2 agonist
b. Centrally acting alpha 2 antagonist
c. Peripherally acting alpha 2 antagonist
d. Centrally peripherally acting alpha 2 agonist and antagonist
Ans. a

Ref: KD Tripathi's Essentials of Medical Pharmacology 7/e p384

40. PPI can cause all except:
a. Hypothyroidism
b. Community acquired pneumonia
c. Clostridium difficile infection
d. Osteoporosis leading to hip fracture
Ans. a

Ref: KD Tripathi's Essentials of Medical Pharmacology 7/e p633

41. Edema is the side effect of all except:
a. Digoxin
b. Cyclosporine
c. Amlodipine
d. Estrogen
Ans. a

Ref: http://www.drugs.com/sfx/digoxin-side-effects.html

42. All are true about Rituximab except:
a. Has dose independent pharmacokinetics
b. Most common side effect is infusion reaction
c. First FD drug approved for resistant lymphomas
d. Chimeric monoclonal antibody against CD 20 B cell antigen
Ans. a

Ref: Harrison's Principles of Internal Medicine 18/e p2749

43. Which of the following drug is Class B: Adequate studies in pregnant women have failed to demonstrate a fetal risk?
a. Brimonidine
b. Latanoprost
c. Dorzolamide
d. Pilocarpine
Ans. a

Ref: http://eyewiki.aao.org/Glaucoma_management_ in_ pregnancy_and_post-partum

44. Time dependent killing and prolonged postantibiotic effect is seen in:
a. Flouroquinolones
b. Beta lactam antibiotics
c. Clindamycin
d. Erythromycin
Ans. c

Ref: Goodman and Gilman 12/e p1332

45. In which of the following condition, cholinomimetics are not used:
a. Glaucoma
b. Post surgical ileus/atony
c. Myasthenia gravis
d. Bradycardia
Ans. d

Ref: Katzung Pharmacology 11/e p106

46. Which of the following antibiotics can be used in the treatment of fungal keratomycosis?
a. Linezolid
b. Vancomycin
c. Silver sulphadiazine
d. Doxycycline
Ans. c

Ref: Clinical Pharmacology by Jill E Maddison, Stephen W Page, David Church p567

47. Which of the following third generation cephalosporin has activity against MRSA?
a. Ceftobiprole
b. Ceftriaxone
c. Cephalexin
d. Aztreonam
Ans. a

Ref: Journal of American Pharmacists Association

48. Which of the following is not atertiary amine derivative:
a. Scopolamine
b. Hyoscine
c. Glycopyrrolate
d. Atropine
Ans. c

Ref: KD Tripathi's Essentials of Medical Pharmacology 7/e p106

49. A person has been consuming 200 ml alcohol per day for last 20 years. Which of the following should be avoided in this patient?
a. Disulfiram
b. Acamprostate
c. Phenytoin
d. Naltrexone
Ans. a

Ref: Niraj Ahuja Textbook of Psychiatry 7/e p41

50. Following serum levels are suggestive of lithium toxicity:
a. 2 mEq/L
b. 4 mEq/L
c. 6 mEq/L
d. 8 mEq/L
Ans. a

Ref: Niraj Ahuja Textbook of Psychiatry 7/e p190

51. Which of the following is incorrect about NSAIDs:
a. Decrease the antihypertensive action of diuretics
b. Used in neuropathic pain
c. Should be avoided in renal failure
d. Can be used topically
Ans. b

Ref: KD Tripathi's Essentials of Medical Pharmacology 7/e p198-199

52. Which of the following drugs is not active against Hepatitis B?
a. Telbivudine
b. Lamivudine
c. Zidovudine
d. Interferon
Ans. c

Ref: KD Tripathi's Essentials of Medical Pharmacology 7/e p803

53. Which of the following is true about Penicillin G?
a. It is effective orally
b. It has a wide spectrum
c. It is used in rat bite fever
d. Probenecid given along with Penicillin G decreases its duration of action
Ans. c

Ref: KD Tripathi's Essentials of Medical Pharmacology 7/e p718-20

54. Which of the following is the drug of choice for antibiotic associated with pseudomembranous enterocolitis?
a. Oral vancomycin
b. Cephalexin
c. Clindamycin
d. Penicillin
Ans. c

Ref: KD Tripathi's Essentials of Medical Pharmacology 7/e p198-99

55. **Which is not true about Paclitaxel:**
   a. It stabilizes the microtubules
   b. It is obtained from E Coli
   c. It is used in Ca ovary, breast and cervix
   d. It most commonly causes myelosuppression and alopecia
   Ans. b

Ref: KD Tripathi's Essentials of Medical Pharmacology 7/e p198-99

56. **Which of the following drug is useful against seudomonas:**
   a. Piperacillin-Tazobactam
   b. Cefotaxime
   c. Streptomycin
   d. Cephalexin
   Ans. a

Ref: KD Tripathi's Essentials of Medical Pharmacology 7/e p198-99

57. **All are caused by Nontypeable Hib except:**
   a. Otitis media
   b. Meningitis
   c. Peurperal sepsis
   d. Exacerbation of COPD
   Ans. b

Ref: Ananthanarayan and Panicker's Textbook of Microbiology 8/e p331

58. **The role played by major histocompatibility Complex 1 and 2 is to:**
   a. Transduce the signal to T-cells following antigen recognition
   b. Mediate immunogenic class switching
   c. Present antigens for recognition by T-cell antigen receptors
   d. Enhance secretion of cytokines
   Ans. c

Ref: Ananthanarayan and Panicker's Textbook of Microbiology 8/e p132-35

59. **A cystic fibrosis patient presented with an episode of pneumonia. On sputum culture mucoid colonies of pseudomonas were seen. What does this indicate?**
   a. It formed a biofilm on bronchial walls
   b. It underwent a mutation
   c. It is resistant to most of the antibiotics
   d. There is a mistake with the culture technique
   Ans. a

Ref: Harrison's principle of Internal Medicine 18/e p1016

60. **A child has neonatal meningitis. CSF examination showed small gram positive bacilli. Which is the likely causative organism?**
   a. Hemophilus
   b. Streptococcus mutans
   c. Listeria
   d. Neisseria
   Ans. c

Ref: Ananthanarayan and Panicker's Textbook of Microbiology 8/e p395, Harrison's Principle of Internal Medicine 18/e p1195

61. **Enterohemorrhagic, Enteroinvasive and Enterotoxic are types of:**
   a. Klebsiella
   b. Shigella
   c. Pneumococcus
   d. E coli
   Ans. d

Ref: Harrison's Principle of Internal Medicine 18/e p276

62. **What is true regarding viral antibodies?**
   a. Appear before interferon
   b. They are formed against viral surface proteins
   c. They are formed against viral nucleic acid
   d. Maximum levels are seen within 1 week
   Ans. b

Ref: Harrison's Principle of Internal Medicine 18/e p1439

63. **Regarding amoebic liver abscess all are true except:**
   a. Trophozoite in stool are essential for clinical diagnosis
   b. Mostly asymptomatic
   c. More common in males than females
   d. It rarely affects brain, eye and skin
   Ans. a

Reference: Harrison's Internal Medicine 18/e Ch 37 p1123

64. **Harakiri is death by:**
   a. Stab in the neck
   b. Stab in the thorax
   c. Stab in the abdomen
   d. Stab in the wrist and neck
   Ans. c

Ref: Parikh's Textbook of Medical Jurisprudence, Forensic Medicine and Toxicology 6/e p 4, 21

65. **A case of suspected homicide comes to a doctor. He is supposed to inform to police under which section of CrPC?**
   a. 174
   b. 176
   c. 37
   d. 39
   Ans. d

Ref: http://indiankanoon.org/doc/164335/Section39 (1) in The Code of Criminal Procedure, 1973, p 34

66. **A female with suspected child abuse comes to the casualty with severe bleeding from perineum. What will be the first step in management?**
   a. Airway
   b. Blood transfusion
   c. First inform the police
   d. Internal iliac artery ligation
   Ans. a

Ref: Schwartz Principles of Surgery 8/e ch6

67. **Fatal dose of arsenic in adults:**
   a. 40–60 mg
   b. 20–30 mg
   c. 60–80 mg
   d. 100–120 mg
   Ans. d

Ref: Parikh's Textbook of Medical Jurisprudence, Forensic Medicine and Toxicology 6/e p99

68. **Calibre is defined as:**
   a. Distance between the two diametrically opposite grooves
   b. Distance between two diametrically opposite lands
   c. Distance between opposite land and groove
   d. Ratio of the length and width of the barrel
   Ans. b

Ref: Parikh's Textbook of Medical Jurisprudence, Forensic Medicine and Toxicology 6/e p4, 26

69. What is the most common cause of para suicide:
a. Drugs
b. Hanging
c. Firearms
d. Wrist cutting
Ans. a

Ref: http://en.wikipedia.org/wiki/Parasuicide

70. According to Galstaun method iliac crest fuses in females at the age of:
a. 13-15 years
b. 15-17 years
c. 17-19 years
d. 19-20 years
Ans. c

Ref: Estimation of Age from Epiphyseal fusion in iliac crest (J Indian Acad Forensic Med Jan-Mar 2011, Vol 33, No1) table no 4

71. A child has a disc battery in the nose. What is the most important consideration in management?
a. Refer the child to a specialist for removal
b. The battery may leak and cause tissue damage
c. It can lead to tetanus
d. Instill nasal drops
Ans. b

Ref: http://www.patient.co.uk/doctor/nasal-injury-and-nasal-foreign-bodies Professional Reference

72. Post adenoidectomy is not seen in:
a. Velopharyngeal insufficiency
b. Hyponasality
c. Retropharyngeal abscess
d. Base of skull fracture/atlantoaxial subluxation/Griesel syndrome
Ans. b

Ref: Disease of Ear, Nose and Throat by Dhingra 5/e p443, 335

73. An elderly male present with T3N0 laryngeal carcinoma. What would be the management?
a. Concurrent chemoradiotherapy
b. Neoadjuvant chemotherapy followed by radiotherapy
c. Radical radiotherapy followed by chemotherapy
d. Radical radiotherapy without chemotherapy
Ans. a

Ref: http://emedicine.medscape.com/article/2047862-overview

74. A patient of head trauma presents with clear nasal discharge. NCCT brain was done which revealed non operable injuries to the frontobasal area. What is the most appropriate management?
a. Wait and watch for 4–5 days to allow for spontaneous healing
b. Do an MRI to localize the leak and control the discharge endoscopically
c. Put a dural catheter to control CSF leaks
d. Approach transcranially to repair the damaged frontobasal region
Ans. a

Ref: Diseases of Ear, Nose and Throat by Dhingra 5/e p179

75. All are true about malignant otitis externa except:
a. ESR is used for follow up after treatment
b. Granulations are seen on superior wall of external auditory canal
c. Severe hearing loss is the chief presenting complaint
d. Pseudomonas is the most common cause
Ans. c

Ref: Diseases of Ear, Nose and Throat by Dhingra 5/e p58

76. Topical steroids are not recommended in:
a. Antrochoanal polyp
b. Ethmoidal polyps
c. Allergic fungal sinusitis
d. Chronic rhinosinusitis
Ans. d

Ref: Scott Brown 7/e p1553, Logan Turner 10/e p55

77. Most common cause of vocal cord palsy:
a. Surgical
b. Inflammatory
c. Trauma
d. Malignancy
Ans. a

Ref: Benninger MS, Gillen JB, Altman JS, Changing Etiology of Vocal Cord Immobility 3/e p233

78. What is true about Meniere's disease?
a. Semont's manoeuvre is used for treatment
b. Electrocochleography is the gold standard for diagnosis
c. Surgery is the mainstay of treatment
d. V shaped audiogram is seen
Ans. b

Ref: Diseases of Ear, Nose, Throat Dhingra 5/e p113

79. Gene commonly indicated in congenital cataract:
a. CRYGS3
b. PAX6
c. PITX3
d. LMX1B
Ans. a

Ref: Ophthalmology Yanoff and Duker 4/e p11

80. Normal value of Arden Index is:
a. 1
b. 1.5
c. Less than 185%
d. More than 185%
Ans. d

Ref: Kanski and Bowling Clinical Ophthalmology 7/e p649

81. There is a retained intraocular iron foreign body. What is the best investigation for monitoring vision?
a. ERG
b. Arden Index
c. Dark adaptometry
d. Serial evoked potentials
Ans. a

Ref: Ophthalmology Yanoff and Ducker 4/e p1088

82. Which diagnostic procedure is not done in a dilated pupil?
a. Fundus examination
b. Gonioscopy
c. Laser inferometry
d. Electroretinography
Ans. b

Ref: Basics and Clinical Science Course, American Academy of Ophthalmology

83. **Which is not a feature of fungal corneal ulcer?**
   a. Fixed hypopyon
   b. Ulcer with sloughing margins
   c. Symptoms are more prolonged than signs
   d. Hyphae are seen on KOH mount
   Ans. c

Ref: Khurana's Comprehensive Ophthalmology 5/e p101

84. **Laser trabeculoplasty is indicated in which of the following?**
   a. Neovascular Glaucoma
   b. Chronic angle Closure Glaucoma
   c. Pseudoexfoliative glaucoma
   d. Uveitic glaucoma
   Ans. c

Ref: Ophthalmology Yanoff and Duker 4/e p1072

85. **A patient presents with painless red eye with an IOP of 60 mm Hg. What is the likely diagnosis?**
   a. Acute anterior uveitis
   b. Glaucomatocyclitic crisis
   c. Angle closure glaucoma
   d. Chronic papilledema
   Ans. b

Ref: Ophthalmology Yanoff and Duker 4/e p773

86. **A distortion increases in both direction on wearing a lens. Which of the following is not true about this?**
   a. It is a type of aniseikonia
   b. It is called as pin cushion effect
   c. Seen on wearing a convex lenses
   d. Cylindrical lenses increase the distortion
   Ans. d

Ref: Ophthalmology Yanoff and Duker 4/e p78

87. **Which is not an absolute contraindication of corneal transplantation?**
   a. TB meningitis
   b. Rabies
   c. SSPE
   d. Death due to unknown cause
   Ans. a

Ref: Ophthalmology Yanoff and Duker 4/e p229

88. **Which of the following is used as a self tonometer?**
   a. Perkins
   b. Rebound
   c. Diaton
   d. Dynamic contour
   Ans. b

Ref: Shields Textbook of Glaucoma 6/e p35

89. **Subretinal demarcation lies (high water marks) indicate:**
   a. Fresh rhegmatogenous RD
   b. Old rhegmatogenous RD
   c. Retinopathy of prematurity
   d. Retinitis pigmentos
   Ans. b

Ref: Ophthalmology Yanoff and Duker 4/e p651

90. Which of the following is not true about rhegmatogenous RD?

a. It is caused due to fibrous bands in the vitreous
b. Presents as floaters
c. Surgery is the primary treatment
d. Can extend up to ora serrate

Ans. a

Ref: Ophthalmology Yanoff and Duker 4/e p649

91. Corneal edema is due to accumulation of:

a. Lactate
b. Pyruvate
c. Glycogen
d. Carbon dioxide

Ans. a

Ref: Ophthalmology Yanoff and Duker 4/e p78

92. Population attributable risk is defined as the difference between:

a. Incidence in exposed and incidence in non exposed compared with incidence in nonexposed
b. Incidence in population and incidence in exposed compared with incidence in nonexposed
c. Incidence in population and incidence in non exposed compared with incidence in population
d. Incidence in population and incidence in exposed compared with incidence in nonexposed

Ans. c

Ref: Park's Textbook of Preventive and Social Medicine 22/e p75

93. A pandemic of H1N1 is never suspected when:

a. Cases are spread over 5 or more cities
b. 25 or more people are affected
c. Cases occur within 2 weeks period
d. At least one or more laboratory confirmed H1N1 case

Ans. a

Ref: mohfw-h1n1.nic.in>Guidelines>Guidelines on objective criteria to determine community spread

94. H5N1 Avian Influenza has not become an epidemic till now. What is the most important reason for this?

a. Seen only in wild birds and not in domestic poultry
b. It has avian influenza genes
c. Human to human transmission is rare
d. It causes serious illness leading to death of the patient

Ans. c

Ref: Robbins 8/e p715

95. School closure is recommended during an outbreak of swine flu. All of the following support this except:

a. Closure of school will not lead to reduction in contact between children
b. Children are the most common affected population by swine flu
c. Increased rates of transmission due to more opportunities of contact
d. Playing together of students increases transmission

Ans. a

Ref: http://www.ncbi.nlm.nih.gov/pubmed/24267871

96. Which is incorrect about inertization?

a. Relatively inexpensive
b. It is done for pharmaceutical waste
c. It involves mixing the waste with cement before disposal
d. It causes water pollution

Ans. d

Ref: Park 22/e p737

97. Which of the following is not a type of VDPV?

a. mVDPV
b. aVDPV
c. iVDPV
d. cVDPV

Ans. a

Ref: Park 22/e p185

98. Which is output indicator of NPCB?

a. Number of cataract surgeries leading to sight restoration
b. Decrease in prevalence of blindness
c. Number of school children provided glasses for retraction
d. Number of eye surgeons trained

Ans. a

Ref: www.ncbi.nlm.nih.gov/pmc/articles/PMC2612994

99. Who is the chairman of District Blindness Control Society?

a. District Collector
b. District eye surgeon
c. District health officer
d. Programme manager

Ans. a

Ref: Park 22/e p406

100. Which of the following is not true about cataract surgery rate?

a. Cataract surgery rate is defined as the total number of cataract surgeries performed per one million population
b. A target cataract surgery rate of 3000/million
c. CSR is a true rate
d. It is an indicator of success of blindness control programmes

Ans. c

Ref: www.ncbi.nlm.nih.gov/pmc/articles/PMC2612994

101. Which of the following is used to compare the two data sets taken on two different scales of measurement?

a. Coefficient of variation
b. Standard deviation
c. Standard error
d. Variance

Ans. a

Ref: http://en.wikipedia.org/wiki/Coefficient_of_variation

102. According to ICDS, supplements given to a pregnant woman are:

a. 200 kcal and 10 g protein
b. 250 kcal and 12 g protein
c. 300 kcal and 15 g protein
d. 330 kcal and 15 g protein

Ans. NONE

Ref: Park 22/e p547

103. A study has been done to establish the relationship between smoking and lung cancer. It was found that the association was more in people who exercise less and less in people who exercise more. In this situation, exercise is a:

a. Confounding factor
b. Effect modifier
c. Collinear factor
d. Bias

Ans. b

Ref: http://sphweb.bumc.bu.edu/otlt/mph-modules

104. Most efficient larval control method to prevent transmission of urban malaria:
- a. Covering overhead tanks
- b. Cleaning of drains
- c. Filling of ditches and cesspools
- d. Uprooting of plants

Ans. b

Ref: Park 22/e p717

105. You are a doctor. You visit a village and want to make a quick estimate of the instant population of the area. Which of the following measures can you use?
- a. No of TT injections in last one year
- b. No of folifer tablets consumed in one year
- c. Female population in reproductive age group
- d. Literacy rate

Ans. b

Ref: Park 22/e p 330

106. Chandler Index is an important tool in epidemiology. Which of the following is at least likely use?
- a. Determining case severity and prognosis
- b. Impact of control programme
- c. Endemicity
- d. Load of infection in the community

Ans. a

Ref: Park 22/e p221

107. All are true about dengue fever except:
- a. Aedes egypti is the vector
- b. Caused by a flavivirus
- c. Malnutrition is protective
- d. Lamivudine is the drug of choice

Ans. d

Ref: Park 22/e p225

108. In a sampling technique every 10th unit of population is chosen. What type of sampling technique is this:
- a. Systematic random
- b. Systematic
- c. Simple random
- d. Cluster

Ans. a

Ref: Park 22/e p792

109. Which of the following is true about ESI act:
- a. Funeral benefit is up to ₹ 50000
- b. The state government's share of expenditure on medical care is 1/8: the ESI corporation's share of expenditure on medical care is 7/8 of total cost
- c. Person with daily wages of ₹ 70 has to contribute ₹ 300 towards ESI
- d. Employee has to contribute 4.75% and employer contributes 8.75%

Ans. b

Ref: Park 22/e p760-762

110. Screening under RNTCP emphasizes on:
- a. Chest X-ray
- b. Sputum microscopy
- c. Sputum culture
- d. PCR

Ans. b

Ref: Park 22/e p394

111. Indicator used in RNTCP to measure the impact of the control measure is:
a. Annual infection rate
b. Incidence of new cases
c. Prevalence of infection
d. Number of people having access to DOTS
Ans. a

Ref: Park 22/e p168

112. Bone dysplasia is invariably seen in:
a. Hyperparathyroidism
b. Osteosarcoma
c. Developmental defect
d. Osteomalacia
Ans. c

Ref: Robbins 8/e p1210

113. A 10-year-old child presented with a mid tibial swelling which on X-ray revealed a lytic lesion with sclerotic margins. What is the most likely diagnosis?
a. Osteoid osteoma
b. Eosinophilic granuloma
c. Fibrocortical defect
d. Fibrous dysplasia
Ans. a

Ref: Robbins 8/e p718

114. A child is diagnosed with osteosarcoma based on sunray appearance on X-ray. This is because of:
a. Calcification along the periosteum
b. Calcification along the blood vessels
c. Periosteal reaction
d. Soft tissue invasion
Ans. b

Ref: Apley's System of Orthopedics and Fractures 9/e p207-208

115. Which of the following displacements is not seen in Colles fracture?
a. Dorsal
b. Supination
c. Volar tilt
d. Radial tilt
Ans. c

Ref: Apley's System of Orthopedics and Fractures 9/e p773

116. Person is hemiplegic and bed ridden for the one year. Changes in bone mineral density are first seen in:
a. Distal radius
b. Lumbar spine
c. Proximal femur
d. Proximal humerus
Ans. d

Ref: Apley's system of orthopedics and fractures 9/e p135

117. A child is spinned around by his father holding his hand. Suddenly the child started crying and did not allow his father to touch his elbow. Which of the following is the likely diagnosis?
a. Supracondylar fracture
b. Pulled elbow
c. Fracture olecranon process
d. Radial head dislocation
Ans. b

Ref: Apley's System of Orthopedics and Fractures 9/e p765

118. A 40-year-old female presents with multiple lytic bone lesions, fracture clavicle, periosteal resorption of 2nd and 3rd metatarsals. What is the most likely diagnosis?
a. Renal osteodystrophy
b. Osteomalacia
c. Hyperparathyroidism
d. Hyperthyroidism
Ans. c

Ref: Harrison's Principle of Internal Medicine 18/e p3102

119. A 40-year-old man presented with acute onset pain and swelling of left great toe. On X-ray a punched out lytic lesion is seen on phalanx with sclerotic margins and overhanging bony edges. The likely diagnosis is:
a. Gout
b. Rheumatoid arthritis
c. Psoriatic arthritis
d. Reiter's syndrome
Ans. a

Ref: Harrison's Principle of Internal Medicine 18/e p2838

120. Which of the following is true about non specific interstitial pneumonia?
a. Common in elderly age group
b. Good prognosis
c. Early honeycombing
d. Males are affected more commonly than females
Ans. b

Ref: Robbin's 8/e p695

121. True about obstructive sleep apnea are all except:
a. Females affected more than males
b. Commonly associated with hypertension
c. Day time sleepiness is seen
d. >5 episodes of apnea per hour
Ans. a

Ref: Harrison's Principle of Internal Medicine 18/e p2186

122. A person starts seizing on a railway station while waiting for a train. A wrist band was found showing he is a patient of epilepsy and has a medicine in his pocket. What will you do next?
a. Put a handkerchief in his mouth and restrain him by holding hands and legs
b. Take him away from the train,give him medicine with small sips of water and wait for seizure to resolve
c. Take him away from the train,give him medicine with small sips of water,raise his legs and wait for seizure to resolve
d. Take him away from the train,make him lie down and refer to the hospital
Ans. d

Ref: http://www.epilepsy.com/get-help/seizure-first-aid/care-and-comfort-first-aid

123. High calcium uptake leads to:
a. Milk alkali syndrome
b. Osteoporosis
c. Osteopetrosis
d. Cardiomyopathy
Ans. a

Ref: Harrison's Principle of Internal Medicine 18/e p3110

124. Female in her twenties presents with abdominal distension and vomiting. On examination she was found to have alopecia and a crepitus in the epigastrium. What is your diagnosis?
a. Trichobezoar
b. Rectus sheath hematoma

c. Intestinal tuberculosis
d. Carcinoma pyloric antrum

Ans. a

Ref: http://en.wikipedia.org/wiki/Rapunzel_ syndrome

125. A 70 year old female suffered from an attack of influenza but refused to take the vaccine. She subsequently developed pneumonia and died within 5 days. What is the most common cause of post influenza pneumonia?

a. CMV
b. Staphylococcus aureus
c. Measles
d. Legionella

Ans. b

Ref: Harrison's Principle of Internal Medicine 18/e p1496

126. A 15-year-old boy came back to his village after a vacation to his relatives. He developed severe headache and purulent nasal discharge and was diagnosed as acute bacterial meningitis. He died 5 days later. Which is the most likely etiological agent?

a. Plasmodium falciparum
b. Toxoplasma
c. Naegleria fowleri
d. Entamoeba histolytica

Ans. c

Ref: Harrison's Principle of Internal Medicine 18/e p1686

127. Which of the following diseases decrease in levels of single neurotransmitter was first identified?

a. Alzheimer's disease
b. Parkinson's disease
c. Huntington's disease
d. Schizophrenia

Ans. b

Ref: http://www.ncbi.nlm.nih.gov/pmc/articles/PMC1736202

128. In which of the following chronic conditions degenerative changes in the brain are seen which are not a part of normal ageing?

a. Dementia
b. Pseudodementia
c. Amnestic syndrome
d. Delirium

Ans. c

Ref: Harrison's Principle of Internal Medicine 18/e p209

129. Which of the following is the most effective treatment of severe malaria?

a. Artesunate
b. Chloroquine
c. Primaquine
d. Doxycycline

Ans. a

Ref: Harrison's Principle of Internal Medicine 18/e p1699-1701

130. Which of the following inflammatory condition has 90% association with HLA-B27?

a. Ankylosing spondylitis
b. Psoriasis
c. Reiters
d. Rheumatoid arthritis

Ans. a

Ref: Harrison's Principle of Internal Medicine 18/e p2774

131. Which of the following is usually not seen in Rheumatic heart disease?
a. PS
b. TS
c. MS
d. AS
Ans. a

Ref: Harrison's Principle of Internal Medicine 18/e p3102

132. A patient has angina, dyspnea and syncope. What is the most likely diagnosis?
a. VSD
b. ASD
c. AR
d. AS
Ans. a

Ref: Harrison's Principle of Internal Medicine 18/e p1939

133. All are seen in chronic MS except:
a. S3
b. Loud S1
c. Opening snap
d. Mid diastolic murmur
Ans. a

Ref: Harrison's Principle of Internal Medicine 18/e p1930

134. Abatacept, a new drug inhibiting costimulation is used for:
a. SLE
b. Scleroderma
c. Rheumatoid arthritis
d. Sjogren syndrome
Ans. c

Ref: Harrison's Principle of Internal Medicine 18/e p2748

135. A known case of bronchial asthma presents with respiratory distress, a respiratory rate of 48 /min and can barely speak 2 words. Nebulised salbutamol was given and patient could speak a sentence but there was fall in SpO2 from 95% to 85%. What could be the possible explanation?
a. Ventilation perfusion mismatch because of increased dead space ventilation
b. Intrathoracic shunting
c. Due to salbutamol
d. Faulty oximeter
Ans. a

Ref: http://copd.about.com/od/glossaryoftermspz/g/vqmismatch.htm

136. Which of the following is diagnostic of acute hepatitis B infection?
a. IgM Anti Hbc
b. IgG Anti Hbc
c. Anti HbS
d. IgM Anti Hbe
Ans. a

Ref: Harrison's Principle of Internal Medicine 18/e p2550-51

137. A nurse has been found to be seropositive for both HbsAg and HbeAg. She is suffering from:
a. Concurrent Hep B and Hep E infection
b. Chronic Hep B infection
c. Acute Hep B infection
d. Past Hepatitis B infection
Ans. c

Ref: Harrison's Principle of Internal Medicine 18/e p2550-51

138. Inability to perform physical activity without discomfort falls under:
a. NYHA Class 1
b. 2
c. 3
d. 4
Ans. d

Ref: Harrison's Principle of Internal Medicine 18/e p1818

139. Which of the following is not an indicator of chronic congestive cardiac failure?
a. Brain natriuretic peptide
b. Troponin
c. CRP
d. Sirtuin
Ans. d

Ref: Harrison's Principle of Internal Medicine 18/e p1906

140. Which of the following pulmonary symptoms don't have the corresponding non pulmonary association?
a. Cyanosis-anxiety
b. Wheezing-CHF
c. Tachypnea-Acidosis
d. Chest pain-pericarditis
Ans. a

Ref: Harrison's Principle of Internal Medicine 18/e p1154

141. 30-year-old man presents to the emergency with complaints of muscle weakness, nausea, vomiting and fatigue. ECG showed all tall peaked T waves, prolonged PR interval, wide QRS and absent P. Which of the following drugs is not used in management?
a. Beta antagonist
b. Calcium gluconate
c. Insulin
d. Sodium bicarbonate
Ans. a

Ref: Harrison's Principle of Internal Medicine 18/e p359

142. H-reflex is done in:
a. L2 radiculopathy
b. L3
c. L4
d. S1
Ans. d

Ref: Harrison's Principle of Internal Medicine 18/e Ebook p 45-46

143. What is the emergent management of tension pneumothorax?
a. Chest X-ray
b. Emergency room thoracostomy if unstable
c. Immediate needle thoracostomy in 2nd intercostal space
d. Tube thoracostomy in 5th ICS
Ans. c

Ref: Harrison's Principle of Internal Medicine 18/e p2181

144. A man presented with bilateral crepitations in the base of the lungs and signs of pneumonintis with a history of exposure to pigeon faeces. What is true about this condition?
a. Diagnosis can be made on the basis of biopsy
b. CT scan is the investigation of choice
c. Chest X-ray will reveal characteristic changes
d. It is a type 1 hypersensitivity reaction
Ans. a

Ref: Harrison's Principle of Internal Medicine 18/e p2118

145. Which of the following is not a component of SIRS:

a. Temperature >38 degree C
b. Urine output < 1 ml/kg/hr
c. SBP< 90 mm Hg
d. RR> 24/min

Ans. b

Ref: Harrison's Principle of Internal Medicine 18/e p2223

146. In case of ascites, Le Veen shunt is done between peritoneum and:

a. SVC
b. Cisterna chili
c. Gall bladder
d. Renal pelvis

Ans. a

Ref: Bailey and Love 26/e p 1077

147. Which of the following drug is useful for treatment of advanced prostate cancer?

a. Ganirelix
b. Abarelix
c. Goserelin
d. Cetrorelix

Ans. c

Ref: Katzung Basic and Clinical Pharmacology 12/e p972

148. All of the following are premalignant except:

a. Peutz Jeghers syndrome
b. Ulcerative colitis
c. FAP
d. Crohn's disease

Ans. a

Ref: Bailey and Love 26/e p1159

149. A 65-year-old man presented with an episode of syncope. He said he felt dizzy during defecation and noticed gross bleeding in the pan. Fecal occult blood test was done 3 months ago as apart of routine screening for colon cancer was negative. There is no history of recurrent weight loss. What is the likely colonoscopic finding?

a. Microscopic colitis
b. Dilated mucosal and submucosal vein in colon
c. Early colonic carcinoma
d. Sigmoid diverticulitis

Ans. b

Ref: http://en.wikipedia.org/wiki/Heyde%27s_ syndrome

150. A 58-year-old female complains of dull aching pain in right iliac fossa. On examination, gross pallor was found and a mass palpable in the iliac fossa. What is the most likely diagnosis?

a. Appendiceal mass
b. Carcinoma ascending colon
c. Ileocaecal TB
d. Diverticulitis

Ans. b

Ref: Bailey and Love 26/e p1181

151. FNAC cannot detect which of the following:

a. Follicular carcinoma
b. Colloid goiter
c. Papillary carcinoma
d. Hahimoto thyroiditis

Ans. a

Ref: Robbin's 8/e p1123

152. A 15-year-old girl with soft painful swelling on posterior aspect of thigh. Color doppler showed multiple venous channels without any major arterial feeder. All of the following are liquid embolizing agents except:

a. Absolute alcohol
b. Sodium tetradecyl sulphate
c. Polyvinyl alcohol
d. Cyanoacrylate

Ans. c

Ref: http://en.wikipedia.org/wiki/Embolization# agents

153. You are a surgeon posted at CHC. A patient of head injury comes to you with rapidly developing sensorium and progressive dilatation and fixation of pupil. No neurosurgeon/CT scan is available. You decide to make a burr hole to emergently relieve the intracranial pressure. Which of the following sites will you choose?

a. In the temporal region contralateral to the side of pupillary dilatation
b. In the midline if both pupils are equal or it is not known which side dilated first
c. In the left temporal region if no localizing sign is found
d. Refer to a higher center if both the pupils are equal or it is not known which side dilated first

Ans. c

Ref: Ramamurthy and Tandon's Textbook of Neurosurgery volume 1 3/e p412

154. A couple presents with infertility. On investigating the husband is found to have azoospermia on semen analysis. Vas was not palpable on per rectal examination. Semen had low volume, high viscosity and fructose was present. What will you do next?

a. CFTR gene mutation analysis
b. Karyotype
c. PSA
d. Transrectal ultrasound

Ans. a

Ref: Nelson Textbook of Pediatrics 19/e p1497

155. Which of the following is the ideal time for repair of cleft palate?

a. 9-12 months
b. 18-24 months
c. 2-3 years
d. 5-6 years

Ans. a

Ref: Nelson Textbook of Pediatrics 19/e p1252-53

156. A Child with cyanosis and chooking on feeding at birth was diagnosed as TEF and had underwent a corrective surgery. He comes to you with complaints of barking cough and expiratory wheeze. What is the most likely diagnosis?

a. Bronchial asthma
b. Croup
c. Tracheomalacia
d. Subglottic stenosis

Ans. c

Ref: Nelson Textbook of Pediatrics 19/e p1452

157. A child complaints of fluid coming out of umbilicus on straining. What is the diagnosis?

a. Patent vitellointestinal duct
b. Urachal Fistula
c. Umbilical fistula
d. Gastroschisis

Ans. b

Ref: Nelson Textbook of Pediatrics 19/e p651

158. A neonate with respiratory distress with enlargement of upper lobe of lung and mediastinal shift towards the right. What is the most likely diagnosis?
a. Congenital lobar emphysema
b. Alpha 1 antitrypsin deficiency
c. Pneumonia
d. Cystic fibrosis
Ans. a

Ref: Nelson Textbook of Pediatrics 19/e p1461

159. A 10-month old-child weighing 5 kg and 65 cm presents with cough and cold. He was found to have a respiratory rate of 48 per minute with no retractions, grunting, cyanosis. There is no history of convulsions. Which is true?
a. No pneumonia, only cough and cold
b. Child has pneumonia
c. Severe pneumonia
d. Very severe disease
Ans. a

Ref: Ghai Essential Pediatrics 8/e p759

160. A female child came with complaints of involuntary movements was diagnosed as a case of sydenham chorea suggestive of a diagnosis of acute rheumatic fever. There is no complaints of carditis or arthritis. Throat culture is negative. Which of the following will mostly suggest any recent streptococcal infection?
a. Antistreptolysin S
b. ASLO
c. PCR for M protein
d. Hyaluronidase
Ans. b

Ref: Ghai Essential Pediatrics 8/e p435

161. A neonate at 48 hours of birth with a history of non passage of meconium. Next step in evaluation will be:
a. Lower GI study
b. Sweat chloride levels
c. CFTR mutation analysis
d. Manometry
Ans. a

Ref: Nelson Textbook of Pediatrics 19/e p1286

162. Which of the following disease is not seen in adults?
a. Susac syndrome
b. Kawasaki disease
c. Takayasu arteritis
d. Henoch Schonlein purpura
Ans. b

Ref: Nelson Textbook of Pediatrics 19/e p865

163. A 6-month-old child presents with episodes of vomiting after ingesting fruit juice. Which of the following enzyme deficiency is likely:
a. Aldolase B
b. Fructokinase
c. Glucose 6 phosphatase
d. Hexokinase
Ans. a

Ref: Ghai Essential Pediatrics 8/e p656

164. A 6-month-old child woke up in the night crying with abdominal pain which got relieved on passing red stools. The diagnosis is:
a. Meckel's diverticulum
b. Inteussusception
c. Malrotation
d. Intestinal obstruction
Ans. b

Ref: Ghai Essential Pediatrics 8/e p287

165. A child presents with pellagra like dermatitis and aminoaciduria. Two siblings have the condition and it is absent in both parents. Which of the following condition is most likely?
a. Alkaptonuria
b. Phenylketonuria
c. Hartnup's disease
d. Von Gierke's disease
Ans. c

Ref: Nelson Textbook of Pediatrics 19/e p446

166. Which is not seen in tuberous sclerosis?
a. Astrocytoma
b. Ependymoma
c. White matter lesions
d. Subependymal nodules
Ans. b

Ref: Nelson Textbook of Pediatrics 19/e p2049

167. Which of the following if seen on day 10 on life is worrisome:
a. Conjugated hyperbilirubinemia
b. No weight gain
c. Dolls Eye reflex
d. Unconjugated hyperbilirubinemia
Ans. a

Ref: Nelson Textbook of Pediatrics 19/e p34

168. A child with Nephrotic syndrome following an episode of diarrhea presented with acute kidney injury with a creatinine of 4.5. All of the following are possible reasons except:
a. Renal vein thrombosis
b. Frusemide
c. Steroid induced diabetes
d. Diarrhoea water depletion
Ans. c

Ref: Nelson Textbook of Pediatrics 19/e p1818

169. All of the following are used for screening cancers in females except:
a. Pap smear-cervical cancer
b. Office endometrial aspirate-Endometrial carcinoma
c. Mammography-breast cancer
d. CA 125-ovary cancer
Ans. b

Ref: Novak's 14/e p1348

170. All of the following are true about augmentation of labor except:
a. Twin pregnancy precludes the use of oxytocin
b. Amniotomy decreases the need for oxytocin use
c. Methods of augmentation does not increase the risk of operational management
d. Associated with a risk of uterine hyperstimulation
Ans. a

Ref: William's Obstretics 23/e p502-4

171. Studies have shown that complications of prematurity IUGR are not affected by the timing of caesarean section. What is the recommended timing of caesarean section?

a. 37 weeks
b. 38 weeks
c. 39 weeks
d. 40 weeks

Ans. c

Ref: American College of Obstreticians and Gynecologists Guidelines 2008 p81

172. Which of the following is not a ligation technique?

a. Parkland
b. Pomeroy
c. Essure
d. Irving

Ans. c

Ref: William's Obstretics 23/e p698-701

173. A girl with normal stature and minimal or absent pubertal development is seen in:

a. Kallman syndrome
b. Testicular feminization syndrome
c. Turner's syndrome
d. Pure gonadal dysgenesis

Ans. a

Ref: Nelson Pediatrics 19/e p1956

174. Which of the following drug is not a first line treatment for an ovulatory abnormal uterine bleeding in a 13 year old?

a. Mefenamic acid
b. Tranexamic acid
c. Estrogen plus progesterone
d. Progesterone

Ans. a

Ref: Shaw's Textbook of Gynecology 15/e p301-4

175. In a patient with APLA syndrome, what treatment is used to prevent further abortions?

a. Aspirin +LMWH
b. Steroids
c. Aspirin
d. LMWH

Ans. a

Ref: Harrison 18/e p2737

176. Which is not true about expected date of delivery?

a. Less than 5% deliver on the expected date of delivery
b. 50% deliver within 1 week
c. 80% deliver within 2 weeks
d. Standard deviation around expected date of delivery is 3 weeks

Ans. d

Ref: Dutta's Textbook of Obstretics 2/e p651

177. All the following factors have been shown to improve fertility except:

a. Vegetarian diet
b. Loss of weight
c. Gain of weight
d. Less exercise

Ans. a

Ref: http://www.cincinnatifertility.com/holistic-treatment/fertility-diet

178. Itchy tense blisters are seen on normal looking skin as well as urticarial plaques as seen in the figure. What is the diagnosis?

a. IgA pemphigus
b. Bullous pemphigoid
c. Dermatitis herpetiformis
d. Pemphigus vulgaris

Ans. b

Ref: Neena Khanna's Illustrated synopsis of dermatology and Sexually transmitted Disease 4/e p67-69

179. A 25-year-old girl presented with erythematous papules on the face. The lesions were exacerbated on excessive sweating, sun exposure and emotional disturbance. What is the diagnosis?

a. SLE
b. Rosacea
c. Acne vulgaris
d. Photodermatitis

Ans. b

Ref: Neena Khanna's Illustrated Synopsis of Dermatology and Sexually Transmitted Disease 4/e p121

180. A patient presented with the lesion as shown in picture. What is the best investigation?

a. Patch test
b. Grattage test
c. Skin sensation testing
d. KOH mount

Ans. d

Ref: Neena Khanna's Illustrated Synopsis of Dermatology and Sexually Transmitted Disease 4/e p291

181. A female patient comes after the holiday with a vulvovaginal discharge and dysuria. Which of the following is most sensitive diagnostic testing?

a. Nucleic Acid Amplification Test
b. Wet mount
c. Gram's staining
d. Blood culture

Ans. a

Ref: Neena Khanna's Illustrated Synopsis of Dermatology and Sexually Transmitted Disease 4/e p313

182. Which of the following is not a type of lichen planus?

a. Lichen planopilaris
b. Lichen pigmentosa
c. Lichen hypertrophica
d. Lichen scrofulosorum

Ans. a

Ref: Neena Khanna's Illustrated Synopsis of Dermatology and Sexually Transmitted Disease 4/e p57'

183. A 24-year-old female presented with complaints of acne. On examination multiple nodules. Cysts and inter communicating sinuses were seen. How will you treat her?

a. Tazarotene
b. Oral isoretinoin
c. Acitretin
d. Doxycycline

Ans. b

Ref: Neena Khanna's Illustrated Synopsis of Dermatology and Sexually Transmitted Disease 4/e p120

184. A 23-year-old male complains of recurret scaly lesion on the glans penis. It always occurred at the same site and healed with slight hyperpigmentation:

a. Syphilis
b. Fixed drug eruption
c. Chlamydia
d. Gonorrhoea

Ans. b

Ref: Neena Khanna's Illustrated Synopsis of Dermatology and Sexually Transmitted Disease 4/e p209

185. Which of the following is used in day care surgeries?

a. Ketamine
b. Diazepam
c. Thiopentone
d. Propofol

Ans. d

Ref: Miller's Anaesthesia 8/e p726

186. The names Bethune and Brethren are associated with which of the following monitoring devices?

a. End tidal capnography
b. Plethysmography
c. Transesophagial echo
d. Precordial Doppler

Ans. a

Ref: Bethune, RWM and Brechner VL (1968)

187. An eye surgery was performed using propofol as the IV anesthetic agent and succinyl choline as muscle relaxant. Recovery from anesthesia was uneventful. However the patient complains of pain in the muscle:

a. Muscle infarction
b. Succinylcholine
c. Propofol
d. None

Ans. b

Ref: Miller's Anaesthesia 8/e p866

188. Which of the following is a plasma expander similar to albumin, has a MW of 30,000 and causes less hypersensitivity reaction but should be used with caution:

a. Dextran
b. HES
c. Polygeline
d. Polypyrrolidone

Ans. c

Ref: KD Tripathi 7/e p645

189. Which of the following is the circuit of choice for spontaneous ventilation?

a. Mapleson D
b. Mapleson C
c. Mapleson B
d. Mapleson A

Ans. d

Ref: Miller's Anaesthesia 8/e p692-95

190. All of the following are methods for improving oxygenation using a ventilator except:

a. ECMO
b. Low tidal volume high PEEP
c. Prone ventilation
d. High frequency ventilation

Ans. d

Ref: Harrison 18/e p2208

191. A neonate presented on day 1 of life with bilious vomiting. What investigation will you do?

a. Ultrasound
b. CT Scan
c. Chest skiagram
d. Babygram

Ans. d

Ref: Nelson Pediatrics 19/e p1278

192. Investigation of choice for acute appendicitis in children:

a. USG
b. MRI
c. CT
d. X-ray

Ans. a

Ref: OP Ghai Pediatrics 8/e p287

193. A person has an injury in forefinger with glass and it is suspected that he has retained piece of glass in his finger. Which is the first investigation that you will do?

a. Ultrasound
b. MRI
c. CT scan
d. Plane radiograph

Ans. d

Ref: http://www.aafp.org/afp/2007/0901/p683.html

194. What is the investigation of choice in a patient with acute head injury?

a. PET
b. MRI
c. CECT
d. Non Contrast CT

Ans. d

Ref: http://emedicine.medscape.com/article/1163653

195. A 3-month-old baby presented with clay Colored stools and dark yellow urine. On further investigations he was found to have a bilirubin of 6 mg%.Which is the most sensitive investigation to diagnose the above condition?

a. Liver Function Tests
b. CT abdomen
c. USG
d. HIDA Scan

Ans. d

Ref: Nelson Pediatrics 19/e p1385

196. Investigation of choice for bronchiectasis:

a. HRCT
b. MRI
c. Chest X-ray
d. Bronchoscopy

Ans. a

Ref: Harrison's Principle of Internal Medicine 18/e p2143

197. A patient was diagnosed with schizophrenia and was started on haloperidol 5 mg. On 3rd day he presented with uprolling of eyes. A complete neurological examination revealed no spasticity or any other abnormalities except uprolling of eye balls. Visual acuity was found to be normal. What is your likely diagnosis?

a. Seizure
b. Akathisia
c. Malingering
d. Acute dystonia

Ans. b

Ref: Harrison's Principle of Internal Medicine 18/e p3544

198. Which of the following is not an objective of mental health act 1987?
- a. Minimal mental health care for all
- b. Application of mental health knowledge in general health care
- c. Promote community participation
- d. Human rights for the mentally ill

Ans. d

Ref: Park 22/e p426

199. Which of the following is the most effective treatment modality for post traumatic stress disorder?
- a. Hypnosis
- b. Rational and emotive therapy
- c. Eye movement desensitization and reprocessing
- d. Cognitive behavioral therapy

Ans. a

Ref: Niraj Ahuja Psychiatry 7/e p112

200. All are true about autism except:
- a. 2/3rd are mentally retarded
- b. Language is impaired
- c. Abnormal dermatoglyphics
- d. Poor eye contact

Ans. c

Ref: Niraj Ahuja Psychiatry 7/e p164

AIIMS SRship Questions 2014 Set A

1. **Term that represent junction between alveolar bone and ramus of mandible where internal oblique ridge originate is?**
   a. Clinical angle of mandible
   b. Anatomical angle of mandible
   c. Surgical angle of mandible
   d. Fracture angle of mandible
   Ans. a

Anatomical angle-Gonion angle of mandible, junction of lower border of mandible and posterior ramal border Surgical angle Junction between body of mandible and ramus. Fracture angle At origin of external oblique line

2. **Champy plate is:**
   a. Rigid
   b. Semirigid
   c. Fixation plate with bicortical screw
   d. Fixation plate with monocortical screw
   Ans. d
   - Discovered by Michelet
   - Popularised by Champy

CASE I	CASE II	CASE III
Behind the mental foramen ↓ Upper border	At angle of jaw	2 Plates between 2 mental foramina

3. **Fracture of mandibular angle heals without complication when?**
   a. 2 plates used in A.O
   b. Compression plate
   c. Single plate functional adaptation
   d. Reconstruction plate
   Ans. c
4. **Type of OKC which has high recurrence and nevoid BCC is seen in:**
   a. Orthokeratinised
   b. Parakeratinised
   c. Not related to keratinisation
   d. Mixed
   Ans. b
   - Classical palisaded,tombstone/picket fence arrangement seen
5. **A female patient came for esthetic improveme nt of her brown teeth, 2 other of 4 brothers have same findings. She has infrequent enamel chipping. No root caries and there is obliteration of root canal and roots were short. What is she suffering from?**
   a. Dentinogenesisimperfecta
   b. Dentin dysplasia
   c. Flourosis
   d. Erythroblastosisfoetalis
   Ans. a

TYPE I	TYPE II now 1	TYPE III now 2
• Not in new class • Associated with Osteogenesis imperfect • Only in decidous	• Both deciduous and permanent • Obliteraton of pulp chamber	• Shell and brandywineteeth • Both dentition involved • Wide pulp chamber

- Mutation in DSSP, Chromosome 4 (4q.21.3)
- Tulip shape in Type 1 D.I
- Partial or total obliteration
- Enamel chipping but not susceptible to caries

6. **The chromosome involved in Dentinogenesis imperfect is:**
   a. 3
   b. 4
   c. 9
   d. 16
   Ans. b
7. **Storiform appearance seen in:**
   a. Malignant fibrous histiocytoma
   b. Recurrentaphthous
   c. Primary herpes
   d. Fibrosarcoma
   Ans. a
   - Both storiform & cartwheel pattern is seen
8. **Gingival involvement not seen in:**
   a. Pyogenic granuloma
   b. Recurrentaphthous
   c. Pemphigoid
   d. Primary herpes
   Ans. b
   - Primary herpes- diffuse gingival enlargement
   - ANUG- Marginal
   - c/c desquamative- attached gingiva and alveolar mucosa: no involvement of marginal gingiva
9. **Oral site involved in lymphogranuloma venereum is:**
   a. Lip
   b. Tongue
   c. Palate
   d. Gingiva
   Ans. b
   - Causes can be Chlamydia trachomatis, STD- anorectal involvement seen
10. **Syphilitic glossitis plummer Wilson syndrome of tongue, mikulikz disease, hepatitis A, SSC is related etiologically to:**
    a. Syphilitic glossitis, P.V syndrome
    b. HepatitisA, Mikulikz syndrome
    c. HSV-1, HPV also associated with SSC
    d. All of the above
    Ans. a
11. **Dermatotropic viral diseases are:**
    a. Hepatitis, Yellow fever, mumps
    b. Rabies, herpes encephalitis

c. Impetigo, scarlet fever, rabies
d. Smallpox, chickenpox, measles

Ans. d

- Viscerotropiceg: yellow fever, jaundice, mumps
- Neurotropic, e.g. polio meningitis, rabies, herpes encephalitis

12. **Fungi seen in healthy oral mucosa is:**
a. Candida
b. Blastomyces
c. Aspergillus
d. Rhinosporidium

Ans. a

13. **A 35-year-old female has 3 teen children, all of them have thickened white corrugated or folded soft texture lesion on cheek. Biopsy points towards:**
a. Leukoplakia
b. Leukedema
c. White sponge nevus
d. Candidiasis

Ans. c

- Also known as Cannon's disease

14. **Rotational forces require for extracting:**
a. Upper molars
b. Lower incisors
c. Maxillary centrals and mandibular second premolars
d. Mandibular centrals and maxillary second premolars

Ans. c

15. **Amongameloblastoma, BCC, ACC and Veruccous carcinoma, which lesions rarely metastasise**
a. Ameloblastoma, BCC, ACC
b. Ameloblastoma, BCC, Veruccous carcinoma
c. BCC, ACC
d. Ameloblastoma,Veruccous carcinoma

Ans. b

- If only BCC+ Veruccous carcinoma is in option,then this will be answer

16. **Which is not true for Adenoid Cystic carcinoma?**
a. Most common timur of parotid gland
b. H/P having both acidophilic and basophilic
c. Neural invasion
d. Reoccur

Ans. a

- Most common location-minor salivary glands, palate most common

17. **Masseteric space infection usually due to:**
a. Molar
b. Parotid space infection
c. Lateral pharyngeal space infection
d. Buccal space infection

Ans. a

18. **Microscopic and radiographic features suggest it central giant cell granuloma, other investigations are needed to rule out:**
a. Hyperparathyroidism
b. Paget's disease

c. Osteosarcoma
d. Hypothyroidism
Ans. a

19. Vitamin D resistant rickets defect is:
a. Osteoid maturation time
b. Bone formation
c. Boneresorption
d. Cutting cone defect
Ans. a

20. Open reduction and fixation of condylar # is done in:
a. More than 4 mm ramal shortening
b. Subcondye # with no reduction
c. Superior 5 mm #
d. Greenstick #
Ans. a

21. Burning tongue is not a feature of:
a. Mucocele
b. Lymphangioma
c. Hemangioma
d. Ranula
Ans. d

22. Internal opening of branchial fistula is located at:
a. Around second premolar
b. Behindpalatoglossal arch
c. Fossa of tonsil
d. Around third molar
Ans. c
- Option B is the external opening

23. SLE, Rheumatoid arthritis, thyroiditis have in common:
a. Arthus reaction
b. Autoimmune
c. Anaphylaxis
d. Immediate hypersensitivity
Ans. b
- SLE-Type I + Type III most common
- R.A- III + IV
- Fever-II
- Scleroderma-Type II
- Good Pasture-Type II

24. Which nerve is associated with Ramsay Hunt syndrome or post herpetic neuralgia?
a. 5th nerve
b. 7th nerve
c. 8th nerve
d. 9th nerve
Ans. b
- Herpes zoster is the viral infection of Geniculate ganglion

25. Incision used for treatment of traumatic telecanthus:
a. Infraorbital
b. Bicoronal

c. Most auricular extending to protect facial nerve
d. Blepharoplasty
Ans. b

- Option D is used for eye lift surgery
- Medial canthus ligament disruption
- Normal- 28 to 35 mm
- Half of interpupillary distance
- Suspected – 35
- Diagnostic- 40

26. An adult patient with prosthetic heart valve undergo tooth extraction, prophylaxisrequired:
a. 1 gmamox 1 hr before procedure
b. 1 gmamox 2 hr before procedure
c. 2 gmamox 1 hr before procedure
d. 2gmamox 2 hr before procedure
Ans. c

27. 10 day after hospitalisation a large incapacitation, myocardialinfarct. A 50-year-old man suddenly develops paralysis of right side. Best explanation of brain damage is:
a. Detachment of bacterial embolus from pulmonary vein
b. Receptor of congenital aneurysm at Circle of Willis
c. Detatchment of mural thrombus from left ventricle
d. Detatchment of mural thrombus from right ventricle
Ans. d

28. Longest acting L. A is:
a. Bupivacaine and Etidocaine
b. Bupivacaine and Lignocaine
c. Bupivacaine and propoxycaine
d. Bupivacaine and mepivacaine
Ans. a

29. The most common cause of pulmonary embolism:
a. Heart failure
b. DVT
c. Cancer lung
d. Pneumonia
Ans..b

30. Odontogenicmyxoma radiographic features:
a. Soap bubble
b. Honey comb
c. Driven snow
d. Jigsaw puzzle
Ans. a

31. Withdrawal line of tooth removal depends upon:
a. Crown pattern
b. Root pattern
c. Thickness of the gums
d. PDL
Ans. b

32. Chromic gut suture is absorbed by:
a. Proteolysis
b. Hydrolysis

c. Saccharolysis
d. Acidolysis

Ans. b

- Generally other sutures by proteolysis

33. **Type VIII Ehlers Danlos syndrome shows:**
    a. Pulpal involvement
    b. Periodontal involvement
    c. Alveolar bone involvement
    d. Radicular involvement

    Ans. b

34. **Five minutes after the administration of L. A for extraction of left second premolar patient was unable to move both upper and lower lips and unable to close the eye on the same side. It is due to:**
    a. Diffusion of L.A into parotid
    b. Paralysis of motor branch supplying to muscle of mastication
    c. Diffusion of L.A into optic nerve ganglion
    d. Ophthalmic division involvement

    Ans. a

35. **In condyle # displacement of condyle is due to:**
    a. Medialpterygoid
    b. Masseter
    c. Lateralpterygoid
    d. Temporalis

    Ans. c

36. **In a patient with body # mandible occlusal loading is applied to fracture site. It will lead to the following change at superior border:**
    a. Traction
    b. Compression
    c. Tension
    d. Splaying

    Ans. c

37. **During L.A administration patient become pale, perspiring and disoriented. The appropriate management:**
    a. Administration of Oxygen
    b. Supine position
    c. Holding head between the knees
    d. Administration of 1: 1000 Adrenaline

    Ans. b

    It's a case of syncope—Leg raise by 10-15 degree

38. **During appropriate execution of IAN block, muscle pierced is:**
    a. Buccinator
    b. Masseter
    c. Medialpterygoid
    d. LateralPterygoid

    Ans. a

39. **Direct surgical access for subcondylar # is gained by which incision:**
    a. Pre auricular
    b. Transparotid
    c. Submandibular
    d. Intraoral

    Ans. b

    - B is the subcondylar best approach for direct access and for high condylar # its preauricular

40. **Exposure of zygomatic arch is best achieved by:**
    a. Preauricular
    b. Directincison over arch
    c. Coronal incision
    d. Submandibular incision
    Ans. c

41. **After reduction of unstable zygoma # with Carrol Gillard screw, the plating should be done firstat which site:**
    a. Frontozygomatic suture
    b. Spheno temporal suture
    c. Zygomaticotemporal suture
    d. Zygomaticomaxillary suture
    Ans. d

Ref: Peterson's Oral & Maxillofacial Surgery 3/e p450-51

- Compression plate can be used
- Carroll Gillard screw is inserted transcutaneously into malar eminence
- A coronal flap is used to gain access to the zygomatic arch

42. **In plane bending is done in:**
    a. Horizontal plane
    b. Vertical plane
    c. Torsion
    d. Plier, bend the plate end
    Ans. a

43. **HBO oxygen is contraindicated in all except:**
    a. Thalassemia trait
    b. Spherocytosis
    c. Glaucoma
    d. Recurrence of tumour
    Ans. c

44. **Management of dry socket aim towards:**
    a. Pain relief
    b. Control of infection
    c. Both
    d. None
    Ans. a

45. **In a transfacialplane, the face is divided into how many planes:**
    a. 2
    b. 3
    c. 5
    d. 7
    Ans. c

46. **In an ideal situation the ratio between 3 proportions of face in vertical plane from abovedownward:**
    a. 34:33:33
    b. 35:30:35
    c. 30:35:35
    d. 25:50:25
    Ans. a

47. Tooth which fails to erupt in oral cavity during its displacement time and is not expected to erupt is:
a. Impacted
b. Submerged
c. Unerupted
d. Ankylosed
Ans. a

48. For third molar surgery to decrease swelling steroid is administered:
a. 8 mg intraoperatively
b. 8 mg one day before surgery, continue 8 mg for 2 days after surgery
c. 8 mg IV at the time of surgery
d. 8 mg intraoperative,continue on the day of surgery and continue for next 2 days
Ans. d

49. Root of third molar 50% complete at age:
a. Birth
b. 6 years
c. 9 years
d. 16 years
Ans. d

50. A patient on dicumarol therapy requiring oral surgery first procedure done is:
a. PT
b. Sedation
c. Vitamin D
d. Vitamin K administration to promote clot formation
Ans. a
- INR up to 3.5, no need to reduce anticoagulant
- PT patient ISI
- PT normal

51. During plating which screw stabilise the plate by compressing it against the bone:
a. IMF
b. Locking
c. Non-locking
d. Lag screw
Ans. c

52. Bone gets # after how much percent elongation:
a. 2 %
b. 4%
c. 6%
d. 8 %
Ans. c

53. In which # there may be a tendency for increase in width of lower face:
a. Guardmans #
b. Bilateralparasymphysis #
c. Bilateral #
d. Symphysis #
Ans. a

54. Middle facial height is measured from:
a. Hairline to subnasale
b. Glabella to menton

c. Glabella to subnasale
d. Subnasale to menton
Ans. c

55. **After maxillofacial trauma, emergency bleeding is usually managed by:**
a. Pressure
b. Suturing
c. Clamping and ligation
d. Facial artery ligation
Ans. a

56. **Open pneumothorax is managed by:**
a. Pressure application with hand
b. Occlusive dressing with all sides closed
c. Dressing with three sides closed
d. Dressing with two sides closed
Ans. c

57. **A patient with sustained mandibular # along with severe chest injury. A chest drain was inserted to relieve pressure. Patient has lost 500 ml blood is lost in 1 hour and become hypotensive. Next step or management to be done is:**
a. Place a second drain to drain more blood
b. Blood transfusion
c. Thoracotomy and exploration
d. This is a cascade in such injury
Ans. c

58. **Structure passing through parotid gland are:**
a. Facial artery, vein and nerve
b. Facial nerve, maxillary artery and veins
c. Facial nerve, retro mandibular vein, transverse facial vein, ECA, post auricular artery
d. All of the above
Ans. c
- Straight pick from NBDE Clinicals

59. **For management of parotid fistula all are used except:**
a. Atropine
b. Suction and dressing
c. Pilocarpine
d. Pterygomandibularraphae
Ans. c

60. **Middle constrictor of pharynx is attached to:**
a. Hyoid
b. Mandible
c. Cricoid
d. Pterygomandibular raphae
Ans. a

61. **In CPR chest compression is done at a rate of:**
a. 1 inch/10 sec
b. 2 inch/sec
c. 2 inch/5 sec
d. 5 inch/sec
Ans. b

62. Miniplate fixation of mandibular fracture is a type of:
- a. Load bearing
- b. Load sharing
- c. Rigid fixation
- d. Non rigid osteosynthesis

Ans. b

63. Which of the following is a non resorbable suture?
- a. Vicryl
- b. PGA
- c. Surgicel
- d. Ethilon

Ans. d

64. Which of the following is the most important virulent factor for P.gingivalis?
- a. Proteases
- b. Fimbriae
- c. Capsule
- d. Polysacharides

Ans. a

65. Which of the following microbial group is associated with Aa?
- a. Yellow
- b. Red
- c. Green
- d. Purple

Ans. c

66. RPP is caused by:
- a. P.gingivalis and T.denticola
- b. P.gingivalis and Aa
- c. P.gingivalis and T.forsythia
- d. P.gingivalis and P.intermedia

Ans. b

67. The Ph of regular non-stimulated saliva is:
- a. 5–6
- b. 6–7
- c. 7–8
- d. >7 always

Ans. b

68. What are calcospherites?
- a. The calcium which is found in supragingival plaque
- b. The calcium found in subgingival plaque
- c. The calcium found at mineralisation front
- d. The calcium bound phosphate in matrix vesicles

Ans. c

69. Which of the following is the long acting anesthesia?
- a. Bupivacaine
- b. Mepivacaine
- c. Articaine
- d. Prilocaine

Ans. a

70. Which of the following is the most potent APC?
a. Macrophage
b. Neutrophil
c. B cell
d. Langerhan cell
Ans. a

71. Most bacterial species of RPP found under:
a. Prevotella group
acteroid group
c. Filamentous
d. Black pigmented
Ans. b

72. The salivary gland acini are lined by:
a. Cuboidal cells
b. Columnar cells
c. Myoepithelial cells
d. Columnar ciliated
Ans. b

73. A father presented his son who is 5 years of age, with swelling in the parotid region. The child is having fever and malaise from last 3 days. He has difficulty swallowing and general malaise. Biopsy of the parotid gland revealed chronic inflammatory cell infiltration and pus discharge. The probable diagnosis would be:
a. Acute bacterial parotitis
b. Mumps
c. Parotid gland
d. Sialolithiasis
Ans. b

74. The artery which loops around superficial temporal artery is:
a. Middle meningeal artery
b. Maxillary artery
c. Masseteric Artery
d. Temporal artery
Ans. a

75. The posterior pillar of the palatine tonsil is formed by which of the following muscle:
a. Palatoglossal
b. Palatophryngeal
c. Buccinators
d. Glossopharyngeal
Ans. a

76. The following is the function of a fixer in the development of radiographic films:
a. It removes the extra silver halids which are unfixed
b. It strengthen/fixes thee silver halids onto the X-ray film
c. It takes away extra developer solution
d. It binds the developer to the film.
Ans. a

77. Which of the antibiotic cannot be given to a pregnant lady?
a. Doxycycline
b. Pencillin

c. Streptomycin
d. Aminoglycosides
Ans. a

78. The most effective and modern diagnostic aid used for the detection of fractures in head and neck region is:
a. CBCT
b. 0.8 mm CT
c. MRI
d. Scans using radio – isotopes
Ans. b

79. Which of the following autogenous bone graft is not preferred for grafting?
a. Tibial graft
b. Sternal graft
c. Rib graft
d. Ileac crest graft
Ans. a

80. Which of the following mineral is essential for wound healing?
a. Selenium
b. Copper
c. Lithium
d. Calcium
Ans. b

81. Which of the following is a diagnostic indicator of viral replication in hepatitis–B?
a. Presence of HbS – Ag in blood
b. Presence of HbS-C in blood
c. Presence of HbS-E in blood
d. Presence of HbS-ab in blood
Ans. c

82. The MMPs most commonly associated with acute periodontitis is:
a. MMP 1
b. MMP 2
c. MMP 9
d. MMP 8
Ans. a

83. A known case of Diabetes mellitus has entered the medical emergency/casulaity in subconscious state, the first step towards the management of this patient would be:
a. Dextrose 5% IV
b. Insulin injection
c. Blood test to monitor the blood glucose
d. HBS IV
Ans. b

84. The time taken for the complete collagen fibers to form during wound healing:
a. 1 week
b. 3 weeks
c. 1 month
d. 6 weeks
Ans. b

85. The bone graft which is best suited for periodontal regeneration is?
a. DMFD
b. FDBG

c. Cortical bone chips from the bone bank
d. Anorganic bone
Ans. a

86. **Which of the following treatment modality is safest for the sinus lift procedure?**
a. Soft lasers
b. Piezoelectric appliances
c. Osteotomes
d. Shwartz membrane lifters
Ans. b

87. **The smooth muscle cells have the following shape:**
a. cylindrical
b. Spindle
c. Flattened
d. Branched fusiform
Ans. b

88. **Which of the following is absent in periodontal fibers?**
a. Dermatan sulphate
b. Mature elastin fibre
c. Chondrotin sulphate
d. Intermediate plexus
Ans. b

89. **The gingival enlargement is the most common finding in what type of leukemia:**
a. AML
b. ALL
c. CML
d. CLL
Ans. a

90. **Which of the following is not a conditioned gingival enlargement?**
a. Pubertal
b. Pregnancy
c. Drug induced
d. Leukemic
Ans. c

91. **Which of the following is the most radiosensitive cells in the body?**
a. Basal cells
b. Lymphoid tissues
c. RBCs
d. Smooth muscles
Ans. a

92. **A child of 5 years of age comes to the Department of Periodontology with necrotic bleeding gingiva, which name can be given to the presenting condition:**
a. ANUG
b. Necrotising gingival enlargement
c. Necrotising gingiva of HIV
d. Necrotising ulcerative periodontitis
Ans. a

93. **Which of the following is not a component of posterior triangle of neck?**
a. Phrenic nerve
b. External jugular vein

c. Subclavian vessels
d. Hypoglossal nerve
Ans. d

94. **A mother brings her daughter of 11 years of age to the clinic with severe gingival recession and acute gingivitis the mother said that she had the same problem when she was of her age and there was complaint of early exfoliation of teeth of her mother. Till the time her mother reached puberty she lost all her teeth. The probable diagnosis would be:**
a. RPP
b. AP
c. Chronic periodontitis associated with systemic illness
d. Chronic periodontitis
Ans. a

95. **The most effective way to clean the root concavities is:**
a. Toothbrush
b. Dental floss
c. Interdental brush
d. Tooth pick
Ans. c

96. **The cells that forms the myelin sheath of cranial nerves:**
a. Schwann cells
b. Oligodendrocytes
c. Glial cells
d. Astral cells
Ans. b

97. **The foam cells in atheromatous plaque is formed by:**
a. Oxidised LDL and macrophages
b. DL and Lymphocytes
c. Macrpophages and cholesterol
d. Smooth muscles and macrophages
Ans. a

98. **Rabies is not caused by:**
a. Cats
b. Dogs
c. Rats
d. Monkeys
Ans. c

99. **The unit to measure the absorbed radiation dose is:**
a. Sieverts
b. Roentgen
c. Joule
d. Rad
Ans. d

100. **The premolar which is commonly found to have only one pulp horn:**
a. Maxillary first
b. Maxillary second
c. Mandibular first
d. Mandibular second
Ans. c

101. The last primary teeth to erupt is:
a. Mandibular second molar
b. Mandibular third molar
c. Maxillary second molar
d. Maxillary third molar
Ans. c

102. Internuclear inclusion bodies are most commonly found in:
a. Condyloma
b. Papilloma
c. CMV
d. HSV
Ans. c

103. Osseous coagulum is formed by:
a. Blood and cortical bone
b. Saline and cortical bone
c. Blood and cancellous bone
d. Saline and cortical bone
Ans. a

104. The best result after periodontal surgery can be expected in:
a. One wall defect
b. Two walled defect
c. Three walled defect
d. Horizontal defect
Ans. c

105. Which of the following local delivery agent is approved by FDA to be used as monotherapy?
a. Chlorhexidine chip
b. Doxycycline gel
c. Minocycline microspheres
d. Tetracycline fibres
Ans. c

106. Lack of primary stability of dental implant will result in:
a. Fibrous encapsulation
b. Anti-titanium antibody formation
c. Peri-implant abscess formation
d. Occasionalosseointegration
Ans. a

107. Which of the following enhances the cytotoxic effect of aldehydes on human gingival fibroblasts?
a. Gelatin
b. Triclosan
c. Polylactic acids
d. Alcohol containing mouthwashes
Ans. d

108. The cementum of periodontally weak root surfaces may exhibit all of the following except:
a. Increased mineralisation
b. Decreased mineralisation
c. Endotoxin adhesion
d. Increased collagen cross bands
Ans. d

109. The commonly occurring species in human gingival crevice are F. nucleatum and:
 a. C. rectus
 b. P.gingivalis
 c. B. forsythus
 d. A. naeslundi
 Ans. d

110. The following antifungal is commonly used in immunocompromised patients for invasive and systemic infections:
 a. Terbinafine
 b. Flucytosine
 c. Griseofulvin
 d. Amphotericin B
 Ans. d

111. Longesthalf life is of:
 a. Diazepam
 b. Lorazepam
 c. Triazolam
 d. Chlorazepam
 Ans. a

112. GTR is contraindicated in:
 a. One walled defect
 b. Two walled defect
 c. Three walled defect
 d. Four walled defect
 Ans. a

113. Purple line which follows the contour of gingiva is seen in position of:
 a. Lead
 b. Bismuth
 c. Arsenic
 d. Mercury
 Ans. b

114. Which of the following are primary colonisers of gingival sulcus:
 a. Streptococcus and actinomyces
 b. Filamentous spirochetes
 c. Gram –ve anerobes
 d. Gram +ve anaerobes
 Ans. a

115. The largest among the tongue papilla are:
 a. Fungiform
 b. Filiform
 c. Foliate
 d. Circumvallate
 Ans. d

116. The patient has high cholesterol strong family history of CHD, smoker and age are all variables of:
 a. Multiple regression model
 b. Multiple logistic regression
 c. Linear logistic regression
 d. Multiple logistic regression
 Ans. d

117. **A test can tell 24 out of 80 positive and P value is <0.0005 which means?**
   a. B is more significant in testing disease than A
   b. There are chances that almost every time the same outcome will occur after testing Both A& B
   c. Test A is more specific than Test B
   d. Both the test will do qualitative analysis
   Ans. b

118. **FDA pregnancy category B NSAID is:**
   a. Tolmetin
   b. Naproxen
   c. Mefanamic acid
   d. Paracetamol
   Ans. d

119. **Where the defect is through and through but covered buy soft tissue what is the kind of furcation involvement?**
   a. Grade I
   b. Grade II
   c. Grade III
   d. Grade IV
   Ans. c

120. **All are synthetic bone grafts except:**
   a. Boplast
   b. Dentogen
   c. Nanogen
   d. Nova-bone
   Ans. a

121. **Which of the following is absent from the intermediate plexus?**
   a. Horizontal
   b. Vertical
   c. Oblique
   d. Wavy
   Ans. d

122. **The first formed bone in an extraction socket is?**
   a. Woven bone
   b. Spongy bone
   c. Cancellous bone
   d. Cortical bone
   Ans. a

123. **Which of the following does not act against Gram negative bacteria:**
   a. Sulphonamides
   b. Macrolides
   c. Extended spectrum beta lactams
   d. Aminoglycosides
   Ans. b

124. **As a part of thumb sucking the intermaxillary width remain constant till:**
   a. 3 years
   b. 5 years
   c. 8 years
   d. 11 years
   Ans. b

125. Which is right with respect to rigidity?
a. SS wire more rigid than TMA
b. TMA twice rigid than SS
c. TMA ten times rigid than SS
d. None of these
Ans. a

126. Comprehensive dental care was started in:
a. Finland
b. Denmark
c. New Zealand
d. Sweden
Ans. d

127. DEJ is formed in which stage?
a. Cap
b. Bell
c. Advanced Bell
d. Bud
Ans. c

128. The muscle related to posterior wall of pharynx is:
a. Palatoglossus
b. Palatopharyngeus
c. Styloglossus
d. Stylopharyngeus
Ans. b

129. The child behaviour theory which have long term benefits was of Frankel and Wright which was modified and accepted in the year?
a. 1996
b. 1997
c. 1998
d. 1999
Ans. d

130. The following are false except:
a. Acute fluoride toxicity depends on body weight of the patient
b. Acute fluoride toxicity depends on body surface area
c. Chronic fluoride toxicity depends on body weight of the patient
d. Chronic fluoride toxicity depends on body surface area
Ans. a

131. Mean alveolar concentration (MAC) refers to:
a. 100 % reflexes in 100 % of the population
b. 100 % reflexes in 50% of the population
c. 50 % reflexes in 100 % of the population
d. 50 % reflexes in 50 % of the population
Ans. b

132. A patient aged 11 years comes for the extraction of right maxillary central incisor, after administering local anaesthetic has complained about burning sensation and pain in the right eye can be attributed to:
a. The alternative course of middle superior alveolar nerve
b. The reaction to the preservative used in the solution

c. Improper entry of solution through the infraorbital pathway
d. Normal occurrence and will be subsided by itself
Ans. b

133. Nitrous oxide levels in Operation Theatres can be best detected using:
a. Dosimeter
b. Infrared spectroscopy
c. High Suction
d. Laminar flow
Ans. b

134. Sensitivity of DMFT increased by which other index:
a. GOSLON Index
b. Stone Index
c. Glass Index
d. ICDAS
Ans. d
- ICDAS –International Caries Detection and Assessment Method

135. Nasal cavity fuses with the palate at:
a. 5 weeks
b. 8 weeks
c. 10 weeks
d. 14 weeks
Ans. c

136. Dental lamina derived from:
a. Mesoderm
b. Endoderm
c. Ectomesenchyme
d. Panniculus
Ans. c

137. Desmoplasti cameloblastoma is mostly seen in:
a. Maxillary anterior region
b. Maxillary posterior region
c. Mandibular anterior region
d. Mandibular posterior region
Ans. a

138. A child was brought by father with frog belly shaped swelling in the floor of mouth. Marsupialisation was done but swelling recurred.The proper intervention needed is:
a. Excision of Unilateral parotids
b. Symptomatic management
c. Marsupialisation again to attempt
d. Bilateral excision of parotids
Ans. d

139. Auriculotemporal nerve encircles:
a. Facial artery
b. Middle meningeal artery
c. Superior thyroid artery
d. Posterior auricular artery
Ans. b

140. Equivalent radiation unit is:
   a. Henry
   b. Curie
   c. Becquerel
   d. Sievert
   Ans. d

141. Spacing seen in the maxillary incisor region should be mostly when no other reasons should be managed:
   a. Wait and watch
   b. Orthodontic treatment
   c. Surgical correction
   d. Supernumerary teeth should be checked
   Ans. a

AIIMS SR Papers 2014 Set B

1. **Which technique create almost parallel retention form to receive master cone?**
   a. Step back technique
   b. Double flare technique
   c. Crown down technique
   d. Modified step back technique
   Ans. d
2. **Third generation apex locators are:**
   a. Frequency based
   b. Resistance based
   c. Impedance based
   d. Capacitance based
   Ans. a
3. **WL determination in elderly patients may be more difficult because of which of the following?**
   a. Increased bone density, making radiograph harder to interpret
   b. Increased cementum deposition, modifying the apical anatomy
   c. Difference in tissue electrical resistance, making apex locator less accurate
   d. Patient unable to sit still for radiograph
   Ans. b
4. **The choice of spreader in obturation is:**
   a. Of the same size, or larger than that of the master cone
   b. Of the same size, or smaller than that of the master cone
   c. Of the same size than that of the master cone
   d. It depends upon convenience
   Ans. a
5. **Fast break rule in IOPA radiograph is to identify:**
   a. Bifurcation
   b. Main canal with apical curves
   c. Main canal which is calcified
   d. Calcification
   Ans. a
6. **In HIV positive endodontic patients if CD4 cell count is less than 200 mm^3:**
   a. Routine endodontic work can be undertaken without premedication
   b. Prophylactic antibiotic is must before endodontic intervention
   c. NSAIDS and Vitamins are given prophylactically
   d. Zidovudine should be given as a measure to increase CD4 cell count.
   Ans. b
7. **According to American Heart Association (AHA) endodontic patients who has VSD should be premedicated with:**
   a. 2 gms amoxicillin
   b. 3 gms amoxicillin
   c. 2.5 gms amoxicillin
   d. 3.5 gms amoxicillin
   Ans. a

8. **In concept of ALARA the maximum permissible dose of radiation a dental team in a year is:**
   a. 50 millisieverts
   b. 25 millisieverts
   c. 12.5 millisieverts
   d. 75.7 millisieverts
   Ans. a
9. **What type of canal is most prone to ledge formation?**
   a. Long, small, and curved
   b. Incomplete apex formation, curved
   c. Large, long
   d. Short, straight
   Ans. a
10. **In access opening through PFM crown which bur is used first:**
   a. Round carbide
   b. Round diamond
   c. Tapered carbide
   d. Tapered diamond
   Ans. b
11. **According to vertucci Type 2 configuration of mesiobuccal root of maxillary first molar is seen in:**
   a. 18% of cases
   b. 12% of cases
   c. 54% of cases
   d. 82 % of cases
   Ans. d
12. **In molars ideal site for EPT electrode placement is:**
   a. Mesiobuccal cusp tip
   b. Occlusal third
   c. Middle third
   d. Cervical third
   Ans. a
13. **Champagne bubble test is used to identify:**
   a. Missed canals
   b. Perforation negotiation
   c. Ledge
   d. Transportation of canal
   Ans. a
14. **What is the optimal preparation/obturation length relative to the radiographic apex with pulp necrosis?**
   a. Flush
   b. .5 to 1 mm short
   c. Slight extrusion of sealer but not GP
   d. 1-3 mm short
   Ans. b
15. **The percent of tooth strength reduction in conservative access opening is:**
   a. 4%–6%
   b. 40%–55%
   c. 20%–25%
   d. 9%–15%
   Ans. a

16. What magnification of dental operating microscopes is used for anatomic details of a root canal?
   a. 3–8X
   b. 8–12X
   c. 14–26X
   d. 30X
   Ans. c

17. What is a recommended rubber dam weight for endodontic procedures?
   a. Light
   b. Medium
   c. Heavy
   d. Extra-heavy
   Ans. b

18. When chlorhexidine is used as an intra canal medicament the substantivity is?
   a. 12 weeks
   b. 3 weeks
   c. 6 weeks
   d. 2 week
   Ans. a

19. The string-out test for root canal sealer is achieved when, using a spatula, the cement can be raised from the glass slab:
   a. 0.5 inches
   b. 2 inches
   c. 1 inches
   d. 3 inches
   Ans. c

20. Which of the following is the most important consideration for temporary restoration.
   a. At least 4 mm thick
   b. At least 2.5–3 mm thick
   c. Antimicrobial action
   d. Placed over cotton pellet
   Ans. a

21. F speed film requires how much less exposure compared to E speed film?
   a. 10–15%
   b. 20–25%
   c. 30–35%
   d. 50%
   Ans. b

22. Best temporary restorative material with least leakage is:
   a. Cavit
   b. TERM
   c. IRM
   d. Kalsogen
   Ans. b

23. Flare-ups occur more often:
   a. Nonvital asymptomatic teeth with periapical radiolucency
   b. In endodontic treatment of vital teeth
   c. In endodontic treatment of maxillary premolar teeth
   d. Irreversible pulpitis with symptomatic apical periodontitis
   Ans. a

24. What is the usual radiographic appearance of condensing osteitis?
   a. Diffuse radio-opaque appearance
   b. Uniform smooth borders
   c. Irregular moth eaten appearance around apex
   d. Presence of radiolucent lesion
   Ans. a

25. What is the best site for an intraosseous injection for a premolar?
   a. Mesial perforation
   b. Apical Perforation
   c. Distal Perforation
   d. lingual perforation
   Ans. c

26. When does onset of pulpal anaesthesia occur after Inferior nerve block injection?
   a. Immediately
   b. 0–5 minutes
   c. 10–15 minutes
   d. 30 minutes
   Ans. c

27. Treatment option in case of intruded teeth with open apex greater than 7 mm is:
   a. Spontaneous eruption
   b. Orthodontic extrusion
   c. Surgical extrusion
   d. Extraction
   Ans. c

28. Major cause of VRF is:
   a. Traumatic occlusion
   b. Heavy biting force
   c. Loss of one or both marginal ridge
   d. Condensation force during obturation
   Ans. d

29. In Hot tooth anesthesia is difficult to obtain because:
   a. Presence of Tetrodoxin resistant channel
   b. Because of acidic Ph due to inflammation
   c. Due to activation of voltage gated Na Channel no 5 and 7
   d. Due to inactivation of Ca channels
   Ans. a

30. The carry over effect of chlorhexidine as ICM is neutralized by:
   a. Sodium thiosulphate
   b. Tween 80 and alpha- lecithin
   c. Citric acid with Tween 80
   d. Citric acid only
   Ans. a

31. Which of the following has a minor role in Passive ultrasonic irrigation for cleaner canals?
   a. Acoustic streaming
   b. Cavitation
   c. Rise in temperature
   d. Shear stress
   Ans. d

32. **Photo Activated Disinfection kills the microorganism:**
    a. Through free radical injury
    b. Through toxic dye tolunium bromide
    c. Disruption of enzyme glycosyl transferase
    d. None
    Ans. c

33. **Rapid disinfection of GP points in clinical settings can be achieved through:**
    a. 2.5% hypochlorite
    b. 0.5% hypochlorite
    c. 5.25% hypochlorite
    d. Betadine 10%
    Ans. c

34. **Obtura 2 utilizes:**
    a. Alpha form of Gutta percha
    b. Beta form
    c. Amorphous form
    d. Both a and b
    Ans. b

35. **Venturii effect is use to minimize:**
    a. Emphysema during root canal therapy
    b. Flow of irrigants through apical foramen
    c. Water canon effect
    d. Positive aspiration during LA administration.
    Ans. a

36. **Trauma related replacement resorption shows transient Ankylosis when?**
    a. Size of injured area is 1–4 mm^2
    b. Size of injured area is > 5 mm^2
    c. Size of injured area is 20 mm^2
    d. Size of injured area is 50 mm^2
    Ans. a

37. **When post is planned how much GP should be retained apically?**
    a. 5 mm
    b. 4 mm
    c. 6 mm
    d. 3–4 mm
    Ans. a

38. **The temperature of thermal bleaching is:**
    a. 125–140°F
    b. 150–160°F
    c. 75–100°F
    d. 100–115°F
    Ans. a

39. **The auto stop and reversal of rotation in Tri Auto ZX is seen when torque threshold of:**
    a. 30 g/cm is exceeded
    b. 40 g/cm is exceeded
    c. 68 gm/cm is exceeded
    d. None
    Ans. a

40. Medically complex endodontic Patients receiving STATINS have:
a. Constricted pulp chamber
b. Broader pulp chamber
c. Chances of resorption are very high
d. Periodontal disease is very common
Ans. a

41. In immature teeth WL determination is more accurately done through:
a. Apex locator
b. Paper point
c. Tactile method
d. Radiographic method
Ans. d

42. Platelet rich plasma in comparison with PRF:
a. Releases its growth factor quickly
b. Slow and sustained release
c. Both
d. None
Ans. a

43. In root fractures the radiograph should be taken at:
a. 90, 110, 130
b. 45, 90, 110
c. 45 and 90
d. 90 and 135 degree
Ans. b

44. MB2 canal is located on an average:
a. At 2.25 mm from MB1 and mesially
b. 3.9 mm MB1 and palatally
c. 4 mm MB1 and palatally
d. 0.5 mm MB1 and palatally
Ans. a

45. Absolute contraindication of LA with adrenaline is:
a. Thyrotoxicosis
b. History of MI
c. Diabetes
d. SLE
Ans. a

46. If a patient is allergic to both ester and amide LA the anesthesia can be achieved through:
a. Diphenhyramine
b. High doses of aminoglycosides
c. Cold application
d. Oxethazaine
Ans. a

47. Which precipitate is formed when hypochlorite interacts with chlorhexidine:
a. Para chloro aniline
b. Para chloro Bromine
c. Para chloro anthraciline
d. Dimethyl chloro bumetinide
Ans. a

48. **Pathgonomic feature of apical periodontitis is:**
    a. Hanging oil drop sign
    b. Pear drop sign
    c. Tear drop sign
    d. Apical PDL widening
    Ans. a
49. **In RCT treated tooth moisture loss is:**
    a. 9%
    b. 12%
    c. 14%
    d. 20 %
    Ans. a
50. **Which sealer is hydrophilic?**
    a. Endorez
    b. Roeko seal
    c. Reibler paste
    d. RC2B
    Ans. a
51. **Fatigue strength of GTX is due to incorporation of which form of NITI alloy?**
    a. M wire
    b. R phase wire
    c. CM wire
    d. Alpha phase wire
    Ans. a
52. **PRF is prepared by choukrons method at:**
    a. 2400 rpm
    b. 1200 rpm
    c. 2700 rpm
    d. 1750 rpm
    Ans. c
53. **After root end resection Cementogenesis begin at:**
    a. 7–8 days
    b. 21–28 days
    c. 14–15 days
    d. 10–12 days
    Ans. d
54. **New bone formation is apparent about ------- after periradicular surgery:**
    a. 3 days
    b. 6 days
    c. 3 months
    d. 1 month
    Ans. b
55. **Recommended CBCT voxel size to clinically diagnose VRF:**
    a. 0.2 mm
    b. 0.125 mm
    c. 0.25 mm
    d. 0.4 mm
    Ans. a

56. 1, 1, 1, 2- tetra fluoroethane used for cold test has a temperature of:
   a. -69°F
   b. -56°C
   c. -26°C
   d. -78°C
   Ans. c

57. In case of necrotic tooth patient still complains of pain because of:
   a. Transmodulation of A Beta type of fiber
   b. Transmodulation of A delta type of fiber
   c. Transmodulation of C type of fiber
   d. Transmodulation of A gamma type of fiber
   Ans. a

58. Tiger clamps are used:
   a. During rubber dam application on severely broken down teeth
   b. During rubber dam application on immature tooth
   c. During rubber dam application on maxillary second Molar
   d. During rubber dam application on mandibular incisors
   Ans. a

59. Photo Fenton reaction occurs through bleaching of vital tooth by:
   a. Zoom 2
   b. Zoom
   c. Pearl
   d. Pearl 2
   Ans. a

60. Most commonly affected teeth by Dentin Hypersensitivity are:
   a. Maxillary premolars
   b. Maxillary molars and premolars
   c. Maxillary and mandibular premolars
   d. Mandibular incisors and molars
   Ans. c

61. Fan's Classification for C shaped category 3 has:
   a. Either angle alpha or beta should be no less than 60 degree
   b. Both angle alpha and beta less than 60 degree
   c. Both angle alpha and beta greater than 60 degree
   d. Angle beta is less than 60 degree.
   Ans. b

62. Sodium Hypochlorite kills microorganism by:
   a. Saponification
   b. Chloramination
   c. Amino acid neutralization
   d. Reduction of sulphydryl groups
   Ans. b

63. International Association of Dental Traumatology number of radiographs in trauma cases should be:
   a. 2
   b. 3
   c. 4
   d. 5
   Ans. c

64. Lamberts beers law is utilized in:
 a. Pulse oximetry
 b. Phlethsymography
 c. Dual wave spectrophotometry
 d. Lazer Doppler flowmetry
 Ans. a

65. All of the following are diagnostic aid in endodonticexcept:
 a. Laser Doppler flowmetry
 b. Pulse oximetry
 c. Kiagnodent
 d. All of the above
 Ans. c

66. Lawaty technique is used in:
 a. MTA obturation
 b. Calcium hydroxide Apexification
 c. C shaped canal obturation
 d. Perforation repair
 Ans. a

67. Which of the following sealer is most satisfactorily used with the silver cones?
 a. Wach paste
 b. AH-26
 c. Rickerts
 d. Tubliseal
 Ans. c

68. During retrograde root canal filling, where removal of root structure leads to an inadequate crown root ration which type of cavity preparation is used?
 a. Class 1 preparation
 b. Class 2 preparation
 c. Figure of 8 preparation
 d. Matsura preparation
 Ans. d

69. Standard files have taper 2% taper. What percentage of taper you create when you step back by 2 mm?
 a. 1 %
 b. 5%
 c. 2%
 d. 4%
 Ans. b

70. Total length of post in molars should not approach:
 a. 8 mm
 b. 4 mm
 c. 6 mm
 d 5 mm
 Ans. a

71. How much root resection is done during periradicular surgery?
 a. 2 mm
 b. 3 mm
 c. 4 mm
 d. 5 mm
 Ans. b

72. **Apicoectomy of MB root of maxillary molar is done up to:**
   a. 6 mm
   b. 5 mm
   c. 4 mm
   d. Till isthmus area is exposed
   Ans. d
73. **Citric acid concentration in MTAD:**
   a. 4.25 %
   b. 3.75%
   c. 1%
   d. 0.5 %
   Ans. a
74. **Root resection in periradicular surgery is:**
   a. Perpendicular to the root surface
   b. At angle of 45 degree
   c. Depends on the curvature of the root
   d. 65 degree
   Ans. a
75. **Which among the following is most longest potent and toxic LA:**
   a. Etidocaine
   b. Mepivacaine
   c. Dibucaine
   d. Tetracaine
   Ans. c
76. **Methemoglobin aemia is caused by which LA?**
   a. Prilocaine
   b. Benzocaine
   c. Articaine
   d. All of the above
   Ans. a
77 **Best LA in Hot tooth anaesthesia in mandibular molars:**
   a. Articaine
   b. Mepivacaine
   c. Lidocaine with hyaluronidase
   d. Tetracaine
   Ans. a
78. **Best storage media for avulsed tooth is:**
   a. Milk
   b. Coconut water
   c. HBSS
   d. Viaspan
   Ans. d
79. **In Chronic renal failure child local anaeshthetic preferred is:**
   a. Bupevacaine
   b. Lignocaine
   c. Chlorprocaine
   d. Articaine
   Ans. d

80. **Free gingival groove is b/w:**
   a. Marginal gingiva & attached gingivae
   b. Attached gingvae and oro non keratinized gingivae
   c. Both of these
   d. None of these
   Ans. a
81. **GCF in pocket:**
   a. 3 to 4 times of that in serum
   b. 8–10 times of that in serum
   c. 30–40 times of that in serum
   d. None
   Ans. a
82. **Sclerotic dentine is usually:**
   a. Intertubular
   b. Intratubular
   c. Peritubular
   d. None
   Ans. b
83. **Pulp has all of the following except:**
   a. Cell free zone of Weil
   b. Weibel Palade bodies
   c. Zone of Rinaggio
   d. Zone of Testut
   Ans. d
84. **A 14-year-old hard boy with swelling in body of mandible raised ESR warm sunray appearance around radiolucency:**
   a. Osteosarcoma
   b. Dentoalveolar abscess
   c. Osteochondroma
   d. Chondrosarcoma
   Ans. a
85. **CREST which is not a part:**
   a. Calcinosis
   b. Ehler danlos
   c. Raynauds disease
   d. Telengectiasia
   Ans. b
86. **Yellow stains are due to:**
   a. Depleted developer
   b. Depleted fixer
   c. Abundant developer
   d. Abundant fixer
   Ans. a
87. **Ma controls:**
   a. Heating of filament
   b. Number of electrons
   c. Cooling of filament
   d. Angulation of the rays
   Ans. b

88. The features of acantholysis and nikolsky positive lesions are seen in:
a. Pemphigoid
b. SLE
c. Pemphigus
d. Lichen Planus
Ans. c

89. Acrodynia due to the minor element:
a. Bismuth
b. Sulphur
c. Silver
d. Mercury
Ans. d

90. Microdontia of all teeth in which type of enamel hypoplasia:
a. Type 1. Localised
b. Type 1 generalized
c. Typc 2
d. Type 3
Ans. b

91. Gene of basal cell nevoid is in which chromosome:
a. 21 q
b. 9 q
c. 10 p
d. 23 p
Ans. b

92. Antigen presenting cell:
a. Macrophage
b. T lymphocytes
c. Langerhan cells
d. Merkel cells
Ans. c

93. Dens in dente is:
a. AD
b. AR
c. X linked recessive
d. None
Ans. a

94. Cowdry Type A Intranuclear inclusion bodies seen in:
a. Papilloma
b. Condyloma
c. Herpes
d. All
Ans. c

95. The form of cell signaling in which a cell secretes a hormone or chemical messenger autocrine that binds to receptors on that same cell, leading to changes in the cell is known as—signalling.
a. Paracrine
b. Autocrine
c. Autologous
d. Paralogous
Ans. b

96. Pair of chromosomes having the same gene sequences, each derived from one parent is called:
a. Heterologous
b. Homologous
c. Isologous
d. All
Ans. b

97. False about Phenotype is:
a. It is modified with passage of time
b. It is influenced by genotype
c. It is the genetic sequence of an individual
d. Associated with morphological appearance
Ans. c

98. Mineral for wound healing:
a. Selenium
b. Calcium
c. Copper
d. Iron
Ans. c

99. Dentinogenesis imperfect is associated with chromosome:
a. 4
b. 5
c. 13
d. 14
Ans. a

100. Which can not be taken orally?
a. Macrolide
b. Sulphonamides
c. Aminogylcosides
d. None
Ans. c

101. Which help in lysis:
a. Lysozyme
b. Leucozyme
c. Zymogen
d. Prozyme
Ans. d

102. Which of the following is the most radiosensitive cell in the body?
a. RBC
b. Muscle
c. Lymphoid tissue
d. Basal layer
Ans. d

103. Radiation absorbed in body:
a. Roentgen
b. Sievert
c. Gray
d. None
Ans. c

104. Least dependent on diagnostic radiation based damage:
a. Mutagenesis
b. Mucosisits
c. Teratogenesis
d. None
Ans. c

105. A laboratory test used to study an individual's chromosome make-up is called:
a. Phenotyping
b. Genotyping
c. Karyotyping
d. Variance
Ans. c

106. Patient with sickle cell anaemia complaint's of pain 2 days mild tenderness. No radiographic changes can be due to:
a. Anachoretic reaction
b. Pulp necrosis
c. Pulp polyp
d. All of the above
Ans. a

107. Patient with pain in tooth from 2 days no radiographic change top + be mild:
a. Acute periodontitis
b. Acute apical abscess
c. Granuloma
d. Osteomyelitis
Ans. a

108. Fast Speed of film:
a. Less movement of patient clearer image
b. Less movement of patient no image
c. More movement of patient blurred image
d. Less movement of patient blurred image
Ans. a

109. Acute osteomyelitis caused by:
a. Staphylococcus aureus
b. Prevotella intermedia
c. Streptococcus mutans
d. Corynebacterium diphtheria
Ans. a

110. Fixer functions to:
a. Used in processing photographic or X-ray film
b. It neutralizes any developer remaining on the film
c. Removes undeveloped silver halides
d. All of the above
Ans. d

111. Film holder used with paralleling technique are all except:
a. Rinn XCP
b. Snap a Ray
c. Stabe bite block
d. Projet bite block
Ans. d

112. PSP is doped with which material usually?
a. Beryllium
b. Tungsten
c. Neodymium
d. Europium
Ans. d

113. TNM stands for:
a. Tumor, necrosis, metastasis
b. Tumor, nevus, metastasis
c. Tumor, node, morphology
d. Tumor, node, metastasis
Ans. d

114. Vascular part of articular disc:
a. Posterior region
b. Centre
c. Anterior
d. None
Ans. a

115. Rate of flow of dentinal fluid is affected by all except:
a. Tubule diameter
b. Tubule length
c. Tubule direction
d. None
Ans. b

116. Stainless steel obeys the law:
a. Hookians elasticity
b. Transformation law
c. Beer Lambert's Law
d. Inverse square law
Ans. a
- C is obeyed by Pulse oximetry

117. Crack is seen in the floor of endodontically treated mandibular molar. Treatment protocol is:
a. To extract it
b. Restore with composite
c. Restore with gic
d. None
Ans. c

118. Orthodontic extrusive force is:
a. 75–100 gms
b. 50–75 gms
c. 25–50 gms
d. 35–60 gms
Ans. d

119. Exchange zone of instruments between operator and assistant:
a. At chin
b. Above chin
c. Above head
d. Below chin
Ans. d

120. Difference between stools used by operator and assistant:

a. Absence of cushion
b. Absence of pedal
c. Absence of foot rest
d. Absence of wheels

Ans. c

121. In a symptomatic tooth with apical periodontitis and tenderness on percussion after complete debridement:

a. Occlusal reduction will not help to reduce postoperative pain
b. Occlusal reduction of functional cusp should be done
c. Reduction of tooth should done
d. All of the above

Ans. a

122. A patient with symptomatic pulp comes to a clinician without appointment. He has to adjust him between two patients. Treatment will be:

a. Perform pulpectomy and give calcium hydroxide dressing
b. Perform pulpectomy of largest canal and give cotton dressing
c. Give antibiotics and pain killers
d. All of these

Ans. b

123. Dentinal microcracks are maximum in:

a. Hand NiTi files
b. Wave one
c. Rotary proTaper
d. Hand Protaper

Ans. c

124. Best protocol to remove triple antibiotic paste is:

a. PUI with NaOCl
b. 10% citric acid
c. Tetracycline
d. Normal saline

Ans. a

125. Direction of Vertical root fractures:

a. Mesiodistal
b. Bucco lingual
c. Corono apical
d. Occlusolingual

Ans. b

126. Best protocol for irrigation of immature teeth that ll save SCAP and other stem cells:

a. 5.25% NaoCl and 2% CHX
b. 2.5% NaoCl and 17% EDTA
c. 0.5% NaoCl and 2% CHX
d. 6% NaoCl and 17% EDTA

Ans. b

127. Incidence of furcation canals in mandibular first molar:

a. 22%
b. 29%
c. 59%
d. 71%

Ans. b

128. The success of orthograde retreatment in teeth with apical periodontitis is:
a. More in anteriors and less in posteriors
b. Less than teeth without apical periodontitis
c. More than teeth without apical periodontitis
d. Equal
Ans. a

129. In a patient having high cholesterol, the factors affecting are diet (a+b), fat (c+d). The combination of these factors, i.e. a+b+c+d is example of:
a. Simple linear regression
b. Multiple linear regression
c. Correlation
d. Permutation
Ans. b

130. The modification for a very dark tooth requiring porcelain veneer are all except:
a. Extend veneer 2–3 mm below gingival
b. Increase thickness of resin layer
c. Increase the opacity of poecelain by 5–10
d. None of these
Ans. b

131. Which is wrong statement?
a. Maximum time for heat testing 15 sec
b. Maximum time for cold testing 15 sec
c. SAF belongs to type 4 instruments
d. Tween 80 is seen in MTAD
Ans. a

132. Which test has least sensitivity?
a. Heat
b. Cold
c. Electric
d. Cavity
Ans. c

133. Main cause of NiTi instrument fracture:
a. Torsoinal and bending alongwith fatigue fracture
b. Manufacturers defects
c. Operators use
d. Angulation
Ans. a

134. McSpadden factor is high, this means that:
a. Instrument will fracture easily
b. Instrument will not fracture easily
c. The instrument is sharp
d. The instrument is not sharp
Ans. b

135. Amitryptalline contraindication lies in:
a. Use with vasoconstrictor
b. Use with analgesic
c. Use with antibiotic
d. None of these
Ans. a

136. Isthmus Classification two or three canal openings without visible connections comes under

a. Type II
b. Type III
c. Type IV
d. Type V

Ans. d

137. TR is needed in:

a. Type 1
b. Type 2
c. Type 3
d. Type 4

Ans. d

138. The factor responsible for bone resorption is:

a. TNF alpha
b. TNF gamma
c. TGF
d. FGF

Ans. a

139. The long-term complication of intentional resorption:

a. Ankylosis
b. Avulsion
c. Fracture
d. All of the above

Ans. a

- Root resorption

140. Acute apical periodontitis can be attributed to:

a. P gingivalis
b. E.foecali
c. Treponema denticola
d. Bdellovibrio

Ans. c

141. Obturation of vital tooth in multivisit procedure should be done:

a. After 1–2 days
b. After 2–3 days
c. After 4–5 days
d. After 5–7 days

Ans. d

142. Maximum conduction velocity:

a. A alpha
b. A beta
c. A delta
d. C fibers

Ans. a

143. Long standing perforations are sterilized by:

a. 2.5 % NaOCl
b. 2% CHX
c. 5% NaOCl
d. 3% saline

Ans. a

144. Safety limit of Hg in clinic:
a. 20 weeks/hr 50 micrograms/mm^3
b. 30 weeks/hr 50 micrograms/mm^3
c. 40 weeks/hr 50 micrograms/mm^3
d. 60 weeks/hr 50 micrograms/mm^3
Ans. c

145. Acc to ALARA principle:
a. Leaded aprons are not necessary but thyroid collars are must
b. Leaded aprons are necessary but thyroid collars are not must
c. Leaded aprons and thyroid collars are must
d. Leaded aprons and thyroid collars are not that necessary
Ans. a

146. Polymerization shrinkage of siloranes:
a. 1%
b. 2%
c. 3%
d. 4%
Ans. b

Ref: Craig 13/e p164 and 175

147. In Munsell color system all of the following colors are used as principal colors except:
a. Blue
b. Red
c. Purple
d. Orange
Ans. d

148. Rubber dam on nose is due to:
a. Off centric punching of holes
b. On centric punching of holes
c. Lateral punching of holes
d. Lack of punching
Ans. a

149. Halo effect is seen in:
a. Amalgam
b. Cements
c. Varnish
d. Composite
Ans. d

150. Wedge placement site for composite:
a. Above Narrow-Regular gingival crest
b. At the gingival crest
c. Below gingival crest
d. Not needed
Ans. c

151. Triangular wedges are indicated in:
a. Shallow occlusal embrasures
b. Deep occlusal embrasures
c. Shallow gingival embrasures
d. Deep gingival embrasures
Ans. d

152. Automatrix are available in all four sizes except:

a. Medium-Thin
b. Narrow-regular
c. Medium-Regular
d. Wide thin

Ans. d Wide regular is the fourth type

153. Pin failure most common type is:

a. Pin tooth
b. Pin restorative
c. Pin fracture
d. Tooth fracture

Ans. b

154. As per Sotokowa classification of instrument fracture type 4 refers to:

a. Bent instrument
b. Partial clockwise twist
c. Cracking along axis
d. Full fracture

Ans. b

155. A working length measured by gen 3 apex locator is smaller when confirmed radiographically cause is:

a. Fluid in canal
b. Lateral canal
c. Accessory canal
d. Calcified canal

Ans. a

156. Rubber dam recommended for endodontic purpose:

a. Small
b. Large
c. Medium
d. Ultra small

Ans. c

157. Knife Line attack all are true except:

a. Intragranular corossiom
b. Seen in SS
c. Intergranular corrosion
d. Occurs in a narrow band adjacent to the weld

Ans. a

158. A viscoplastic material that behaves as a rigid body at low stresses but flows as a viscousfluid at high stress:

a. Pseudoplastic
b. Newtonian
c. Bingham
d. Thixotropic

Ans. c

159. Identify what the arrow is pointing in this IOPA ?

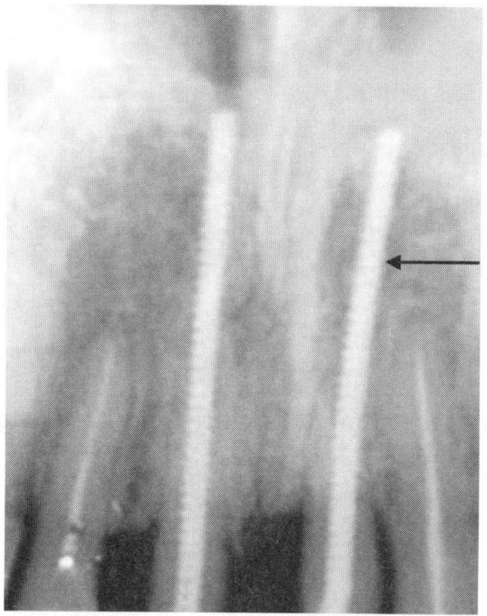

Ans. POST

160. Identify which type of defect this clinical photograph shows?

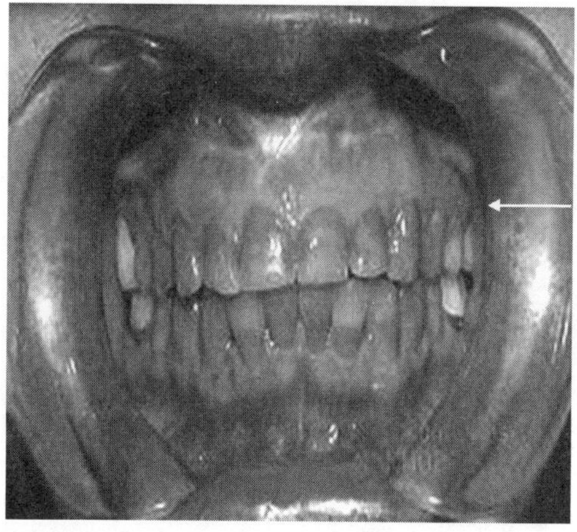

Ans. Dentinogenesis Imperfecta

161. Identify the clinical condition with this IOPA in tooth # 36, #37:

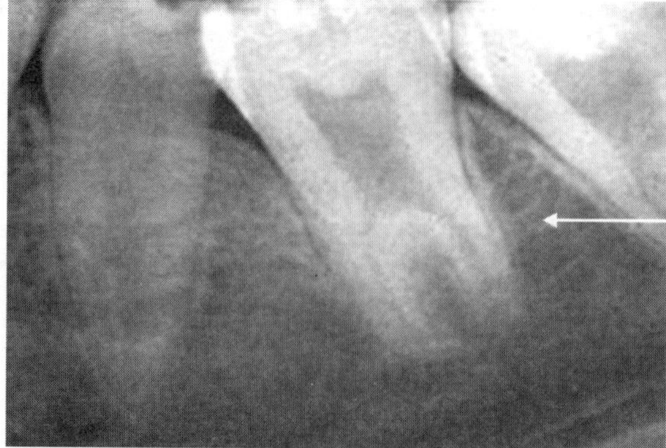

Ans. Dilaceration

162. **Identify what this clinical photograph and IOPA shows?**

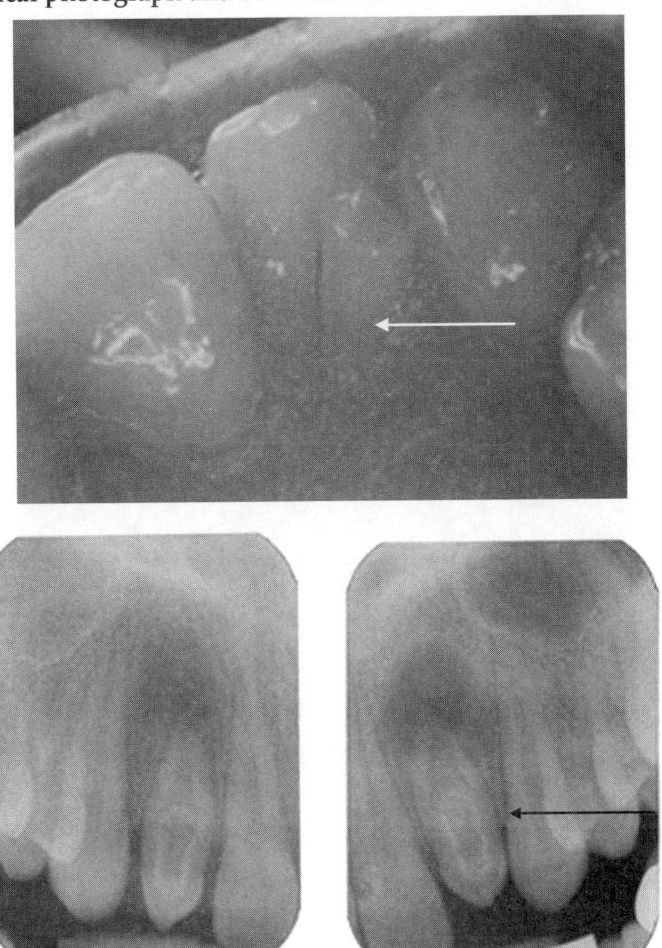

Ans. Internal Resorption

163. **Identify what this clinical photograph shows?**

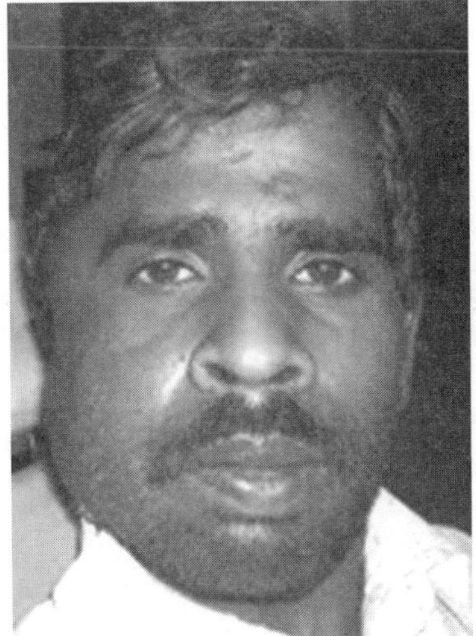

Ans. Buccal Space Infection

164. Identify in this radiograph what type of endo perio lesion is this?

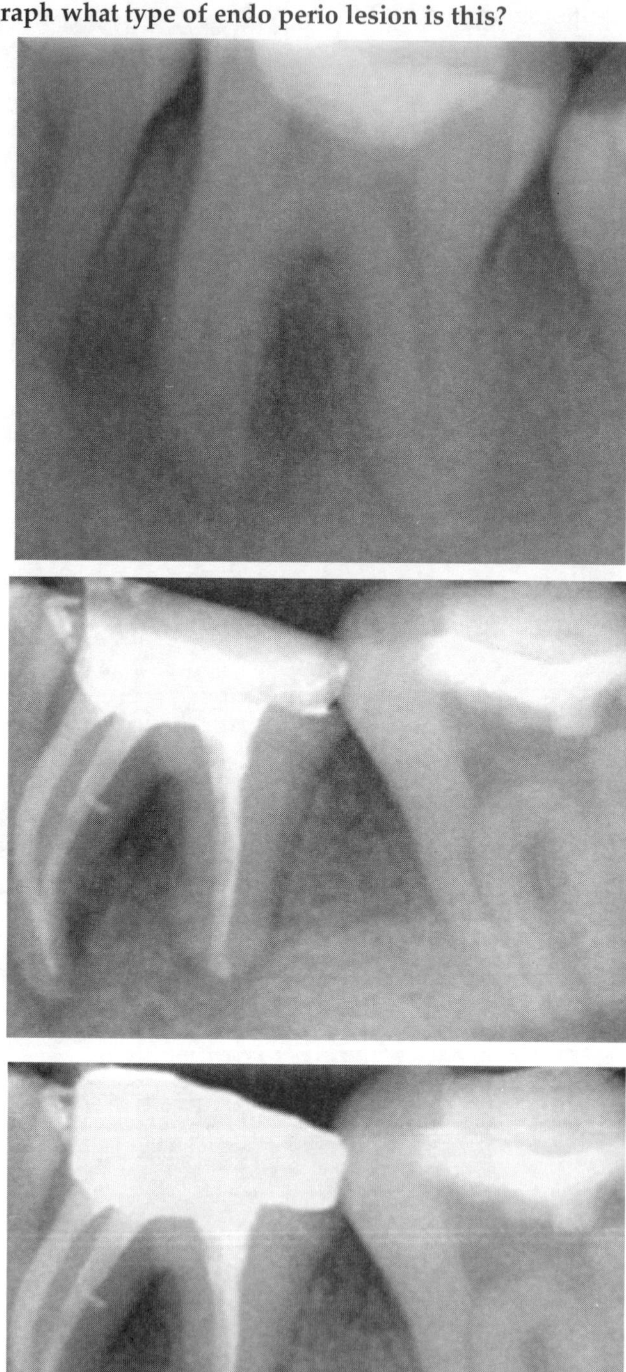

Ans. Type III

AIIMS Unreleased SR Papers

1. **The term 'Mortality Rate' in epidemiology means:**
   a. Measure of death in a population due to a disease
   b. Characterizes the rapidity with which deaths from the disease occur over time
   c. Characterizes the rapidity with which deaths from the disease occur without time frame
   d. Most frequent cause of death
   Ans. b
2. **The 'Incubation period' is defined as:**
   a. The time from the disease outbreak to disease manifestation
   b. The time difference between two observational studies
   c. Time between exposure to risk factor to actual onset of symptoms
   d. Time between exposure to risk factor to actual end of symptoms
   Ans. c
3. **The term 'odds ratio' is used commonly in statistics. It means:**
   a. Odds of getting one condition in one group as compared to other group
   b. Relative chances of acquisition of symptoms after exposure to risk factor
   c. Causes of death cumulated
   d. Causes of death unaccumulated
   Ans. a
4. **While finding out oral pre cancerous conditions using dyes, we should use the dye which gives?**
   a. Least sensitivity and highest specificity
   b. High specificity and low sensitivity
   c. High specificity and high sensitivity
   d. Low specificity and low sensitivity
   Ans. c
5. **When a particular test gives results negative while actually it is positive then it is called as?**
   a. True Negative
   b. True Positive
   c. False Positive
   d. False Negative
   Ans. d
6. **The common notation used to describe the likelihood of a type II error is?**
   a. Alpha
   b. Beta
   c. Gamma
   d. Delta
   Ans. b
7. **When study results give false positive results, which type of error it is called:**
   a. Type–I
   b. Type–II
   c. False negative
   d. True Negative
   Ans. a

8. **The study of one time examination of oral health status in children who were born with low birth weight will be termed as:**
   a. Retrospective study
   b. Case control study
   c. Observational study
   d. Cohort study
   Ans. c
9. **The Rate Ratio is can be calculated by:**
   a. Rate of outcome among unexposed persons divided by rate of outcome among exposed persons
   b. Rate of outcome among exposed persons divided by rate of outcome among unexposed persons
   c. Rate of outcome among exposed persons plus by rate of outcome among unexposed persons
   d. Rate of outcome among exposed persons minus by rate of outcome among unexposed persons
   Ans. b
10. **During sample selection for an oral health survey a Karnataka state one particular school is selected in a particular village by lottery method for examination of all the schoolchildren, this selection methods will be called as:**
   a. Individual randomization
   b. Block randomization
   c. Multi stage randomization
   d. Sample randomization
   Ans. c
11. **The 5% level of statistical significance, the observed result is most appropriately interpreted as indicating a:**
   a. Significant hazard
   b. Significant benefit
   c. Non significant hazard
   d. Non significant benefit
   Ans. a
12. **In a drug trial study plan, when the observer an well as pharmacist dispensing the medicines do not know about the drug/placebo and neither the patient know, what is he being given, it will be called as?**
   a. Triple blind study
   b. Association study
   c. Double blinded study
   d. Case control study
   Ans. a
13. **The popularly used term 'confidence Interval' means:**
   a. The relative chances of occurrence of an event
   b. The relative chances of non occurrence of an event
   c. Certainity of happening of an event with a specified level
   d. Certainity of happening of an event with a non specified level
   Ans. c
14. **The average probing force required to record CPITN index is:**
   a. 10 gms
   b. 25 gms
   c. 50 gms
   d. No force required
   Ans. b
15. **The code 'X' in CPI index is used for denoting:**
   a. Extracted tooth
   b. Excluded tooth

c. Excavated tooth
d. Examined tooth
Ans. b

16. **The spectrum of health does not include:**
a. Social dimension
b. Physical dimension
c. Vocational dimension
d. Psychological dimension
Ans. d

17. **Dental caries can be defined as:**
a. Contagious disease
b. Communicable disease
c. Non communicable disease
d. Potentially communicable disease
Ans. d

18. **During waste disposal, excess temporary filling material removed from patients mouth should be thrown into:**
a. Red bad
b. Yellow bag
c. Black bag
d. Blue bag
Ans. a

19. **The best method to sterilize piezo endo hand piece is:**
a. Hot air oven
b. Autoclave
c. UV Chamber
d. Formalin chamber
Ans. c

20. **The community water fluoridation was first started in USA in the year:**
a. 1945
b. 1947
c. 1951
d. 1957
Ans. a

21. **The recommended water fluoride level in a middle school for school water fluoridation plan should be:**
a. 1 ppm
b. 2 ppm
c. 4 ppm
d. 12 ppm
Ans. a

22. **The common oral finding in HIV positive 8-year-old child with CD4 counts of about 1300 would be:**
a. Bilateral painless parotid swellings
b. Oral Thrush
c. Hairy leukoplakia
d. Kaposi's sarcoma
Ans. a

23. **A 24-year-old female fashion designer weighing about 38 kg reports to you with unusual loss of tooth enamel for anterior teeth, the most probable diagnosis would be:**

a. Dental caries
b. Root caries
c. Abrasion
d. Erosion
Ans. d

24. **The primary preventive programme named Tattle tooth – II was first started in which province of USA:**
a. North Carolina
b. California
c. Texas
d. Amazon
Ans. c

25. **The Special Olympics International (SOI) committee planned a programme for oral health of the athletes participating in special Olympics in year:**
a. 1999
b. 1995
c. 1993
d. 1970
Ans. c

26. **The Dentists Act was introduced in India in the year:**
a. 1942
b. 1950
c. 1956
d. 1945
Ans. b

27. **Which of the following country is not member country for the SEARO office of the World Health Organization?**
a. Pakistan
b. Srilanka
c. Bangladesh
d. Thailand
Ans. a

28. **Out of the following, relatively highest rate of dental caries incidence (non rampant) should be anticipated in which age group:**
a. 3-4 years
b. 0-2 years
c. 6-7 years
d. 10-12 years
Ans. a

29. **UN agency which works exclusively for children is?**
a. WHO
b. UNAIDS
c. UNICEF
d. UNFPA
Ans. c

30. **The action of Fluoride varnish can not be explained by:**
a. Effect on bacteria directly
b. Remineralization of incipient caries
c. Inhibition of production of extra cellular products by the bacteria
d. Alteration in tooth morphology
Ans. a

31. According to the malocclusions survey which type of malocclusion in commonest?
a. Class I
b. Class II
c. Class III
d. Class II subdivision
Ans. a

32. Class III malocclusion is more common in:
a. Indians
b. Black Americans
c. Japanese
d. Caucasians
Ans. c

33. Assume that a 53-year-old woman demands that her new dentures restore a more youthful appearance. You decrease the interocclusal distance to improve esthetics. The patient finds the dentures esthetically acceptable. What possible difficulty you might not expect the patient to encounter?
a. Loss of muscle tone
b. Premature striking of the teeth causing a clicking sound
c. Angular cheilitis
d. Loss of centric occlusion
Ans. a

34. Which is a true statement concerning injury to the supporting tissues of a patient who has been wearing dentures?
a. The extent of injury to the tissues can be directly correlated with occlusal interferences
b. The extent of injury to the tissues can always be correlated with the accuracy of the dentures
c. The use and care of the dentures are seldom related to the extent of injury to the tissues
d. Because of a systematic condition, the injury may be disproportionately severe
Ans. b

35. Which of the following conditions can cause abrasions on the mucosa of the cheek and lips?
a. Cheek biting
b. Irregular occlusal anatomy on the teeth
c. Unpolished denture bases
d. Any of the above
Ans. d

36. You have made a centric relation record for the purpose of articulating the dentures prior to equilibration. Which of the following would suggest an accurate record?
a. Cusp penetration through the recording material.
b. Contact of the denture base plastic between the retromolar pad areas and the maxillary tuberosity areas
c. Record made at a slightly increased vertical dimension of occlusion
d. Inability to have the patient close perfectly into the record after it has been chilled, trimmed, and returned to the mouth
Ans. a

37. On examination of a patient who has worn new dentures for two months, irritation is noted on the lingual side of the mandibular residual ridge from canine to canine. Retention of the mandibular denture is adequate. What treatment procedure should be instituted to correct the problem?
a. Shortening the lingual flange
b. Relining the mandibular denture
c. Remaking the mandibular denture
d. Remounting and equilibrating the dentures
Ans. a

38. The most likely tissue reaction to gross overextension of a complete denture that has been worn for a long time is:
a. Epulis fissuratum
b. Pyogenic granuloma
c. Papillary hyperplasia
d. Giant cell reparative granuloma
Ans. a

39. Speech difficulties related to complete dentures can be avoided by:
a. Moving the maxillary incisors anteriorly
b. Moving the maxillary incisors posteriorly
c. Placing the artificial teeth as nearly as possible to the position of the natural teeth
d. Providing spaces or diastama between the incisors
Ans. c

40. At the 24 hour recall adjustment appointment, your patient complains of a sore throat, particularly when swallowing. Use of disclosing wax indicates that the mandibular lingual denture flange extends too far distally. What muscle contracts during swallowing, forcing the mucous membrane of the throat against the overextended area?
a. Superior constrictor of pharynx
b. Tensor velli palatine
c. Platoglossus
d. Platopharyngeous
Ans. a

41. One of your patient have poor neuromuscular control which technique you will use to correct the occlusal error:
a. Correct by direct method because it is difficult to take jaw relation records
b. You will just ask the patient to grind on carborandum paste
c. You will take interocclusal records and then do the correction on the articulator
d. In such patients occlusal correction is not required
Ans. c

42. If a patient come to you for relining and rebasing you can do the relining in which situation?
a. When an excessive amount of bone resorption has taken place
b. There is discrepancy in centric relation and Centric occlusion
c. There is need to raise the vertical dimension more then two mm
d. Your patient is poor he can not afford the cost of new denture
Ans. d

43. A complete denture patient come to you, next day after the delivery of denture with a complained, he has pain in his throat during swallowing, First thing will come in your mind:
a. Overextended posterior palatal seal area
b. Inflammation of tonsils
c. Overextended sublingual crescent area in mandibular denture
d. Overextended lingual flange in retromylohyoid region
Ans. d

44. New inter occlusal record of centric and eccentric relations should be made at the time, new dentures are 1st placement in oral cavity:
a. To eliminate the occlusal error other then processing error
b. To eliminate the processing error
c. This procedure is required if there is gross discrepancy in occlusion
d. This procedure is not required as minor occlusal discrepancy can be settle it self due to resiliency of underlying soft tissue.
Ans. b

45. After the processing of complete denture if the upper and lower teeth are nearly end-to-end in centric occlusion to correct this:
  a. The centric holding cusp of maxillary and mandibular teeth should be shortened
  b. The central fossa of upper and lower teeth should be depend
  c. Inclines of maxillary and mandibular cusp grind in such a way to move the upper cusp incline buccally and lower cusp incline lingually
  d. Inclines of maxillary and mandibular cusp grind in such a way to move the upper cusp incline lingually and lower cusp incline buccally

  Ans. c

46. High density (D1) bone is favorable for implant placement is usually found in:
  a. Anterior maxillary region
  b. Posterior maxillary region
  c. Anterior mandibular region
  d. Posterior mandibular region

  Ans. c

47. Osseointegration of implants placed in mandibular interforamina region usually takes:
  a. 1.0–2 months
  b. 2.3–4 months
  c. 4–6 months
  d. 6–12 months

  Ans. b

48. According to envelop of "Limits of Treatment" by Profitt and Ackerman, combined orthodontic and surgical treatment can bring about a maximum of:
  a. 6 mm of buccal segment intrusion in the maxilla
  b. 5 mm of sagittal advancement in maxilla
  c. 4 mm of buccal segment extrusion in mandible
  d. 3 mm of buccal segment expansion in mandible

  Ans. d

49. Spacing in dentition will cause distortion of which of following speech sounds?
  a. Lingual alveolar phonemes (S, Z)
  b. Lingual palatal phonemes (J, Sh, Ch)
  c. Both 1 and 2
  d. Sibilant and alveolar speech sounds.

  Ans. c

Ref: Textbook of Orthodontics by OP Kharbanda 1/e p118

50. According to available studies on prevalence of class II malocclusion, its prevalence is known to be highest in:
  a. Europeans/Caucasians
  b. Negros
  c. Asians
  d. French Polynesians of Puka Puka Island

  Ans. a

51. Which of following classifications of malocclusion uses premolars as a reference point?
  a. Simon's law
  b. Ballard and Wayman - classification
  c. Ackerman and Proffit classifications
  d. Katz's classification

  Ans. d

52. **Which of the following about affected dentin is not true?**
    a. It is remineralizable
    b. The discoloration is slight
    c. It is hard in consistency
    d. It is irreversible
    Ans. d
53. **The disadvantages of composite restorations are all of the following:**
    a. Greater localized wear
    b. Technique sensitive
    c. Increased recurrent caries
    d. Required more time for placement
    Ans. d
54. **Which of the following statements is not true; In epidemiological studies indices used?**
    a. Should have clarity, simplicity and objectivity
    b. Should be amenable to statistical
    c. Reversible is a more dependable
    d. Cumulative index measures all evidence of a disease condition
    Ans. c
55. **Limitations of DMFT include all the following except:**
    a. Can be considered invalid in older adults and children, because teeth could be lost for reasons other than caries
    b. It can over estimate caries experience
    c. Is very useful to measure root causes
    d. It is not related to number of teeth at risk
    Ans. c
56. **Unit of surface energy is:**
    a. Erg/cm^2
    b. Dyne/cm
    c. Modulus
    d. Jaules m^{-3}
    Ans. b
57. **Hue describes the:**
    a. Saturation of color
    b. The basic color of the object
    c. Change of color in different light
    d. Lightness or darkness of object
    Ans. b
58. **The temperature of carbon dioxide snow is:**
    a. + 4°C
    b. -78 °C
    c. -1 °C
    d. -89 °C
    Ans. b
59. **In deciduous teeth, formocresol pulpotomy is preferred over calcium hydroxide pulpotomy because:**
    a. Formocresol is a strong bactericide
    b. Internal resorption is not found
    c. The entire pulpal tissue is devitalized and fixed
    d. Desposition of secondary dentin is faster and thicker
    Ans. b

60. Which of the following conditions is characterized by abnormally large pulp chambers?
   a. Amelogenesis inperfecta
   b. Regional odontodysplasia
   c. Dentinogenesis imperfecta
   d. Dentinal dysplasia Type –I

   Ans. b

61. Protection from radiaton exposure in a dental operatory is determined by all the following except:
   a. Radiography work load
   b. Distance from the path of direct beam
   c. Direction of the primary beam
   d. Lead lining of the walls is mandatory

   Ans. a

62. Which of the following about mouth protectors is not ture?
   a. Made from laminate polymers are stronger than single material sheet
   b. Thickness of sheet varies between 1.6-3 mm
   c. They may be custom-made stock available or fabricated inside the mouth
   d. As the content of ethylene increases, hardness of the polymer increases

   Ans. a

63. The age of the child considered to be in 'pre-cooperative stage' of development is:
   a. 9 years old
   b. 8 years old
   c. 2 years old
   d. 5 years old

   Ans. c

64. Peg shaped teeth are formed in which stage of 'Life of the tooth'?
   a. Initiation
   b. Histo-differentiation
   c. Morpho-differentiation
   d. Apposition

   Ans. c

65. Change is dietary system or a child from candies, cookies and aerated surgery drinks to non Cariogenic snacks is advised because:
   a. Less calories
   b. Taste of non Cariogenic snacks makes children less interested in the food
   c. Elimination of sucrose from diet
   d. There is more dextrose in non Cariogenic diets

   Ans. d

66. A history of Rubella virus infection in a mother may cause which of the following condition in the offspring?
   a. Congenital development anomalies
   b. Diabetes Mellitus
   c. Cerebral palsy
   d. Down's syndrome

   Ans. a

67. Which of the following is the most appropriate denominator of Need for orthodontic treatment?
   a. Ackerman and Profitt's Venn Diagram
   b. Index of Orthodontic Treatment and Need (IOTN)
   c. Index of Complexity Outcome and Need (ICON)
   d. Simon's 3D classification

   Ans. c

68. Irreversible pulpitis is often characterized by:
a. A moderate response to percussion
b. A strong painful response to cold that lingers
c. A strong painful response to cold
d. A response
Ans. b

69. Pulpal pain response is:
a. Dull and throbbing when carried by myclinated `c` fibers
b. Dull and throbbing when carried by unmyuelinated `c` fibers
c. Quick and sharp when carried by myelinated c fibers
d. Quick and sharp when carried by unmyelinated c fibers
Ans. b

70. Radiographic contrast can be directly affected by altering:
a. Millamperage
b. Exposure time
c. Killovoltage
d. Angulation
Ans. c

71. Gutta-percha is best starililzed in:
a. An auto clave
b. Dry heat
c. 5.5% sodium hypochlorite for 1 minute
d. Paraformaldehyde for 1 minute
Ans. c

72. The fourth canal is ofter found in:
a. The mesiobuccal root of the maxillary first molar
b. The mesial root of maxillary second molar
c. The palatal root of maxillary first molar
d. The distobuccal root of maxillary first molar
Ans. a

73. The crown-down prepration advocates beginning radicular access with:
a. A smaller instrument first
b. Precurvature of a smaller instrument
c. A larger instrument first
d. Removal of the clinical crown
Ans. c

74. To achieve the objective of vertical condensation, it is necessary to produce:
a. A cylindrical canal
b. A conical canal
c. A tapering conical canal
d. A straight canal
Ans. c

75. The 'string-out test' for root canal sealer is achieved when, using a spatula, the cement can be raised from the gloss slab:
a. ½ inch
b. 2 inch
c. 1 inch
d. 3 inches
Ans. c

76. **Volume of blood flow in the pulp:**
   a. Is least in the regions of the pulphorn
   b. Is greater in the root position than in the crown position
   c. Is greater than the blood flow in the most visceral organs
   d. Is largely under the control of the adregenic sympathetic system
   Ans. d
77. **The presence of which component of complement in the inflamer periapex suggests that the complement system participates in the pathogenesis?**
   a. C1
   b. C3
   c. C7
   d. C9
   Ans. b
78. **The endodontic broach is used to:**
   a. Locate the ositices of the root canals
   b. Remove pulp tissue from the pulp space
   c. Smooth the walls of root canals
   d. Enlarge the root canal space
   Ans. b
79. **The basic difference between K-type files and Reamers is:**
   a. The number of spirals or flutes per unit length
   b. The Geometric cross section
   c. The depth of the flutes
   d. The direction of the spirals
   Ans. a
80. **A disadvantage of Cavit composed to IRM as a temporary restoration is that Cavit:**
   a. Has less compressive strength
   b. Does not seal as well with time
   c. Is more susceptible to thermal change
   d. Shrinks while setting
   Ans. a
81. **Relatively few bacteria are found in a pulp abscess because of the:**
   a. Immune response of pulp tissue
   b. High tissue ph is the adjacent inflammation
   c. Mechanical blockage of sclerotic dentin
   d. Antibacterial production of neutrophil
   Ans. a
82. **Which of the following radiographic film exposuses is best for diagnosing root fractures in the apical third?**
   a. Parallel
   b. Bisecting angle
   c. Occlusal
   d. Panoramic
   Ans. c
83. **Neonatal teeth are:**
   a. Teeth present at the time of birth
   b. Teeth erupt within 30 days of birth
   c. Teeth erupt within 180 days of birth
   d. Teeth erupt during first year
   Ans. b

84. A 7-year-old child, resident of Bhavnagar, Gujarat presents to you with yellowish discolored spot of left central incisor. The mother gives history of injury to the milk tooth in that area and subsequent recurrent infection swelling about 3 years back. What will be your most probable diagnosis?

a. Dental Fluorosis
b. Syphilitic Hypoplasia
c. Hypomineralization of teeth due to deficiency of Calcium
d. Turner's Hypoplasia

Ans. d

85. Deficiency of which component of food will definitely cause generalized hypoplasia in permanent dentition?

a. Vitamin B
b. Lipids
c. Vitamin A
d. Carbohydrates

Ans. c

86. Digital fiber optic transillumination (DIFOTI) is a method of:

a. Detecting bone loss in children
b. Detecting calcium concentration in Enamel
c. Detecting proximal caries
d. Detecting Occlusal caries

Ans. c

87. A single tooth germ splits or shows an attempt at splitting to from two completely or partially separated crowns, the process is called:

a. Fusion
b. Gemination
c. Concrescence
d. Dens in dente

Ans. b

88. Supernumerary tooth/teeth can be most commonly found at:

a. Mandibular incisor area
b. Pre-maxilla and Maxillary incisor area
c. Mandibular molar area
d. Maxillary molar area

Ans. b

89. The permanent teeth show calcification at the age of:

a. At birth
b. One month
c. Four months
d. One year

Ans. a

90. Tooth is formed from more than one lobe. What is the minimum number of lobes from which any tooth may develop?

a. Two
b. Three
c. Four
d. Five

Ans. c

91. Orthodontic implications of inter-proximal caries of deciduous molars are:

a. Loss of tooth structure
b. Loss of Arch length

c. Increase in arch length
d. Constriction in transverse width of the arch
Ans. b

92. Which of the following would suggest a maxillary prognathism?
a. An SNA angle of approximately 82
b. An SNA angle greater than 86 degrees
c. An SNA angle less than 78
d. An SNA of 72 degrees
Ans. b

93. Which of the following theories most likelyexplains why there is a strong tendency for mandibular anterior crowding in the late adulthood?
a. Lack of leeway space
b. Pressure from third molars
c. Late mandibular growth
d. Late maxillary growth
Ans. c

94. Which cusp listed below of the maxillary first molar serves as a reference point in identifying Angle's Class I, II and III occlusions?
a. Distobuccal
b. Mesiobuccal
c. Mesiolingual
d. Distolingual
Ans. b

95. Which type of cementum is found on the apical third of the root?
a. Cellular
b. Acellular
c. No cementum dentine is exposed
d. There is no definite pattern
Ans. a

96. Bilateral contraction of the posterior fibers of the temporalis muscles results in which of the following mandibular movements?
a. Retrusion
b. Protrusion
c. Opening
d. Closing
Ans. a

97. When a patient attempts protrusion, the mandible deviates markedly to the right. Which muscle listed below is unable to contract?
a. Left lateral pterygoid
b. Right lateral pterygoid
c. Temporalis muscle
d. Buccinator
Ans. b

98. The nerve for the motor function to the buccinator muscle is:
a. Facial nerve
b. Trigeminal nerve
c. Glossopharyngeal nerve
d. Hypoglossal nerve
Ans. a

99. **Which of the following nerve provides major sensor innervations to the TMJ?**
 a. Masseteric nerve
 b. Auriculotemporal nerve
 c. Facial nerve
 d. Buccal Nerve
 Ans. b

100. **Long acting local anesthetic agent are:**
 a. Bupivacaine and Propoxycaine
 b. Bupivacaine and Mepivacaine
 c. Bupivacaine and Etidocaine
 d. Bupivacaine and Lignocaine
 Ans. c

101. **In 1844 nitrous oxide was introduced in dentistry by:**
 a. Horace wells
 b. Van der Woude
 c. Wyburn-Mason
 d. Garcia Ballesta
 Ans. a

102. **Ill defined margin in the radiograph is seen in following all conditions except:**
 a. Giant cell lesions
 b. Fissural cysts
 c. Multiple myeloma
 d. Adenoameloblastoma
 Ans. b

103. **Stuart-Prower factor is:**
 a. Factor V
 b. Factor VII
 c. Factor X
 d. Factor XII
 Ans. c

104. **This is bactericidal drug which interfere with the formation of peptidoglycan layer so that bacterial wall absorbs water and bursts:**
 a. Erythromycin
 b. Penicillin
 c. Rifampicin
 d. Tetracycline
 Ans. b

105. **This graft denotes that the graft has been derived from another species of different genetic disposition:**
 a. Heterograft
 b. Allograft
 c. Isograft
 d. Homograft
 Ans. a

106. **Radiographic picture of a dentigerous cyst is:**
 a. Soap- bubble appearance
 b. Unilocular radio lucent lesion
 c. Unilocular radio opaque lesion
 d. Unilocular or multilocular lesion with an unerupted.
 Ans. d

107. Which is a true statement concerning injury to the supporting tissues of a patient who has been wearing dentures?

a. The extent of injury to the tissues can be directly correlated with occlusal interferences
b. The extent of injury to the tissues can always be correlated with the accuracy of the dentures
c. The use and care of the dentures are seldom related to the extent of injury to the tissues
d. Because of a systematic condition, the injury may be disproportionately severe

Ans. b

108. Which of the following conditions can cause generalized abrasions on the mucosa of the cheek and lips?

a. Cheek biting
b. Irregular occlusal anatomy on the teeth
c. Unpolished denture bases
d. Any of the above

Ans. d

109. Mean, Mode and Median all three are measurement of central tendency in a data. The Mode is defined as:

a. Measure of average in a group
b. Number of values closest to the arithmetic mean
c. When values are arranged in ascending or descending order, the most centrally place value
d. Most frequently occurring observation

Ans. d

110. A Perfect normally distributed data will be found when it fulfills following condition:

a. The data is equally distributed in whole range
b. When mean, mode and median coincide at one point
c. When positive values are double the negative so as to have positive mean
d. When positive values are four time the negative to have positive mean

Ans. b

111. During an epidemiological study of malaria in coastal areas of Maharashtra, the investigators decide to keep small sample, it will:

a. Give Adequate precision
b. Not be representative data for the population
c. The standard error will be very high
d. The standard deviation will come higher than expected

Ans. b

112. In biostatitstics, a sampling unit is:

a. A group of sample
b. A sub-set of a sample
c. The unit which represent each member of a sample
d. The arithmetical units being used to represent a sample like Kg, mm, litre, etc.

Ans. c

113. When we report a correlation between an infectious disease and risk factor, the data is presented with confidence interval. When p=0.05, it can be concluded that?

a. All the values will fall in the confidence interval
b. 95% of the values will be out side the mean 1SD
c. 99% of the value will be out side the mean 1SD
d. 99.1% of the value will be out side the mean 1SD

Ans. a

114. When the sample is small and the observations are independent of each other, which test will be applied to find out the significance of difference in the means?

a. Fisher's test
b. Z test

c. Unpaired t test
d. Paired t test
Ans. d

115. **Children's day is worldwide celebrated on:**
a. November 20
b. November 11
c. November 14
d. April 4
Ans. a

116. **Salivary viscosity is:**
a. 1.002
b. 1.003
c. 1.005
d. 1.008
Ans. b

117. **For examining a 15-year-old child for periodontal disease using CPITN scores will be:**
a. 0,1
b. 0,1,2
c. 0,1,2,3
d. 0,1,2,3,4
Ans. c

118. **Oral dose of diazepam for pediatric sedation is:**
a. 0.05-0.1 mg/kg
b. 0.15-0.5 mg/kg
c. 0.45-0.89 mg/kg
d. 0.9-1.1 mg/kg
Ans. b

119. **In a 10-year-old child for extraction of permanent tooth, final decision will rest with:**
a. Patient
b. Dentist
c. Owner of clinic
d. Hospital authority
Ans. b

120. **Delayed eruption occurs in:**
a. Cerebral palsy
b. Autism
c. Down's syndrome
d. Beckwith weidmann syndrome
Ans. c

121. **Synonym for neurilemmoma is:**
a. Nasolipoma
b. Schwannoma
c. Neurofibroma
d. Cylindroma
Ans. b

122. **A 6-year-old child reported with typical umbilicated white lesion on face, the first differential diagnosis that comes to your mind is:**
a. Leukoplakia
b. Lichen Planus

c. Molluscum contagiosum
d. Scleroderma

Ans. c

123. Body temperature is controlled by:

a. Thalamus
b. Hippocampus
c. Limbic System
d. Hypothalamus

Ans. d

124. Fever is caused by:

a. Leukotrienes
b. Prostaglandins
c. Interferons
d. Interleukins

Ans. d

125. The preferred method of determining working length in a blunderbuss canal is:

a. Guttapercha
b. Radiographs
c. Paper points
d. EAL

Ans. c

126. The condition commonly called as bronchiectasis by pediatrician refers to:

a. Collapse of bronchi
b. Constriction of bronchi
c. Relaxation of bronchi
d. Dilatation of bronchi

Ans. d

127. Hypoglossal nerve injury causes:

a. Paralysis of tongue
b. Paralysis of soft palate
c. Sensory loss of tongue
d. Sensory loss of soft palate

Ans. a

128. Metallic sound on percussion is seen in:

a. Lateral luxation
b. Subluxation
c. Extrusion
d. Avulsion

Ans. a

129. An 8-year-old child with carious distal pit extending into enamel in 46, the treatment should be:

a. Pit and fissure
b. PRR
c. Flouride varnish
d. Observation only

Ans. b

130. A child reported with bird face or fish face, cleft palate, malar hypoplasia with bilateral blind fistula, the diagnosis of syndrome is:

a. Pierre Robin
b. Treacher Collins
c. Prader Willi

d. Angelmann
Ans. b

131. **A 6-year-old child reported with trauma to upper central incisor with intruded incisor, treatment is:**
   a. Reposition and splint
   b. Wait and watch
   c. Extraction
   d. Pulpectomy
   Ans. c

132. **Which of the viral infection cannot occur parenterally?**
   a. HCV
   b. HIV
   c. HEV
   d. HDV
   Ans. c

133. **Pulp has collagen fibers belonging to:**
   a. Type IV
   b. Type III
   c. Type V
   d. Type VII
   Ans. b

134. **In a child with sickle cell anemia the prophylaxis to prevent S.pneumonia is:**
   a. Penicillin
   b. Clotrimazole
   c. Ofloxacin
   d. Metronidazole
   Ans. a

135. **Hair on end appearance is seen in:**
   a. Plummer Wilson syndrome
   b. Cushing syndrome
   c. Addison syndrome
   d. Sickle cell anemia
   Ans. d

136. **In a child with secretion of GH after fusion of epiphysis can be:**
   a. Hyperpituitarism
   b. Gigantism
   c. Dwarfism
   d. Acromegaly
   Ans. d

137. **In minimal sedation, verbal command:**
   a. Child responds purposefully
   b. Child responds to pain only
   c. Child responds to touch only
   d. Child responds normally
   Ans. d

138. **3D seen in deficiency of:**
   a. Cyanocobalamine
   b. Pantothenic Acid

c. Riboflavin
d. Niacin
Ans. d

139. In recurrent herpes zoster which branch mostly involved:
a. Ophthalmic of trigeminal
b. Mandibular of trigeminal
c. Maxillary of trigeminal
d. Stapedial of facial
Ans. a

140. Branchial cyst occurs due to non fusion of:
a. 3rd and 4th branchial pouches
b. 2nd and 3rd branchial arches
c. 4th and 5th branchial arches
d. 1st and 3rd branchial arches
Ans. b

141. In subgingival calculus maximum concentration of which is seen?
a. $CaCo_3$
b. $CaPO_4$
c. $MgPO_4$
d. $Al\,2O_3$
Ans. b

142. Endodontically treated teeth are:
a. More prone to caries
b. Less prone to caries
c. Same as other teeth
d. None of the above
Ans. c

143. Xylitol inhibits:
a. Glycolysis
b. Gluconeogenesis
c. Glycogenesis
d. Rapaport leubering shunt
Ans. b

144. OSMF occurs in:
a. Oral mucosa
b. Oral mucosa and pharynx
c. Oral mucosa and pharynx and 2/3rd of oesophagus
d. Oral mucosa and tongue
Ans. c

145. Predominant demineralization occurs mainly at:
a. Tail of enamel rods
b. Head of enamel rods
c. Head of periphery
d. Uniform
Ans. b

146. Long face syndrome occurs in:
a. Mouth breathing
b. Tongue thrusting

c. Lip biting
d. Thumb sucking
Ans. a

147. Excessive callus formation occurs in:
a. Amelogenesis imperfect
b. Dentin dysplasia
c. Fibrous dysplasia
d. Osteogenesis imperfecta
Ans. d

148. In maxilla intercanine width increases with eruption of:
a. Incisors
b. Canines
c. Premolars
d. Molars
Ans. a

149. In salivary reductase test, high caries activity shown by color change to:
a. Orchid
b. Red
c. Yellow
d. Blue
Ans. b

150. Popliteal artery is present in:
a. Wrist
b. Medial malleolus
c. Cubital fossa
d. Behind the knee
Ans. d

151. Submandibular gland is:
a. Highly serous
b. Highly mucous
c. Predominantly serous
d. Predominantly mucous
Ans. c

152. If both parents have cleft lip and palate the chances of children to have that is:
a. 1:10
b. 1:5
c. 3:5
d. 4:9
Ans. c

153. Pulp vascularity best detected by:
a. LDF
b. Pulse oximetry
c. EPT
d. Cold test
Ans. a

154. Which cry is not a true cry?
a. Compensatory
b. Obstinate

c. Hurt
d. Defiant
Ans. d

155. According to WHO classification of handicap which is not included:
a. Diabetes
b. Juvenile periodontitis
c. Autism
d. Mental retardation
Ans. a

156. In a 15-year-old normal adolescent true is:
a. Lingual embrasure filled with gingiva
b. Occlusal embrasure is larger than gingival embrasure
c. Occlusal embrasure is the largest embrasure
d. All of the above
Ans. a

157. Best Evidence can be obtained from:
a. Controlled trials
b. Meta analysis
c. RCT
d. Cohort study
Ans. b
Note: *As per recent concept if CPG or Clinical Practice Guidelines in option go for that then second next will be meta analysis in the evidence pyramid*

158. Reparative dentin is formed by:
a. Ameloblasts
b. Odontoblasts
c. Cementoblasts
d. Fibroblasts
Ans. b

159. In RME a quarter turn actually opens:
a. 0.05 cm
b. 0.04 cm
c. 0.01 cm
d. 0.02 cm
Ans. d

160. Fluorescent antibody test is used for condition where interepithelial antibodies are seen:
a. Pemphigus vulgaris
b. Bullous mucous membrane pemphigoid
c. Erythema multiforme
d. Cicatricial pemphigoid
Ans. a

161. In SABE most commonly involved valve is:
a. Mitral
b. Bicuspid
c. Tricuspid
d. Pulmonary
Ans. a

162. Disadvantage of disclosing agent is:
a. Stains teeth
b. Stains operator's hands
c. Stains clothes
d. Stains silicate restorations
Ans. d

163. The disadvantage of cone shift technique is:
a. Lingual structures are more blurred than buccal structures
b. Contrast between radiopaque and radiolucent structures high
c. Buccal and lingual canals could not be seen
d. Normal anatomic structure can superimpose on root apices
Ans. d

164. True about Sjogren's syndrome is:
a. Excessive lacrimation
b. Excessive salivation
c. Higher incidence in males than females
d. May be autoimmune in nature
Ans. d

165. Notched incisors seen in:
a. Mulberry incisors
b. Moon incisors
c. Hutchinson incisors
d. Robinson incisors
Ans. c

166. Complete isthmus belongs to:
a. Class I
b. Class II
c. Class III
d. Class IV
Ans. b

167. Two or three canals and both alpha and beta angles less than 60 degrees belongs to which class of C shaped canals:
a. Class II
b. Class III
c. Class IV
d. Class V
Ans. b

168. Stabident and X-tip are which type of anesthesia?
a. Intraarterial
b. Intraligamentary
c. Intrapulpal
d. Intraosseous
Ans. d

169. Time period of substantivity of chlorhexidine is:
a. 6 weeks
b. 9 weeks
c. 12 weeks
d. 18 weeks
Ans. c

170. Best plane to view CBCT for vertical fractures:
a. Transverse
b. Axial
c. Sagittal
d. Coronal
Ans. a

171. Letter resembling vertical fracture is:
a. L
b. I
c. V
d. J
Ans. d

172. Alkaline phosphate level increased in A/E:
a. Osteomyelitis
b. Paget's disease
c. Hyperparathyroidism
d. Fibrous dysplasia
Ans. a

173. Angle fracture of mandible is diagnosed by:
a. OPG
b. OPG+ PA view
c. Reverse towne's view
d. SMV
Ans. b

174. Generally normal space in healthy persons contain:
a. Water
b. Air
c. Loose areolar tissue
d. Fibrous tissue
Ans. c

175. Malignant cell resembling with primitive undifferentiated cell is called as:
a. Metaplastic
b. Anaplastic
c. Metastatic
d. Hypoplastic
Ans. b

176. Joint space examination with contrast media is called as:
a. Arthroscopy
b. Arthrography
c. Arthroplasty
d. Thermography
Ans. b

177. Tetanic contraction is due to summation of:
a. Sub threshold potential
b. Action potential
c. Local excitatory stimulation
d. Neural stimulation
Ans. b

178. Nasal fossa floor formed by:
- a. Maxillary process and vertical process of palatine bone
- b. Maxillary process and horizontal process of palatine bone
- c. Maxillary process only
- d. Palatine process only

Ans. b

179. Patient having Class III occlusion and increased length of mandible and increased interdental spacing:
- a. Hyperthyroidism
- b. Hyperpituitarism
- c. Hyperparathyroidism
- d. Hypergonadism

Ans. b

180. True about dry socket is:
- a. Eugenol dressing is contraindicated
- b. Blood supply and dislodgement of clot is not responsible only
- c. Trismus is usual
- d. Pain aggravated after removal of suture on 5th postoperative day

Ans. d

181. Submasseteric space infection is due to:
- a. Peritonsillar infection
- b. IANB
- c. Spread of infection from ear
- d. Mandibular molar

Ans. d

182. Most common oral manifestation seen in leukemia is:
- a. Myelocytic
- b. Lymphocytic
- c. Acute lymphoid
- d. Chronic lymphoid

Ans. a

183. SABG should be done:
- a. After maxillary expansion and cross bite correction & before cuspid eruption
- b. After maxillary expansion and cross bite correction & after cuspid eruption
- c. Before maxillary expansion and cross bite correction & before cuspid eruption
- d. Before maxillary expansion and cross bite correction & after cuspid eruption

Ans. a

184. To see foreign body embedded in soft tissue:
- a. 1/4th exposure time as compared to normal
- b. 1/8th exposure time as compared to normal
- c. Same as compared to normal
- d. Don't have to change exposure time, alter Kvp and Ma

Ans. d

185. Setting strength of MTA between 7 and 28 days of mixing will come in range of:
- a. 34 MPa
- b. 67 MPa
- c. 99 MPa
- d. 134 MPa

Ans. b

186. Taurodontism is associated with all except:
- a. Smith Mclean syndrome
- b. Down's syndrome
- c. Apert's syndrome
- d. Klinefelter's syndrome

Ans. a

187. Etching time in case of flourosed tooth is:
- a. 10–20 seconds
- b. 20–30 seconds
- c. 60–90 seconds
- d. More than 360 seconds

Ans. c

188. ADA number for setting time of sealers is:
- a. 55
- b. 56
- c. 57
- d. 58

Ans. c

189. While negotiating canals all can be useful except:
- a. DG 16
- b. H_2O_2
- c. NaOCl
- d. Dentinal map

Ans. b

190. In case of acute apical abcess the irrigant used is:
- a. Normal saline
- b. EDTA
- c. Tetraclean
- d. MTAD

Ans. a

191. Radiopacity of Retroplast is:
- a. 3.08 mm of Al
- b. 4 mm of Al
- c. 6 mm of Al
- d. 9 mm of Al

Ans. c
- Option A is the answer if MTA is being asked

192. The freshly mixed MTA has a pH of:
- a. 9
- b. 10
- c. 11
- d. 12

Ans. b

193. Dentin plug is seen in the root canal of:
- a. Maxillary first molar and premolar
- b. Maxillary lateral incisor and mandibular canine
- c. Mandibular first premolar and maxillary first molar
- d. Mandibular canine and Maxillary first molar

Ans. b

194. Shortest root of maxillary first molar is:
a. Distobuccal
b. Mesiobuccal
c. Palatal
d. All are same
Ans. a

195. The care to be taken after intraoral zygoma elevation is:
a. IMF for 6 weeks
b. IMF for 2 weeks
c. Restrict mouth opening
d. Avoid pressure on the operated side
Ans. d

196. In humans Hb consists of:
a. 4 heme group and 4 peptide chain
b. 2 alpha and 2 gamma chains
c. 3 gamma and 2 beta chains
d. 2 Alpha and 2 beta chains
Ans. d

197. Multilocular radiolucency and negative aspiration test with all vital teeth extending from 44 to 36 region could be:
a. Periapical granuloma
b. PGCG
c. CGCG
d. Aneurysmal bone cyst
Ans. c

198. Oral and dermal erythematous lesion along with patient having photophobia joint pain raynoud s disease symptoms can be:
a. Erythema multiforme
b. DLE
c. SLE
d. Erythroplakia
Ans. c

199. Melanoneuroectodermal tumor most seen in:
a. Ethmoid
b. Mandible
c. Maxilla
d. Cervical spine
Ans. c

200. The TMJ ankylosis in systemic sclerosis patient is managed by:
a. Interpositional arthroplasty
b. Gap arthroplasty
c. No treatment
d. Bone resection with aggressive muscle stripping
Ans. a

201. The joint having slight movement and joined together with ligament or fibrous disc is called as:
a. Gomphosis
b. Pseudoarthrosis
c. Diarthroses
d. Fibrosis
Ans. c

202. The type of OKC having maximum recurrence is:
a. Orthokeratotic
b. Parakeratotic
c. Orthoparakeratotic
d. None of these
Ans. b

203. Fracture angle mandible with minimal displacement case, the radiograph will show radiopaque line due to:
a. Increased bone formation
b. Overlapping
c. Hard callus
d. Normal in angle region
Ans. b

204. Compression osteosynthesis tension band is given to avoid:
a. Lingual fraying
b. Lingual splicing
c. Alveolar separation
d. Inferior border flaring
Ans. c

205. Differential diagnosis for periapical cemental dysplasia and periapical granuloma can be by:
a. Radiography
b. Vitality testing
c. Aspiration
d. Symptom
Ans. b

206. In thrombocytopenia the most important complication is:
a. Hemorrhage
b. Eccymosis
c. Swelling
d. Purpura
Ans. b

207. Burning mouth syndrome is present in all except:
a. Diabetes Mellitus
b. Epidermolysis bullosa
c. Ranula
d. Pernicious anemia
Ans. c

208. To detect vertical root fractures best angulation is:
a. 45,90
b. 45,110
c. 45
d. 45,90,110
Ans. d

209. Best material for RC treated teeth:
a. Lathe cut
b. Spherical
c. Admixed
d. None
Ans. c

210. The percentage reduction in tooth stiffness as a result of conservative access cavity preparation is:
a. 5
b. 9
c. 13
d. 21
Ans. a
Loss of moisture due to change in free water as result of endo treatment is 9%

211. Chromosome affected in Dentinogenesis imperfecta:
a. 3
b. 4
c. 5
d. 6
Ans. b

212. SnF2 subgingival irrigation concentration is:
a. 0.56
b. 0.67
c. 0.64
d. 0.98
Ans. c

213. Spirochetes seen in which zone of ANUG?
a. Zone 3
b. Zone 4
c. Zone 5
d. Zone 6
Ans. b

214. Which organism produces trypsin like enzyme?
a. A.acomitans
b. Capnocytophaga
c. Treponema pallidum
d. Tannerella forsythia
Ans. b

215. The brushing technique in progressive recession cases is:
a. Modified stillman
b. Leonard
c. Scrub
d. Charters
Ans. a

216. In PSR which site is seen?
a. Only facial
b. Only lingual
c. Only faciolingual
d. Only mesiodistal
Ans. c

217. Monobloc effect is seen with:
a. GP
b. AH 26
c. Resilon+Epiphany
d. All of the above
Ans. c

218. High flow AVM in mandible, line of treatment is:
a. Wait and watch as it gets involute with time
b. CNA glue intralesionally
c. Embolisation of feeding vessel
d. Aspiration
Ans. c

219. Leucocytes which are more involved in periodontitis are:
a. Neutrophils
b. Basophils
c. Eosinophils
d. Lymphocytes
Ans. a

220. PDL adaptive remodeling seen in stage:
a. I
b. II
c. III
d. IV
Ans. c

221. An initial colonizer is:
a. Strep.sanguis
b. P.gingivalis
c. Capnocytophaga
d. Tannerella
Ans. a

222. Gene associated with invasion and progression of ameloblastoma:
a. bcl2
b. P53
c. MMP
d. FGF
Ans. c

223. Ledge can be considered as:
a. Positive architecture
b. Reverse architecture
c. Negative architecture
d. All of these
Ans. b

224. Cul de sac comes under:
a. Grade I
b. Grade II
c. Grade III
d. Grade IV
Ans. b

225. Moderate for desquamative gingivitis, what clinical changes are seen:
a. Patches of redness and epithelium is smashed
b. Fiery red appearance
c. Erythematous with pathogen
d. None of the above
Ans. a

226. Blue black staining is due to
a. Lead
b. Copper
c. Mercury
d. Bismuth
Ans. d

227. 1: 2,00000 solution is better than 1:80,000 solution for LA due to:
a. Profound anesthesia
b. Increased duration of anesthesia
c. Relatively less toxicity
d. Early onset of action
Ans. c

228. Crestant tooth refers to:
a. Regional odontodysplasia
b. Dens evaginatus
c. Dens in dente
d. Dentin dysplasia
Ans. c

229. Lymphogranuloma venerum most commonly is seen in:
a. Lip
b. Tongue
c. Palate
d. Nasopharynx
Ans. c

230. Lymphoepithelioma most commonly is seen in:
a. Lip
b. Tongue
c. Palate
d. Nasopharynx
Ans. d

231. High difficulty happens when extreme curvature is about:
a. 20 degrees
b. 25 degrees
c. 30 degrees
d. 35 degrees
Ans. c

232. Occlusal reduction helps in reducing:
a. Pain
b. Sensitivity
c. Bleeding
d. None of these
Ans. a

233. Cracked tooth syndrome is treated by:
a. Extraction
b. Bonded tooth restoration
c. Wait and watch
d. A or B
Ans. d

234. Ideally preferred rubber dam is:
a. Hard
b. Medium
c. Soft
d. Resilient
Ans. b

235. Thyroid collar works on:
a. Isometry rule
b. Rule of truncation
c. Inverse square law
d. ALARA principle
Ans. d

236. Partial clockwise twist belongs to which type of Sotokowa's Classification:
a. Type II
b. Type III
c. Typc IV
d. Type V
Ans. c

237. Vertical root fracture is happening usually which direction:
a. Lateral
b. Buccolingual
c. Mesiodistal
d. None
Ans. b

238. Maxillary premolars show striking difference in:
a. Asians
b. Orientals
c. Polynesians
d. Africans
Ans. d

239. To completely dissolve pulp the temperature needed is:
a. 40 degrees
b. 45 degrees
c. 55 degrees
d. 65 degrees
Ans. b

240. Tubliseal is based on:
a. Calcium
b. Sodium
c. Rocksalt
d. Flouride
Ans. a

241. Endodontic panacea refers to:
a. Calcium hydroxide
b. RC files
c. Gutta percha
d. Normal saline
Ans. a

242. White knuckle syndrome refers to:
a. Vibration finger
b. Type of Raynaud's syndrome
c. Type of Carpal tunnel syndrome
d. Both A and B
Ans. d

243. Water trees refers to:
a. Porosities in adhesive layer
b. Cracks in adhesive layer
c. Porosities in non adhesive layer
d. Cracks in non adhesive layer
Ans. a

244. The local anesthesia used in chronic renal failure case:
a. Bupivacaine
b. Procaine
c. Lignocaine
d. Articaine
Ans. d

245. Gene of basal cell nevoid is seen in which chromosome?
a. 21 p
b. 21q
c. 9 p
d. 9 q
Ans. d

246. Microdontia of all teeth is seen in which type of enamel hypoplasia?
a. Type I localized
b. Type II generalized
c. Type III
d. Type IV
Ans. b

247. Dens in dente is:
a. Autosomal dominant
b. Autosomal recessive
c. Polygenic
d. Multifactorial
Ans. a

248. Yellow stains are due to:
a. Depleted developer
b. Depleted fixer
c. Overcooled water
d. All of these
Ans. a

249. Mineral that helps in wound healing is:
a. Zinc
b. Selenium
c. Calcium
d. Sodium
Ans. c

250. Incidence of furcation canals in mandibular molars is:

a. 14 %
b. 23%
c. 43%
d. 66%

Ans. b

251. According to recent research the origin of Pindborg tumor is:

a. Stratum intermedia
b. Dental lamina
c. Stratum granulosa
d. Stellate reticulum

Ans. b

252. In Grand Rapids the control used was:

a. Kingston
b. Muskegon
c. Oakpark
d. Culemberg

Ans. b

253. Crowe's sign is seen in:

a. Cholecystitis
b. Von Recklinghausen disease
c. Mandibular fracture
d. Herpetiform ulcer

Ans. b

254. APDI value is:

a. 81.4
b. 89.3
c. 78
d. 91.2

Ans. d

255. 100% artificial fluoridation is seen in:

a. Spain and France
b. Thailand and Germany
c. Singapore and Hongkong
d. Switzerland and Malaysia

Ans. c

256. The canalization theory of growth was by:

a. Pankey
b. Schuyler
c. Waddlington
d. Luca

Ans. c

257. The distance between 2 miniplates in the symphyseal region is:

a. 3.5 mm
b. 4.5 mm
c. 5.5 mm
d. 7.5 mm

Ans. b

258. Best anesthetic for teeth with TTXR Channels are:
a. Articaine
b. Mepivacaine
c. Bupivacaine
d. Cinchocaine
Ans. c

259. ICON has all false except:
a. Aesthetic component weightage-4
b. Cross bite weightage-2
c. Crowding/spacing weightage-4
d. Buccal segment Ap relationship weightage-3
Ans. d

260. Bird's eye photograph is taken at:
a. 15 degrees
b. 35 degrees
c. 45 degrees
d. 75 degrees
Ans. c

261. The total height of both casts in occlusion should be about:
a. 2.5–5 cm
b. 7–7.5 cm
c. 8–8.35 cm
d. 9.15–9.7 cm
Ans. b

262. The orifices of the root canals are always located at the junction of walls and the floor. This is called:
a. First law of orifice location
b. Second law of orifice location
c. Third law of orifice location
d. Law of centrality
Ans. a

263. Cubic interpolatory spline was given by:
a. Currier
b. Begole
c. Merrifield
d. Stolzenberg
Ans. b

264. The incidence of two canals one foramina configuration in mandibular central incisors is:
a. 24%
b. 70%
c. 44%
d. 6%
Ans. a

265. The average distance between the main and the minor mesio buccal canal of the maxillary first molar is:
a. 1.8 mm
b. 0.8 mm
c. Mid way between the Mesio buccal- palatal canal orifices
d. Mid way between the Mesio buccal- distal l canal orifices
Ans. a

266. Which is the most characteristic radiographic feature suggestive of vertical root fracture?
a. Dual intra oral sinus
b. Persistent periodontal defect
c. A radio opaque lesion at the site of the fracture
d. A radiolucent lesion surrounding the fractured root
Ans. d

267. What type of collagen is the most prominent found in the dental pulp?
a. Type I
b. Type II
c. Type III
d. Type IV
Ans. a

268. All are preferred hemostatic agent for perforation repair except:
a. Ferric sulphate
b. Calcium hydroxide
c. Collagen
d. Freeze dried bone
Ans. a

269. Preferred method for working length measurement in blunderbuss canals with open apex is:
a. EAL
b. Radiographic method
c. Tactile method
d. Paper point method
Ans. d

270. If adhesive repair for perforation is planned the barrier material preferred is:
a. Collagen
b. Calcium sulphate
c. No barrier is required
d. Freezed dried bone
Ans. b

271. In endodontics the highest level of evidence (LOE) is gained from:
a. Case series
b. Uncontrolled trials
c. Randomized clinical trials
d. Controlled clinical trials
Ans. c

272. Recommended method for gutta-percha removal during preparation of a post space:
a. Chemical method
b. Thermal
c. Mechanical
d. Thermal combined with mechanical
Ans. d

273. How much gutta–percha should be ideally retained to preserve the apical seal during post space preparation?
a. 2 mm
b. 4 mm
c. 5 mm
d. 3 mm
Ans. c

274. Endodontically treated teeth are:
a. Not susceptible to development of caries
b. Are as susceptible as healthy teeth to development of caries
c. More susceptible to development of caries
d. Only root caries can develop
Ans. c

275. The Stropto flexi tip needle is a:
a. 23 gauge
b. 27 gauge
c. 30 gauge
d. 21 gauge
Ans. c

276. Residual antimicrobial activity of CHX in the root canal system remains for up to:
a. 6 weeks
b. 12 weeks
c. 6 days
d. 12 days
Ans. b

277. Optimal location for intra osseous anesthesia for mandibular second molars is:
a. Distal to the molar
b. Mesial to the molar
c. In the furation area
d. Apical perforation and injection
Ans. b

278. The best protocol for detection of Vertical Root Fractures by Using Cone Beam Computed Tomography is achieved at:
a. 0.125 mm Voxel Sizes
b. 0.2 mm Voxel Sizes
c. 0.3 mm Voxel Sizes
d. 0.4 mm Voxel Sizes
Ans. b

279. If the size of the furcal perforation is doubled, the surface area to be repaired becomes:
a. Half
b. Double
c. Remains same
d. Four times
Ans. d

280. Advantage of using 1, 1, 1, 2–tetrafluoroethane for cold testing is:
a. It does not cause craze lines
b. It has increased sensitivity
c. Has zero ozone depletion potential
d. It has increased specificity
Ans. c

281. The method of choice for assessing pulp vitality in luxation injuries is:
a. Pulse Oximetry
b. Laser Doppler flowmetry
c. Electric pulp test
d. Cold test
Ans. b

282. In 'C' shaped configuration category III is:
   a. Uninterrupted 'C' with no separation
   b. Only one round or oval canal
   c. Two or three separate canals and both angles, alpha and beta are less than 60 degree
   d. Semicolon canal shape buteither angles alpha and beta should be no less than 60 degree
   Ans. c

283. Working length determination in elderly patients may be more difficult because of which of the following?
   a. Increased bone density, making radiographs harder to interpret
   b. Increased cementum deposition, modifying the apical anatomy
   c. Differences in tissue electrical resistance, making apex locators less accurate
   d. Patients unable to sit still for the radiographs
   Ans. b

284. The healing capacity of older patients is significantly less than younger patients because of a decrease in periradicular vascularity. The vascularity of the periradicular tissues is a critical determinant in healing.
   a. The first statement is false, and the second statement is true
   b. The first statement is true, and the second statement is false
   c. Both statements are true
   d. Both statements are false
   Ans. a

285. A patient presents for a post treatment examination after three years with no complaint of symptoms except the apical radiolucency that was present before treatment, although it appears smaller. Treatment for this patient would be classified as which of the following?
   a. Healed
   b. Healing
   c. Diseased
   d. A clinical success but radiographic failure
   Ans. b

286. Profound anesthesia is difficult to attain before incision for drainage. What is a preferred approach for a maxillary cuspid with extensive swelling?
   a. Start with an infraorbital block and then infiltrate at the margins of the swelling
   b. Start with posterior superior alveolar block and then use refrigerant spray
   c. Inject buffer and anesthetic directly into the swelling
   d. Use topical anesthetic and then refrigerant spray. No anesthetic is needed.
   Ans. a

287. Which of the following is not true regarding the removal and retreatment of hard- setting pastes?
   a. They are more difficult to remove than a soft paste
   b. They may be impossible to remove
   c. Solvents have been shown to soften hard-setting pastes
   d. Use of ultrasonics is the most predictable method
   Ans. c

288. What solvent has been shown to be the most efficient (fastest) in softening gutta-percha?
   a. Chloroform
   b. Halothane
   c. Methylchloroform
   d. Xylene
   Ans. a

289. The following steps are used to attempt removal of a canal ledge during non surgical treatment except which one?

a. Remove all obstructions coronal to the ledge
b. Bypass the ledge with a flexible nickel-titanium hand file
c. File in a circumferential motion after bypassing the ledge
d. Proceed from small size file to larger size files
Ans. b

290. Which of the following scenarios yields the most favourable prognosis in cases with a separated instrument?
a. A small instrument short of the working length
b. A small instrument beyond the apical foramen
c. A large instrument at an early stage of instrumentation
d. A large instrument close to the working length
Ans. d

291. What type of perforation has the poorest long term prognosis?
a. Zipping (apical third) root perforation
b. Stripping perforation in the apical third of the root
c. Stripping perforation in the coronal third of the root below the crest
d. Direct floor to furcation perforation in a multi-rooted tooth
Ans. c

292. What type of canal is most prone to ledge formation?
a. Long, small and curved
b. Incomplete apex formation, curved
c. Large, long
d. Short, straight
Ans. a

293. If a lateral root perforation does occur, what is the most favourable location for perforation repair?
a. At or above the height of crestal bone
b. Below the crestal bone in the coronal third of the root
c. On the furcal side of the coronal root surface
d. A zipping perforation at the apex of the root
Ans. a

294. What pulp and periapical diagnosis may have completed the treatment in a single visit?
a. Symptomatic (acute) apical periodontitis
b. Asymptomatic apical periodontitis (chronic apical periodontitis)
c. Acute apical abscess
d. Painful irreversible pulpitis
Ans. d

295. What is the optimal preparation/obturation length relative to the radiographic apex with pulp necrosis?
a. Flush
b. 0.5–1 mm short
c. Slight extrusion of the sealer but not gutta-percha
d. 1.0 to 3.0 mm short
Ans. b

296. EDTA is most effective for which of the following uses?
a. Decalcifying small canals to allow instruments to negotiate to length
b. Lubricating canals to facilitate instrumentation
c. Bacterial elimination in canals
d. Removing smear layer after cleaning and shaping
Ans. d

297. For the irrigating solution to effectively reach the apical third of the canal, the apical canal should be enlarged to at least a No.......... file.

a. 25 or 30
b. 20 or 25
c. 35 or 40
d. 45 or 50

Ans. c

298. What is the recommended rubber dam weight for endodontic procedures?

a. Light
b. Medium
c. Heavy
d. Extra heavy

Ans. b

299. What is torsional limit?

a. Amount of apical pressure that can be applied to a file to the point of breakage
b. The beginning of plastic deformation of the instrument
c. Amount of rotational torque that can be applied to a locked instrument to the point of breakage
d. Amount of force necessary so that a file does not return to its original shape upon unloading of the force.

Ans. c

300. Nickel-titanium alloy has increased flexibility over stainless steel. How does the modulus of elasticity for nickel-titanium alloy compare to that of stainless steel?

a. Similar to stainless steel
b. One-fourth to one fifth that of stainless steel
c. Half that of stainless steel
d. 2–3 times that of stainless steel

Ans. b

301. What is the disadvantage to the cone shift image?

a. Lingual objects become more distorted than buccal objects
b. There is a excessive contrast between radiolucent and radiopaque objects
c. It may superimpose normal anatomic structures over the root apices
d. It does not reveal additional canals within a root

Ans. c

302. F speed film requires how much less exposure compared to E speed films?

a. 10% to 15%
b. 20% to 25%
c. 30% to 35%
d. 50%

Ans. b

303. What factor should be considered that determines the treatment of an intrusive luxation injury?

a. Depth of intrution
b. Stage of root development
c. Availability of adjacent tooth for stabilisation
d. Amount of soft tissue injury

Ans. b

304. Does increasing the volume of anesthetic solution affect the duration of pulpal anesthesia?

a. For mandibular anesthesia, increasing the volume improves the success rate with the inferior alveolar nerve block
b. For maxillary infiltration, increasing the volume increases the depth of pulpal anesthesia

c. For maxillary infiltration, increasing the volume increases the duration of pulpal anesthesia
d. For maxillary infiltration, increasing the volume has no effect on the success rate of pulpal anesthesia

Ans. c

305. Does the direction of the needle bevel affect the effectiveness of the inferior alveolar nerve block?
a. Needle bevel toward the mandibular ramus improves success
b. Needle bevel away from the mandibular ramus improves success
c. Half cartridge should be injected with the bevel toward the ramus, the needle rotated, and the second half of the cartridge injected with the bevel away from the ramus
d. Direction of the needle bevel does not affect success

Ans. d

306. What is the allodynia phenomenon?
a. Inflamed tissue has an increased threshold of pain
b. Inflamed tissue has a decreased threshold of pain
c. Inflamed tissue is much less sensitive to a mild stimulus
d. Inflamed tissue responds mildly to a stimulus that would otherwise be very painful

Ans. b

307. What is the common direction that fractures extend in cracked teeth?
a. Mesiodistal
b. Faciolingual
c. Apical to coronal
d. Horizontal

Ans. a

308. During a review of the patient's healthy history, it is noted that the patient is on a regimen of intravenous bisphosphonate medication. What significance does this hold for the patient and their treatment plan?
a. Possible side effect of bleeding disorder
b. Possible side effect of osteonecrosis of the jaw
c. Lowered pain threshold
d. Inability to obtain adequate anesthesia

Ans. b

309. What type of collagen is the most prominent found in the dental pulp?
a. Type I
b. Type II
c. Type III
d. Type IV

Ans. a

310. Which of the following is not a major component of the odontoblast?
a. Cell body
b. Basal located nucleus
c. Cell process
d. Synaptic junction

Ans. d

311. Fluoride sealers is seen maximum with:
a. Resin Modified Glass Ionomer
b. Polyacid Glass Ionomer resin Composite
c. Conventional Glass Ionomer
d. Cermet

Ans. c

312. Standard Light curing tip has a diameter of:
a. 3 mm
b. 11 mm
c. 5 mm
d. 8 mm
Ans. b

313. The acid dissolution process occurs more in which part of the enamel rod?
a. Head region
b. Tail region
c. Periphery of head region
d. Equal in all regions
Ans. a

314. At what pH, the enamel surface remains intact while the subsurface mineral is lost?
a. 3
b. 4
c. 5
d. 5.5
Ans. c

315. Which zone of dentinal caries is characterized by demineralization of the intertubular dentin and formation of very fine crystals in the tubule lumen?
a. Sub transparent dentin
b. Transparent dentin
c. Infected dentin (outermost zone)
d. Normal dentin
Ans. a

316. Which phase acts as the strongest cathode in low Cu amalgam?
a. Residual amalgam alloy particle
b. Sn-Hg phase
c. Cu-Sn phase
d. Ag-Hg phase
Ans. a

317. Application of what concentration of phosphoric acid results in formation of dicalcium phosphate monohydrate precipitate that cannot be removed easily and consequently may interfere with adhesion:
a. 85%
b. 50%
c. 37%
d. 25%
Ans. d

318. Nd:YAG laser operates at which wavelength?
a. 10.60 μm
b. 2.06 μm
c. 1.06 μm
d. 308 μm
Ans. c

319. LCTE of hybrid glass ionomer is:
a. Less than conventional glass ionomer
b. Equal to tooth
c. 2 times that of tooth
d. 3 times that of tooth
Ans. c

320. Slow heating of the tooth produces no response until the temperature reaches approximately:
a. 39 degree Celsius
b. 45 degree Celsius
c. 55 degree Celsius
d. 65 degree Celsius
Ans. b

321. For approx. How much time the 4% buffered gluteraldehyde is applied over the pulp stump during pulpotomy?
a. 10 sec
b. 60 sec
c. 2 min
d. 4 min
Ans. d

322. In 'salivary reductase' test the color change indicating high caries activity is:
a. Blue
b. Orchid
c. Red
d. Colorless
Ans. d

323. 'Miller index' is an objective systems used to determine:
a. Mobility of the tooth
b. Periodontal pocket depths
c. Efficacy of anesthesia
d. Tooth surface temperature
Ans. a

324. The usual range of temperature for bleaching vital teeth with a heat or light source is:
a. 100–115 degrees F
b. 115–140 degrees F
c. 140–160 degrees F
d. 160 degrees to as high the patient can tolerate
Ans. b

325. Type II isthimus is characterized as:
a. Faint communication between two canals
b. Definite connection between two canals
c. Very short, complete isthmus between two canals
d. Complete or incomplete isthmus between three or more canals
Ans. b

326. For endodontic retreatment through a Zirconia based crown the access should be gained with:
a. Round coarse diamond bur
b. Carbide bur
c. Steel bur
d. Medium or fine grit diamond bur
Ans. d

327. The incisal edge of the access cavity of maxillary anterior teeth:
a. Should have a long bevel
b. Should have a short bevel
c. Should not be beveled
d. Should have a partial bevel
Ans. c

328. The interaction between NaOCl and CHX results in an insoluble neutral salt as a precipitate. This can be prevented by:
a. Using absolute alcohol between two irrigants
b. Using 17% EDTA between two irrigants
c. Using saline and distilled water as intermediate flushes.
d. Their formation cannot be prevented and hence this irrigation regimen should not be used
Ans. a

329. Chemical that can be effectively used as an adjunct to dissolve set White MTA is:
a. Chlorhexidiene gluconate
b. Carbonic acid
c. EDTA
d. Absolute alcohol
Ans. b

330. Ideal depth of root end cavity preparation is:
a. 3 mm
b. 1 mm
c. 2 mm
d. 4 mm
Ans. a

331. The detergent used in Tetraclean irrigant is:
a. Poly sorbate 80
b. Polypropylene glycol
c. Sodium Lauryl Sulfate
d. Alkyl Polyglycoside and N, N'-bis (3-aminopropyl) Propane-1, 3- Diamine
Ans. b

332. A metallic percussion sound is usually seen in:
a. Lateral Luxation
b. Extrusive luxation
c. Subluxation
d. Concussion
Ans. a

333. All statements regarding Gates-Glidden drills are true except:
a. Used to open orifices
b. They are available in sizes 1-6
c. They are available in 15–19 mm length
d. They have parallel cutting sides
Ans. d

334. Maximum perforation that occur are:
a. Pathological
b. During access opening
c. During post space preparation
d. During canal preparation
Ans. c

335. All are indicators for bicuspidization except:
a. Furcation perforation
b. Furcation pathosis from periodontal disease
c. Deep furcation (thick floor of pulp chamber)
d. Bucco lingual cervical caries
Ans. c

336. What is the incidence of interappointment flare-ups?
a. Primarily after obturation at a range of 4.4 to 6.0%
b. Overall at a range of 1.8 to 3.2%
c. Overall at a range of 10.7 to 21.3%
d. Primarily after vital pulp removal at a range of 7.5 to 10.7%
Ans. b

337. Using the Case Difficulty Assessment system developed by the American Association of Endodontists, cases in which any factors score 3 should be:
a. Treated by a general dentist
b. Treated by an endodontist
c. Should be referred to endodontist for opinion only
d. Tooth is not treatable and hence extracted
Ans. b

338. How does electric pulp testing determine the degree of pulpal inflammation?
a. A shorter response indicates a healthier pulp
b. A mid range response indicates pulp inflammation
c. A mid range response indicates partial necrosis
d. It can only be used to determine the presence or absence of vital tissue
Ans. d

339. Which of the following has not been demonstrated with MTA when used in apexification?
a. Good biocompatibility
b. Good sealability
c. High pH value
d. Adjacent zone of necrosis
Ans. d

340. What is dentin 'blushing'?
a. The color of newly erupted teeth due to large pulp chambers
b. Use of a masking color during restorative procedures
c. Vascular hemorrhage of pulp tissue, often during crown preparation
d. An esthetic concern requiring laminate restorations
Ans. c

341. Fewer tooth fractures have been recorded in laboratory studies when what type of post has been used?
a. Cobalt chromium alloy post
b. Stainless steel post
c. Titanium post
d. Carbon fiber post
Ans. d

342. Of the following, which is the most important consideration of a temporary restoration?
a. Antimicrobial
b. Placed over a cotton pellet
c. Resistant to acids
d. At least 4 mm thick
Ans. b

343. Dens invaginatus (dens in dente) occurs most commonly in which teeth?
a. Maxillary canines
b. Maxillary lateral incisors
c. Maxillary and mandibular lateral incisors
d. Mandibular first premolar
Ans. b

AIIMS Endodontics Question Bank

THE DENTAL PULP AND PERIRADICULAR TISSUES

1. **What is the primary function of the dental pulp?**
   a. Induction
   b. Formation
   c. Nutrition
   d. Defense
   Ans. b
2. **Which of the following is not a stage of tooth formation?**
   a. Bud
   b. Cap
   c. Bell
   d. Basal
   Ans. d
3. **From what cells are odontoblasts derived?**
   a. Undifferentiated basal
   b. Undifferentiated ectomesenchymal
   c. Undifferentiated cartilage
   d. Dental papilla
   Ans. b
4. **Where does deposition of unmineralized dentin matrix begin and in what direction does it proceed?**
   a. It begins at the cusp tip and progresses laterally
   b. It begins at the cusp tip and progresses cervically
   c. It begins at the cementoenamel junction and progresses laterally.
   d. It begins at the cementoenamel junction and progresses coronally
   Ans. b
5. **The cervical loop is the location of which of the following?**
   a. The apical constriction
   b. Formation of the pulp horn
   c. Formation of the furcation
   d. Where inner and outer dental epithelium meet
   Ans. d
6. **What is the first thin layer of dentin that is formed?**
   a. Predentin
   b. Primary dentin
   c. Mantle dentin
   d. Root sheath
   Ans. c
7. **Epithelial cell rests of Malassez are remnants of what?**
   a. Odontoblasts
   b. Cementoblasts
   c. Epithelial root sheath
   d. Teeth of the deciduous dentition
   Ans. c

8. **Why are lateral canals clinically significant?**
   a. Symptoms may persist if not treated
   b. They allow pulp disease to extend to periodontal tissues
   c. They effectively block periodontal disease from extending to the pulp
   d. They contain the greatest amount of pulp tissue
   Ans. b
9. **What morphological changes occur to the dental pulp over time?**
   a. Root canal diameter increases in size
   b. Pulp horns grow higher into the cup tips
   c. Overall size of the pulp chamber is reduced
   d. Mesiodistal dimension of pulp space is reduced more than apical-occlusal dimension in molars
   Ans. c
10. **The cementodentinal junction (CDJ) is which of the following?**
    a. The area where cementum contacts dentin inside the canal
    b. Located at the same level for each tooth type
    c. Usually located 1.0 to 2.0 mm coronal to the apical constriction
    d. The widest portion of the canal
    Ans. a
11. **What is the defensive function of the dental pulp?**
    a. Odontoclast activation for resorption of dentin from areas of inflammation
    b. Odontoblast formation of enamel to increase enamel thickness
    c. Odontoclast differentiation into macrophages
    d. Odontoblast formation of dentin in response to injury
    Ans. d
12. **Which of the following is not a major component of the odontoblast?**
    a. Cell body
    b. Basally located nucleus
    c. Cell process
    d. Synaptic junction
    Ans. d
13. **What cell type is primarily related to the immune system in the dental pulp?**
    a. Dendritic
    b. Macrophages
    c. Neutrophils
    d. All of the above
    Ans. a
14. **What type of collagen is the most prominent found in the dental pulp?**
    a. Type I
    b. Type II
    c. Type III
    d. Type IV
    Ans. a
15. **Which of the following is not a type of pulp stones?**
    a. Free
    b. Attached
    c. Embedded
    d. Floating
    Ans. d

PROTECTING THE PULP, PRESERVING THE APEX

1. **What is a 'pulp cap'?**
   a. An early stage of tooth development
   b. Capping the exposed pulp with a thin layer of lining or base material
   c. Capping exposed necrotic tissue by placing a layer of mineral trioxide aggregate (MTA)
   d. A method of isolation used during root canal treatment
   Ans. c
2. **What is the effect on blood flow to the pulp when anesthetics with vasoconstrictors are used during restorative procedures?**
   a. Reduced by 10% its normal rate
   b. Reduced to less than half its normal rate
   c. Unchanged
   d. Increased by 25% because of stress on the pulp tissue
   Ans. b
3. **What is dentin 'blushing'?**
   a. The color of newly erupted teeth due to large pulp chambers
   b. Use of a masking color during restorative procedures
   c. Vascular hemorrhage of pulp tissue, often during crown preparation
   d. An esthetic concern requiring laminate restorations
   Ans. c
4. **Why are deeper carious lesions more injurious to the dental pulp?**
   a. Increased dentin permeability in deeper areas
   b. Increased length of the dentinal tubule in deeper areas
   c. Decreased density of dentinal tubules in deeper areas
   d. Decreased diameter of dentin tubules in deeper areas
   Ans. a
5. **Why does a blast of compressed air directed at freshly exposed dentin create a sensation of pain?**
   a. Frightens the patient
   b. Air is cold
   c. Rapid outward movement of fluid in patent dentinal tubules
   d. Rapid inward movement of fluid in patent dentinal tubules
   Ans. c
6. **What is the most important characteristic of any restorative material in determining its effect on the pulp tissue?**
   a. Heat generated by the material
   b. Speed the material sets
   c. Ability to form a marginal seal
   d. Life expectancy of the restorative material
   Ans. c
7. **What effect does orthodontic tooth movement have to the dental pulp?**
   a. No clinically significant changes
   b. Continued reliability to electric pulp testing
   c. Extrusion reduces pulpal blood flow for a few minutes
   d. Intrusive forces have no effect on pulpal blood flow
   Ans. a
8. **Should bases be used to protect the pulp beneath metallic restorations?**
   a. Yes, a thin cement base should be used
   b. Yes, a thick layer of varnish should be used

c. No, a base is only necessary if the tooth is to be crowned
d. No, additional thermal insulation is rarely needed
Ans. d

9. **Vital pulp therapies have variable rates of success. What is the most significant determinant of the success of vital pulp therapy?**
a. Periapical status before the procedure
b. Periodontal status before the procedure
c. Pulp status before the procedure
d. Type of restorative material to be used
Ans. c

10. **Which of the following steps are used in step-wise evacuation of caries?**
a. Removing all the caries in a single visit
b. Placing a calcium hydroxide base at the initial visit
c. Placing a glass ionomer base at each visit
d. Removing only a superficial layer of caries at the first visit
Ans. c

11. **How does a direct pulp cap for an accidental mechanical pulp exposure differ from a direct pulp cap for an exposure caused by caries?**
a. Pulp is likely to be severely inflamed beneath a deep carious lesion
b. Long-term success for a mechanical exposure is low
c. Long-term success for a carious exposure is high
d. A mechanical exposure should be immediately root canal treated
Ans. a

12. **When does apical closure occur in the developing root?**
a. At the time of eruption
b. Approximately 1 year after eruption
c. Approximately 3 years after eruption
d. Approximately 5 years after eruption
Ans. c

13. **If the pulp becomes necrotic before root growth is complete, the resultant root is:**
a. Short with thick dentin walls
b. Short with thin dentin walls
c. Normal length with thick dentin walls
d. Normal length with thin dentin walls
Ans. b

14. **What is apexogenesis?**
a. Induction of a calcific barrier across an open apex
b. Removal of the necrotic pulp
c. Determination of corrected working length
d. Continued physiological root formation
Ans. d

15. **Which of the following has not been demonstrated with MTA when used in apexification?**
a. Good biocompatibility
b. Good sealability
c. High pH value
d. Adjacent zone of necrosis
Ans. d

ENDODONTIC MICROBIOLOGY

1. **Which of the following is not a main portal of entry for microorganisms to enter the dental pulp?**
   a. Dentinal tubules
   b. Di
   c. Periodontal disease
   d. Occlusal grooves
   Ans. d
2. **Why is there greater dentin permeability near the pulp?**
   a. Increased thickness of dentin
   b. Smaller diameter dentinal tubules
   c. Higher density of dentinal tubules
   d. Longer length of dentinal tubules
   Ans. c
3. **Exposed dentin provides an unimpeded access for bacteria to enter the pulp.**
   a. True
   b. False
   Ans. b
4. **What is anachoresis?**
   a. Artificial formation of an apical barrier
   b. Induction of a biologic calcific apical barrier
   c. Microorganism transport from blood vessels into damaged tissue
   d. Systemic infection resulting from infected pulp tissue
   Ans. c
5. **Root canals can become infected through anachoresis?**
   a. True
   b. False
   Ans. b
6. **Which of the following is not a category of intraradicular infections?**
   a. Primary
   b. Secondary
   c. Tertiary
   d. Persistent
   Ans. c
7. **The most common microorganisms in primary endodontic infections are:**
   a. Gram-negative bacteria
   b. Gram-positive bacteria
   c. Facultative anaerobes
   d. Facultative aerobes
   Ans. a
8. **Which of the following is not a source of nutrients for bacteria within the root canal system?**
   a. Necrotic pulp tissue
   b. Inflamed vital pulp tissue
   c. Proteins and glycoproteins seeping into the root canal system
   d. Components of saliva penetrating into the pulp tissue
   Ans. b
9. **Which of the following microorganisms are commonly present in large percentages of root canal–treated teeth that present with persistent apical periodontitis, indicative of failed treatment?**
   a. Enterococcus faecalis
   b. Pseudoramibacteralactolyticus
   c. Tannerella forsythia
   d. Dialisterinvisus
   Ans. a

10. **Gram-positive bacteria have been demonstrated to:**
    a Have a higher occurrence in post-instrumentation samples
    b. Are more resistant to antimicrobial treatments
    c. Are able to adapt to harsh environmental conditions
    d. All of the above
    Ans. d

PULP AND PERIAPICAL PATHOSIS

1. **A direct pulp exposure of a carious lesion is necessary to have a pulpal response and inflammation.**
    a. True
    b. False
    Ans. b
2. **What factor is the most important in determining if pulp tissue becomes necrotic slowly or rapidly after carious pulp exposure and pulpal inflammation?**
    a. Virulence of bacteria
    b. Host resistance
    c. Amount of circulation
    d. Lymph drainage
    Ans. d
3. **What is necessary for pulp and periradicular pathosis to develop?**
    a. Exposure of pulp tissue
    b. Exposure of dentin
    c. Presence of bacteria
    d. Trauma
    Ans. c
4. **Which of the following statements is true regarding mechanical irritants?**
    a. Changes to the underlying pulp, such as odontoblast aspiration, are irreversible
    b. Potential for pulp injury decreases as more dentin is removed
    c. Operative procedures without water coolant cause more irritation than those performed under water spray
    d. There is decreased permeability and constriction of blood vessels in the early stages of pulpitis
    Ans. c
5. **What nonspecific inflammatory mediators are not present when the dental pulp is irritated?**
    a. Histamine
    b. Epinephrine
    c. Bradykinin
    d. Arachidonic acid metabolites
    Ans. b
6. **What cell type associated with immune response is not present in severely inflamed dental pulp?**
    a. T lymphocytes
    b. B lymphocytes
    c. Macrophages
    d. Odontoclasts
    Ans. d
7. **What is the cause of pain during the progression of pulpal injury?**
    a. Elevation of the sensory nerve threshold
    b. Decrease of arteriole vasodilatation
    c. Increase of venule vascular permeability
    d. Decrease of pulp tissue pressurerect pulp exposure
    Ans. c

8. **What is reversible pulpitis?**
   a. Severe inflammation of pulp tissue
   b. Yields a negative response to electric pulp testing
   c. Yields a positive response to thermal pulp testing
   d. Requires root canal treatment
   Ans. c
9. **What is irreversible pulpitis?**
   a. A severe inflammatory process
   b. Precedes reversible pulpitis
   c. Resolves when the causative agent is removed
   d. Yields a negative response to thermal pulp testing
   Ans. a
10. **Which of the following is not a hard tissue change that may result from pulpal irritation or inflammation?**
    a. Calcification of pulp tissue spaces
    b. Resorption of pulp tissue spaces
    c. Formation of pulp stones
    d. Thickening of periodontal ligament
    Ans. d
11. **What are the signs and symptoms associated with symptomatic apical periodontitis (acute apical periodontitis)?**
    a. Normal sensation on mastication
    b. Normal sensation on finger pressure
    c. Marked or excruciating pain on tapping with a mirror handle
    d. Presence of a large periapical lesion
    Ans. c
12. **What histologic feature differentiates a periapical granuloma from a periapical cyst?**
    a. Presence of mast cells
    b. Presence of lymphocytes
    c. Presence of plasma cells
    d. Presence of an epithelial lined cavity
    Ans. d
13. **Which of the following is not associated with acute apical abscess?**
    a. Moderate to severe discomfort
    b. Intense and prolonged response to thermal stimulus
    c. Negative response to electric pulp testing
    d. Tenderness to percussion and palpation
    Ans. b
14. **What factors may impact and influence whether periradicular lesions heal completely or incompletely?**
    a. Size of the lesion
    b. Blood supply
    c. Systemic disease
    d. All of the above
    Ans. d
15. **What is the most important aid in distinguishing between endodontic and nonendodontic periradicular lesions?**
    a. Radiographic location
    b. Radiographic appearance
    c. Pulp vitality testing
    d. Patient's history
    Ans. c

DIAGNOSIS AND TREATMENT PLANNING

1. **Which of the following is not one of the five basic steps in the diagnostic process?**
   a. Chief complaint
   b. Medical and dental history
   c. Oral examination
   d. Review of insurance coverage
   Ans. d
2. **Are patients that seek endodontic treatment usually younger or older than the general population?**
   a. Age has not been shown to be a factor
   b. Patients seeking endodontic treatment are usually younger
   c. Patients seeking endodontic treatment are usually older
   Ans. c
3. **During a review of the patient's healthy history, it is noted that the patient is on a regimen of intravenous bisphosphonate medication. What significance does this hold for the patient and their treatment plan?**
   a. Possible side effect of bleeding disorders
   b. Possible side effect of osteonecrosis of the jaw
   c. Lowered pain threshold
   d. Inability to obtain adequate anesthesia
   Ans. b
4. **When pain is one of the patient's complaints, what question is less relevant regarding their pain and does not need to be asked of the patient?**
   a. When did the pain begin?
   b. Is the pain always in the same place?
   c. Why did you not seek treatment when the pain began?
   d. Once initiated, how long does the pain last?
   Ans. c
5. **Why is it important to use control teeth during the clinical tests?**
   a. To calibrate the patient's response
   b. So the patient can predict which tooth is being tested
   c. So teeth can be tested repeatedly
   d. To test whether isolation is adequate
   Ans. a
6. **A painful response obtained by pressing or by tapping on the crown indicates the presence of which of the following?**
   a. Periapicalinflammation.
   b. Pulpal inflammation.
   Ans. a
7. **What is palpation testing used to determine?**
   a. Pulpal inflammation
   b. Periapical inflammation
   c. Periodontal inflammation
   d. Periapical histology
   Ans. b
8. **Which of the methods of cold testing are preferred for pulp testing?**
   a. Regular ice (frozen water)
   b. Refrigerant spray or CO_2
   c. Flooding the arch with chilled water
   d. Blast of air from the air/water syringe
   Ans. b

9. **How does electrical pulp testing determine the degree of pulpal inflammation?**
   a. A shorter response indicates a healthier pulp
   b. A midrange response indicates pulp inflammation
   c. A midrange response indicates partial necrosis
   d. It can only be used to determine the presence or absence of vital tissue
   Ans. d
10. **What are the four characteristics of a periapical lesion of endodontic origin?**
    a. The lamina dura of the tooth socket is intact
    b. The lucency remains at the apex in radiographs made at different cone angles
    c. The lucency tends to resemble a round circle
    d. It is usually associated with an irreversible pulpitis
    Ans. b
11. **In which situation is caries removal necessary to obtain a definitive pulpal diagnosis?**
    a. Deep caries with no symptoms and negative pulp testing
    b. Deep caries with no symptoms and positive pulp testing
    c. Shallow caries with mild symptoms and positive pulp testing
    d. Shallow caries with mild symptoms and negative pulp testing
    Ans. b
12. **How may selective anesthesia be an aid in diagnosis?**
    a. It can localize a painful tooth to a specific arch
    b. It can localize an individual painful tooth in the mandibular arch
    c. It can confirm the tooth the patient identifies as the offending tooth
    d. It can be used to start posterior and work toward the anterior teeth
    Ans. a
13. **Using the Case Difficulty Assessment system developed by the American Association of Endodontists, cases in which any factors score 3 should be?**
    a. Treated by a general dentist
    b. Treated by an endodontist
    Ans. b
14. **Which of the following is not a category of external resorption?**
    a. Inflammatory
    b. Replacement
    c. Regenerative
    d. Surface
    Ans. c
15. **If a patient is to be referred to an endodontist for treatment, when is the most appropriate time for the referral?**
    a. Before beginning treatment
    b. During treatment when expected difficulties arise
    c. Before weekends or holidays
    d. After obturation when separated instruments are present
    Ans. a

ENDODONTIC AND PERIODONTAL INTERRELATIONSHIP

1. **Which of the following are potential avenues for communication between the dental pulp and periodontium?**
   a. Dentinal tubules
   b. Apical foramen
   c. Lateral/accessory canals
   d. All of the above
   Ans. d

2. **What characterizes the diameter of dentinal tubules in radicular dentin?**
   a. The diameter is 1 µm on the root surface, 3 µm at the pulp
   b. The diameter is constant
   c. The diameter is 3 µm on the root surface, 1 µm at the pulp
   d. The diameter increases with age.
   Ans. a
3. **Patent accessory canals are characterized by which of the following?**
   a. They serve as a pathway for microorganisms from pulp to periodontium
   b. They can be the result of scaling and root planing
   c. In the apical third, they may lead to pulp necrosis if exposed to oral environment
   d. All of the above
   Ans. d
4. **A narrow, vertical probing depth associated with pulp necrosis, but only mild periodontal disease is probably:**
   a. A vertical root fracture
   b. A fistula
   c. A sinus tract
   d. A periodontal abscess
   Ans. c
5. **The effect of periodontal disease on the pulp is thought to occur by migration of...............through dentinal tubules, accessory canals, or the apical foramen.**
   a. Dental plaque
   b. Saliva
   c. Microorganisms
   d. Exudates
   Ans. c
6. **Poor endodontic treatment can allow reinfection of the canal, leading to treatment failure and subsequent inflammatory response of the periodontal tissues.**
   a. True
   b. False
   Ans. a
7. **Periodontal inflammation resulting from primary endodontic disease may mimic periodontal disease by which of the following?**
   a. Generalized increase in probing depths in the affected quadrant
   b. An apical radiolucency
   c. A narrow deep solitary probing defect associated with an affected tooth
   d. All of the above
   Ans. c
8. **A patient presents with a chief complaint of pain to cold temperatures. Examination and testing reveal a maxillary left premolar exhibiting severe lingering pain in response to cold. No caries or fractures are noted. Periodontal probings are 6 to 9 mm around that specific tooth and 6 to 7 mm around the other posterior teeth in the quadrant. The patient reports having a "deep cleaning" (root planing) three times per year. What would the diagnosis in this case be?**
   a. Primary endodontic disease with secondary periodontal involvement
   b. Primary periodontal disease with secondary endodontic involvement
   c. Separate and unrelated endodontic and periodontal disease
   d. A true combined endodontic-periodontic (endoperio) disease process
   Ans. b

9. **What will the long-term prognosis for the patient described in question 8 primarily depend on?**
   a. Successful periodontal treatment
   b. Successful endodontic treatment
   c. Treatment sequencing
   d. Timing of treatment
   Ans. a
10. **Which of the following best represents similarities between endodontic apical and periodontal pathosis?**
   a. Both are often the result of traumatic occlusion
   b. Both are usually symptomatic
   c. Both are mediated by microorganisms
   d. Both are associated with loss of attachment
   Ans. c
11. **The best description of the effect of moderate periodontal disease (loss of attachment in the apical/middle third) on the underlying pulp is usually characterized by:**
   a. No or slight regional inflammation
   b. Generalized acute inflammation
   c. Generalized chronic inflammation
   d. Necrosis
   e. Bacterial invasion through tubules into the pulp
   Ans. a
12. **Which of the following is characteristic of the true combined endoperio lesion?**
   a. It occurs much less frequent than the primary endodontic lesion
   b. It is usually the end result of a severe endodontic lesion that causes loss of attachment
   c. It is usually the end result of a severe periodontal lesion
   d. It is usually successfully managed with both endodontic and periodontal treatment
   Ans. a
13. **What is the best means of differentiating endodontic from periodontal pathosis?**
   a. Pulp vitality testing
   b. Percussion
   c. Radiographs
   d. Probing patterns
   e. Location of swelling
   Ans. a
14. **Treatment sequencing for primary endodontic disease with secondary periodontal involvement includes:**
   a. Scaling and root planing followed by endodontic treatment
   b. Endodontic treatment followed by scaling and root planing
   c. Endodontic treatment followed by periodontal surgery
   d. Endodontic treatment followed by reevaluation of periodontal status in 2 to 3 months
   Ans. d

LONGITUDINAL TOOTH FRACTURES

1. **What category of longitudinal tooth fractures is most severe?**
   a. Craze lines
   b. Fractured cusp
   c. Cracked tooth
   d. Vertical root fracture
   Ans. d

2. **What clinical conditions or situations are often associated with cusp fractures?**
   a. Teeth with minimal caries
   b. Strong support of the remaining cusps
   c. Missing marginal ridge
   d. Occlusal composite restorations
   Ans. c
3. **What is the common direction that fractures extend in cracked teeth?**
   a. Mesiodistal
   b. Faciolingual
   c. Apical to coronal
   d. Horizontal
   Ans. a
4. **Which of the following is true as related to pulp tissue involvement in a cracked tooth?**
   a. The fracture always includes the pulp tissue
   b. The fracture never includes the pulp tissue
   c. The more centered the fracture, the greater chance for pulp exposure
   d. The more facial or lingual oriented the crack, the greater the chance for pulp exposure
   Ans. c
5. **Are pulp and periapical tests for cracked teeth consistent and reliable?**
   a. Both pulp and periapical testing are consistent
   b. Pulp testing is consistent, but periapical testing is variable
   c. Pulp testing is variable, but periapical testing is consistent
   d. Both pulp and periapical testing are variable
   Ans. d
6. **How can transillumination be used to distinguish between a craze line and a crack line?**
   a. It cannot be used to distinguish between the two entities
   b. Transmitted light readily passes through the air space of a fracture
   c. Transilluminated light is blocked by craze lines
   d. Transilluminated light is blocked by a cracked tooth
   Ans. d
7. **After access preparation of a suspected cracked tooth, the crack line is seen to extend through the chamber floor. In this case, what is the prognosis and recommended treatment?**
   a. Prognosis is favorable and continue with root canal treatment
   b. Prognosis is questionable, inform patient and continue with treatment
   c. Prognosis is hopeless, and extraction is recommended
   d. It does not change the original prognosis, and the treatment plan is not altered
   Ans. c
8. **What is the preferable restoration of a cracked tooth?**
   a. Post and core and crown
   b. Amalgam core
   c. Cast inlay
   d. Full coverage crown
   Ans. d
9. **How does a split tooth differ from a cracked tooth?**
   a. A split tooth precedes a cracked tooth
   b. A split tooth has an incomplete fracture
   c. A split tooth has separable tooth segments
   d. A cracked tooth has the fracture extending faciolingually
   Ans. c

10. What direction does a vertical root fracture (VRF) primarily occur?
 a. Mesiodistal
 b. Faciolingual
 c. Coronal and extending apically
 d. No primary direction
 Ans. b

11. What is a demonstrated major cause of VRFs?
 a. Traumatic occlusion
 b. Occlusal biting habits
 c. Loss of one or both marginal ridges
 d. Condensation forces during obturation
 Ans. d

12. Which is not a possible treatment of a VRF in a multirooted tooth?
 a. Tooth extraction
 b. Nonsurgical retreatment of the affected root
 c. Root amputation of the affected root
 d. Hemisection and extraction of the affected root
 Ans. b

LOCAL ANESTHESIA

1. What is the allodynia phenomenon?
 a. Inflamed tissue has an increased threshold of pain
 b. Inflamed tissue has a decreased threshold of pain
 c. Inflamed tissue is much less sensitive to a mild stimulus
 d. Inflamed tissue responds mildly to a stimulus that would otherwise be very painful
 Ans. b

2. Which of the following is not a component of the psychologic approach to pain management?
 a. Control
 b. Communication
 c. Conservation
 d. Confidence
 Ans. c

3. What is the effect of warming the anesthetic solution on the amount of pain during the injection?
 a. Warmed anesthetic results in less pain during injection
 b. Warmed anesthetic solution results in greater pain during injection
 c. There is no difference in pain perception regardless of warming
 Ans. c

4. What is a two-stage injection?
 a. Injection of one cartridge of anesthetic, waiting 5 minutes followed by injection of a second cartridge of the same anesthetic solution
 b. Injection of one cartridge of anesthetic, followed by injection of a second cartridge of a different anesthetic solution
 c. Injection of a quarter cartridge of anesthetic under the mucosal surface, waiting until regional anesthesia, then injection of the remainder of the cartridge to full depth
 d. Injection of a quarter cartridge of anesthetic under the mucosal surface, waiting until regional anesthesia, then injection of a cartridge of different anesthetic solution to full depth
 Ans. c

5. When does the onset of pulpal anesthesia occur after the inferior alveolar injection?
 a. Immediately
 b. 0 to 5 minutes

c. 10 to 15 minutes
d. 30 minutes
Ans. c

6. **Does the direction of the needle bevel affect the effectiveness of the inferior alveolar nerve block?**
a. Needle bevel toward the mandibular ramus improves success
b. Needle bevel away from the mandibular ramus improves success
c. Half the cartridge should be injected with the bevel toward the ramus, the needle rotated, and the second half of the cartridge injected with the bevel away from the ramus.
d. Direction of the needle bevel does not affect success.
Ans. d

7. **Is anesthesia of the maxilla commonly more or less successful than anesthesia in the mandible?**
a. More successful
b. Less successful
c. Comparable success rates
Ans. a

8. **Does increasing the volume of anesthetic solution affect the duration of pulpal anesthesia?**
a. For mandibular anesthesia, increasing the volume improves the success rate with the inferior alveolar nerve block
b. For maxillary infiltrations, increasing the volume increases the depth of pulpal anesthesia
c. For maxillary infiltrations, increasing the volume increases the duration of pulpal anesthesia
d. For maxillary infiltrations, increasing the volume has no effect on the success rate of pulpal anesthesia
Ans. c

9. **What additional anesthesia procedure should be administered if the classic signs of anesthesia are present after a standard injection, but the patient still has sharp pain when the bur enters the dentin?**
a. Repeat the initial injection
b. Wait an additional 15 minutes and attempt access again
c. Repeat the injection using a different type of anesthetic solution
d. Use a supplemental injection technique for a second injection
Ans. d

10. **What is a consideration of the intraosseous (IO) injection?**
a. It has not been proved effective
b. It has been recommended as the primary injection technique
c. It allows the anesthetic solution to be deposited directly into the pulp tissue of the tooth
d. It allows the anesthetic solution to be deposited directly into the cancellous bone adjacent to the tooth
Ans. d

11. **What is the best site for an IO injection of a premolar?**
a. Mesial perforation and injection
b. Apical perforation and injection
c. Distal perforation and injection
d. Site of injection not important
Ans. c

12. **What is an important requirement for effectiveness when using a periodontal ligament (PDL) injection?**
a. Back-pressure during injection
b. Direction of the needle bevel toward the root surface
c. Direction of the needle bevel away from the root surface
d. All four line angles receive the injection
Ans. a

13. **Can a PDL injection be used for individual tooth selective anesthesia as an aid in diagnosis?**
    a. PDL injection is useful for single tooth anesthesia
    b. PDL injection is not useful for single tooth anesthesia
    Ans. b
14. **Which of the following is an important consideration of the intrapulpal injection (IP)?**
    a. The injection should be given with back-pressure
    b. It will take several minutes for the injection to take effect
    c. A long- acting anesthetic should be used
    d. Another supplemental injection should not be attempted first
    Ans. a
15. **What are the most difficult teeth to anesthetize with irreversible pulpitis?**
    a. Maxillary molars
    b. Mandibular molars
    c. Maxillary anterior teeth
    d. Maxillary premolars
    Ans. b
16. **Why should an anesthetic agent not be injected directly into a swelling before an incision for drainage?**
    a. The anesthetic will cause a decreased flow of exudate following incision
    b. A direct injection will spread the infection
    c. There is an increased chance of aspirating blood
    d. The swelling has increased blood supply so the anesthetic is transported quickly into systemic circulation, diminishing the effect
    Ans. d

ENDODONTIC EMERGENCIES AND THERAPEUTICS

1. **What is the difference between a true endodontic emergency and urgency?**
    a. A true emergency is a condition requiring an unscheduled office visit
    b. A true emergency may be rescheduled for convenience of the patient
    c. An urgency indicates a more severe problem
    d. An urgency may need to be seen after normal office hours
    Ans. a
2. **How many teeth are usually involved in a true emergency?**
    a. One tooth
    b. Two teeth
    c. Often several teeth throughout the mouth
    d. Often teeth in only one quadrant
    Ans. a
3. **Which of the following is not an important factor in assessing the quality and quantity of pain?**
    a. Spontaneity
    b. Intensity
    c. Time of day of occurrence
    d. Duration
    Ans. c
4. **Which of the following is not an immediate goal of the emergency treatment plan?**
    a. Pharmacotherapeutic management of swelling
    b. Reducing the irritant
    c. Reduction of pressure
    d. Removal of the inflamed pulp or periradicular tissue
    Ans. a

5. **What is the most critical factor in a pretreatment emergency?**
   a. Adequate health history
   b. Pain management
   c. Patient management
   d. Adequate provisional restoration
   Ans. c
6. **What is the preferred treatment for an emergency appointment with a diagnosis of irreversible pulpitis with symptomatic apical periodontitis?**
   a. Caries excavation with provisional restoration
   b. Trephination through the mucosa and bone
   c. Partial or total pulpectomy
   d. Pharmaceutical management of swelling
   Ans. c
7. **What is the emergency treatment of choice for pulp necrosis without swelling?**
   a. Trephination for drainage
   b. Pulpotomy
   c. Canal débridement to corrected working length
   d. Single visit root canal treatment
   Ans. c
8. **A patient may present with localized swelling; incision for drainage may be indicated. What does drainage accomplish?**
   a. Patient reassurance and management
   b. Decrease in blood flow to the area
   c. Allows administration of anesthetic solution to the apex
   d. Removal of a very potent irritant—purulence
   Ans. d
9. **At an emergency appointment, should teeth be left open to drain?**
   a. Yes, only if there is swelling
   b. Yes, only if there is no swelling
   c. No, teeth should have an interappointment temporary restoration placed
   Ans. c
10. **What is the most important consideration of administering antibiotics with a localized apical abscess?**
    a. The dosage should be for 10 days
    b. It should be a broad-spectrum antibiotic
    c. The dosage levels should be higher than usual
    d. Antibiotics are ineffective and should not be prescribed
    Ans. d
11. **What is the incidence of interappointment flare-ups?**
    a. Primarily after obturation at a range of 4.4 to 6.0%
    b. Overall at a range of 1.8 to 3.2%
    c. Overall at a range of 10.7 to 21.3%
    d. Primarily after vital pulp removal at a range of 7.5 to 10.7%
    Ans. b
12. **Which of the following has been identified as significant factor related flare-ups?**
    a. Teeth with vital pulps
    b. Teeth without periradicular radiolucency
    c. Patient presenting with preoperative pain or swelling
    d. Completing endodontic treatment in a single visit
    Ans. c

13. What is a consideration of postobturation emergencies?
  a. More common than flare-ups following cleaning and shaping
  b. Infrequent and usually resolve spontaneously
  c. Approximately 10% to 15% occurrence
  d. Often require nonsurgical root canal retreatment
  Ans. b

MANAGEMENT OF TRAUMATIC DENTAL INJURIES

1. Why is age a 'good news/bad news' situation with dental trauma?
  a. Pulps have an incomplete and decreased blood supply
  b. Pulps are better able to recover and have a better repair potential
  c. Poor development will continue in teeth with damaged necrotic pulps
  d. Dentin has more strength in younger teeth
  Ans. b

2. Which of the following factors does not need to be considered when evaluating a crown fracture with pulp exposure?
  a. Extent of fracture
  b. Stage of root development
  c. Position in the arch
  d. Length of time since the injury
  Ans. c

3. Which of the following is not a step as part of the technique for a shallow (partial) pulpotomy?
  a. Rubber dam isolation
  b. Pulp tissue removed to about 2 mm below the exposure
  c. Use of a large round carbide bur in the slow-speed handpiece to remove tissue
  d. Restoration of the cavity with a hard-setting cement
  Ans. c

4. How long should horizontal root fractures be splinted if the coronal section was displaced and repositioned?
  a. Not indicated
  b. 7 to 10 days
  c. 4 to 6 weeks
  d. 3 months
  Ans. c

5. Which of the following are types of luxation injuries?
  a. Concussion
  b. Intrusion
  c. Extrusion
  d. All of the above
  Ans. d

6. What is recommended with pulp testing for teeth with traumatic injuries?
  a. Use of electric pulp testing or carbon dioxide ice to test the injured and adjacent teeth
  b. Opposing teeth also be tested
  c. Retesting is done in 4 to 6 weeks
  d. All of the above
  Ans. d

7. What information does the color change of the clinical crown provide?
  a. There has been a pulp exposure
  b. The initial change is gray in color, which always indicates pulp necrosis
  c. Discoloration may be reversed without treatment
  d. Calcific metamorphosis discoloration tends to be yellow to brown and always indicates pulp necrosis
  Ans. c

8. **What factor should be considered that determines the treatment of an intrusive luxation injury?**
   a. Depth of intrusion
   b. Stage of root development
   c. Availability of adjacent teeth for stabilization
   d. Amount of soft tissue injury
   Ans. b
9. **Of the following, what is the best transport medium to use for transporting an avulsed tooth?**
   a. Saliva
   b. Distilled water
   c. Wrapped in a tissue
   d. Milk
   Ans. d
10. **Which type of medication is indicated for patients with avulsed teeth?**
   a. Narcotic analgesic
   b. Steroid
   c. Tetanus booster if more than 5 years since last administered
   d. All of the above
   Ans. c
11. **What additional treatment should be used on the root surface if an avulsed tooth is replanted after more than 1 hour after avulsion?**
   a. Thorough scrubbing with antimicrobial soap for disinfection
   b. Scaling of the root surface
   c. Soaking the tooth in 2.4% doxycycline for 5 to 20 minutes
   d. Soaking the tooth in a 2.4% solution of sodium fluoride for 5 to 20 minutes
   Ans. d
12. **Which of the following types of external resorption has not been identified with replanted avulsed teeth?**
   a. Surface
   b. Inflammatory
   c. Refractory
   d. Replacement
   Ans. c
13. **When is root canal treatment indicated in a mature avulsed, replanted tooth?**
   a. At the time of replantation
   b. Within 7 to 10 days after replantation
   c. After 3 months if there is no response to pulp testing
   d. When periapical pathosis is noted
   Ans. b
14. **A deciduous tooth that has suffered an intrusive luxation should be extracted if what occurs?**
   a. The child cries but is compliant
   b. The permanent successor is partially erupted
   c. The intruded tooth appears foreshortened on the radiograph
   d. The intruded tooth appears elongated on the radiograph
   Ans. d

ENDODONTIC RADIOGRAPHY

1. **Diagnostic radiology is helpful in all of the following except:**
   a. Identifying pathosis
   b. Determining root anatomy
   c. Determining pulp anatomy
   d. Determining pulp responsiveness
   Ans. d

2. **What are working length radiographs?**
   a. Radiographs made by removing the rubber dam
   b. Radiographs placed using an XCP positioning device
   c. Radiographs that help establish an estimated working length
   d. Radiographs determine the distance from the radiographic apex to a reference point
   Ans. d
3. **Radiographs are useful to evaluate the following qualities of an obturation except which of the following?**
   a. Length
   b. Density
   c. Sealer thickness
   d. Canal configuration
   Ans. c
4. **Radiographs are useful in evaluating success and failure at recalls because they do which of the following?**
   a. Record subjective symptoms
   b. Show pulp vitality
   c. May show failures that often occur without adverse signs or symptoms
   d. Accurately diagnose apical pathosis
   Ans. c
5. **The most accurate radiographs are made by doing which of the following?**
   a. Having the patient hold the film in place with their index finger
   b. Using a paralleling device
   c. Increasing/decreasing the vertical angulation to move superimposed objects out of the field of vision
   d. Having the rubber dam in place for isolation
   Ans. b
6. **Use of a paralleling technique may not be feasible when which of the following occurs?**
   a. There is a high palatal vault
   b. There are maxillary tori
   c. A fixed prosthesis is present
   d. There are exceptionally short roots
   Ans. b
7. **F Speed film requires how much less exposure compared to E Speed film?**
   a. 10% to 15%
   b. 20% to 25%
   c. 30% to 35%
   d. 50%
   Ans. b
8. **What does the cone-image shift do?**
   a. It gives a clear 2 dimensional image
   b. It superimposes facial and lingual structures
   c. It assists in identifying superimposed canals
   d. It moves apical endodontic lesions away from the root apex
   Ans. c
9. **What occurs as the cone position moves away from parallel?**
   a. Objects on the film shift toward the direction of the cone
   b. The facial or buccal object shifts less than the lingual object
   c. The lingual object moves relatively in the same direction as the cone
   d. The buccal object moves relatively in the same direction as the cone
   Ans. c

10. **What is a disadvantage to the cone-image shift?**
    a. Lingual objects become more distorted than buccal objects
    b. There is excessive contrast between radiolucent and radiopaque objects
    c. It may superimpose normal anatomic structures over the root apices
    d. It does not reveal additional canals within a root
    Ans. c
11. **Which of the following is a distinguishing characteristic of a radiolucent lesion of endodontic pathosis?**
    a. Apical/radicular lamina dura is present and intact
    b. A round ball shape is characteristic
    c. The radiolucency stays at the apex regardless of cone angulation
    d. There is no apparent cause of pulpal necrosis
    Ans. c
12. **A radiolucency of endodontic origin is usually present with what type of pulpal diagnosis?**
    a. Normal pulp
    b. Reversible pulpitis
    c. Irreversible pulpitis
    d. Necrotic pulp
    Ans. d
13. **What is the usual radiographic appearance of condensing osteitis?**
    a. Diffuse radiopaque appearance
    b. Uniform smooth borders
    c. Irregular moth-eaten appearance around the apex
    d. Presence of a radiolucent inflammatory lesion
    Ans. a
14. **A mesial projection cone adjustment during working length radiographs is indicated for what?**
    a. Maxillary anterior teeth
    b. Maxillary molars with a mesiolingual canal
    c. Mandibular incisors
    d. Mandibular molars with a second distal canal
    Ans. b
15. **Digital radiography has not been proven to do which of the following?**
    a. Provide superior image quality
    b. Reduce radiation to the patient
    c. Increase speed of obtaining an image
    d. Accurately and reliably be transmitted between computers
    Ans. d

ENDODONTIC INSTRUMENTS

1. **What must an instrument do to completely clean the canal space?**
    a. Be deflected at the canal orifice
    b. Be 2 to 3 mm short of the radiographic apex
    c. Fit loosely into the canal
    d. Contact all walls and surfaces
    Ans. d
2. **What motion is employed with a hand instrument to clean and shape canal walls?**
    a. Pushing
    b. Broaching
    c. Reaming
    d. Vibration
    Ans. c

3. Nickel-titanium alloy has increased flexibility over stainless steel. How does the modulus of elasticity for nickel-titanium alloy compare to that of stainless steel?

a. Similar to stainless steel
b. One-fourth to one-fifth that of stainless steel
c. Half that of stainless steel
d. 2 to 3 times that of stainless steel

Ans. b

4. What is a disadvantage as a result of the increased flexibility of nickel-titanium instruments?

a. Diffculty in negotiating curvatures
b. Inability to rotate in the canals
c. Cannot precurve the files to bypass ledges
d. Tendency to bind in small canals

Ans. c

5. According to ADA Specification No. 28, what is the rate of increase in file diameter per running millimeter of length for a K-type file from point D 0 to point D 16?

a. 0.02 mm per running millimeter of length
b. 0.04 mm per running millimeter of length
c. 0.06 mm per running millimeter of length
d. Parallel sided so no increase in diameter

Ans. a

6. What is torsional limit?

a. Amount of apical pressure that can be applied to a file to the point of breakage
b. The beginning of plastic deformation of the instrument
c. Amount of rotational torque that can be applied to a 'locked' instrument to the point of breakage
d. Amount of force necessary so that a file does not return to its original shape upon unloading of the force

Ans. c

7. Which is a stronger metal alloy: carbon steel or stainless steel?

a. Carbon steel is stronger
b. Stainless steel is stronger

Ans. b

8. How do Gates-Glidden drills differ from Peeso reamers?

a. Gates-Glidden drills are a greater length of cutting surface
b. Gates-Glidden drills are more aggressive cutters
c. Gates-Glidden drills have an elliptical-shaped cutting area
d. Gates-Glidden drills are less flexible

Ans. c

9. How are broaches intended to be used in the canal?

a. Planing of canal walls by a push-pull motion
b. Planing of canal walls by a reaming motion
c. Placed to the corrected working length around canal curvatures
d. Entangling and removing canal contents by rotation

Ans. d

10. Which of the following describes the filing motion?

a. A single-step motion
b. Used only on the furcation side of a molar root canal
c. With a 360-degree rotation motion
d. Circumferential movement around the canal walls

Ans. d

11. Regular inspection of hand files may aid in avoidance of instrument separation. What file defects should be looked for on inspection?

a. Unwinding of the flutes
b. Rolling up or tightening of the flutes
c. Distortion of the tip
d. All of the above
Ans. d

12. What are the characteristics of finger spreaders and pluggers compared to handled instruments when used for lateral condensation?
a. They are annealed to give them greater strength
b. They are best suited for straight canals
c. They are more rigid to access the canal orifice
d. They have greater flexibility
Ans. d

13. Is pressure sterilization superior to dry heat sterilization for sterilization of sharp-edged instruments?
a. Both are equal and comparable and effective
b. Neither should be used for sterilization
c. Yes, pressure sterilization is superior
d. No, dry heat sterilization is superior
Ans. d

14. What are the time, temperature, and pressure necessary for sterilization of gauze-wrapped instruments using pressure sterilization?
a. 10 minutes at 121°C and 15 psi
b. 10 minutes at 100°C and 15 psi
c. 20 minutes at 121°C and 15 psi
d. 20 minutes at 100°C and 15 psi
Ans. c

INTERNAL ANATOMY

1. Lack of knowledge of pulp anatomy is the_______ common cause of treatment failure.
a. Least
b. Second most
c. Third most
d. Fourth most
Ans. b

2. Of the following, which is the best technique to determine if a root contains two canals?
a. Apex locator
b. Viewing access with a microscope
c. Searching with an explorer
d. Interpreting angled radiographs
Ans. d

3. The shape of the canal in cross-section is variable but is almost always round in the apical third.
a. Both parts of the sentence are true
b. The first part of the sentence is false, the second part is true
c. The first part of the sentence is true, the second part is false
d. The entire sentence is false
Ans. c

4. Multiple canals in mandibular premolars occur most often in which population?
a. Asians
b. African- Americans
c. Caucasians
d. No difference by ethnicity
Ans. b

5. **Alterations in the anatomy of the pulp space occur because of which of the following?**
   a. Resorption
   b. Age
   c. Calcifications
   d. All of the above
   Ans. d
6. **Calcifications encountered in the pulp space do which of the following?**
   a. Represent additional dentin formation
   b. Can always be detected by radiograph
   c. Are always attached to the chamber or canal walls
   d. Often prevent instruments from negotiating canals
   Ans. a
7. **Which of the following is not associated with the radicular pulp?**
   a. Lateral canals
   b. Apical foramen
   c. Pulp horns
   d. Canal orifices
   Ans. c
8. **Accessory canals are more common in the apical third, and more common in posterior teeth.**
   a. The entire sentence is true
   b. The first statement is true, the second is false
   c. The first statement is false, the second is true
   d. The entire sentence is false
   Ans. a
9. **Which of the following are true regarding the apical foramen?**
   a. The diameter remains constant throughout life
   b. The position of the apical foramen is often visible on radiograph
   c. The foramen is most commonly located 0.5 mm to 1.0 mm away from the anatomic root apex
   d. None of the above
   Ans. c
10. **Dens invaginatus (dens in dente) occurs most commonly in which teeth?**
   a. Maxillary canines
   b. Maxillary lateral incisors
   c. Maxillary and mandibular lateral incisors
   d. Mandibular first premolars
   Ans. b
11. **The lingual groove defect is (1) found most frequently in maxillary central incisors and (2) has a poor prognosis for treatment.**
   a. Statements 1 and 2 are true
   b. Statement 1 is true, statement 2 is false
   c. Statement 1 is false, statement 2 is true
   d. Statements 1 and 2 are false
   Ans. c
12. **A C-shaped canal is characterized by which of the following?**
   a. Has complex internal anatomy
   b. Is most commonly found in Asian populations
   c. Usually occurs in mandibular second molars
   d. Should be referred to an endodontist for treatment
   e. All of the above
   Ans. e

13. **Of the following, which tooth or root is the most likely to have two canals?**
    a. Maxillary second premolar
    b. Mandibular first molar mesial root
    c. Mandibular lateral incisor
    d. Maxillary first molar mesiobuccal root
    Ans. b
14. **The lingual root of the maxillary first molar often has a curvature in the apical third to which of the following?**
    a. Buccal
    b. Lingual
    c. Mesial
    d. Distal
    e. None of the above, the root is usually straight
    Ans. a

ISOLATION, ENDODONTIC ACCESS, AND LENGTH DETERMINATION

1. **What is true of the rubber dam?**
   a. The rubber dam is elective for endodontic treatment
   b. The rubber dam allows irrigating solution to contact and disinfect surrounding soft tissues
   c. The rubber dam protects the patient from swallowing or aspirating instruments and materials
   d. The rubber dam injures soft tissue from the pressure of the clamp
   Ans. c
2. **What is the recommended rubber dam weight for endodontic procedures?**
   a. Light
   b. Medium
   c. Heavy
   d. Extra heavy
   Ans. b
3. **Why are plastic rubber dam frames recommended over metal frames?**
   a. They are radiolucent
   b. They are easier to remove during exposure of interim radiographs
   c. They are more comfortable for the patient
   d. They are easier to place
   Ans. a
4. **Which of the following clamps is designed for an anterior tooth?**
   a. No. 8
   b. No. 212
   c. No. 0
   d. No. 24/25
   Ans. b
5. **What is an advantage of a provisional crown used to replace missing tooth structure before root canal treatment?**
   a. It accurately reproduces tooth anatomic landmarks
   b. It maintains tooth orientation for access and canal location
   c. It is easily removed and replaced during root canal treatment appointments
   d. It increases visibility of the root canal chamber
   Ans. c
6. **What is the preferred method for rubber dam placement on molars?**
   a. Placement as a unit
   b. Placement of a clamp and rubber dam, followed by attachment of the frame

c. Placement of a clamp, followed by the dam and then the frame
d. Placement of the rubber dam and frame, followed by placement of the clamp
Ans. a

7. **What is a major objective of the access opening?**
a. Locate the primary or largest canal
b. Achieve unimpeded straight-line access of the instruments to the first canal curvature or apical one third
c. Expose the pulp horns
d. Remove all restorative materials
Ans. b

8. **Outline form for access is described best by which of the following?**
a. It mimics the shape of the canal or canals
b. It is toward the distal in the occlusal surface in molars
c. It is a projection of the internal tooth anatomy onto the external surface
d. It is a constant and unchanging shape regardless of age
Ans. c

9. **What is an advantage of caries removal during access?**
a. It enhances the effectiveness of NaOCl
b. It reduces inter appointment pain
c. It strengthens tooth structure
d. It allows assessment of the restorability prior to the endodontic treatment
Ans. d

10. **Estimated depth of access is a measurement from which of the following?**
a. Incisal edge of anterior teeth to the coronal portion of the pulp chamber
b. Occlusal reference of posterior teeth to the coronal portion of the pulp chamber
c. Incisal edge of anterior teeth to the radiographic apex of the tooth
d. Occlusal reference of posterior teeth to the radiographic floor of the chamber
Ans. b

11. **What is the shape of the access opening of a maxillary central incisor in a young patient?**
a. Round
b. Triangular
c. Trapezoidal
d. Square
Ans. b

12. **What is the outline shape of the access for a maxillary first molar?**
a. Round
b. Triangular
c. Trapezoidal
d. Square
Ans. b

13. **What is the outline shape of the access for a mandibular first molar with four canals?**
a. Round
b. Triangular
c. Trapezoidal
d. Square
Ans. c

14. **To obtain an accurate measurement, how should the working length radiographs be made?**
a. They should be made with a loosely fitting file in place
b. They should be made with a minimum of a No. 20 file

c. They should be made with a positioning device and a parallel technique
d. They should be made with the rubber dam removed for visibility and access
Ans. b

15. **An apex locator is helpful in patients with which of the following?**
a. With high palatal vaults
b. With implanted cardiac pacemakers
c. With missed canals
d. With a strong gag reflex
Ans. d

CLEANING AND SHAPING

1. **What is the preferred method to evaluate if a canal has been adequately cleaned?**
a. The canal is three file sizes larger than the initial master apical file
b. The canal walls are 'glassy smooth' when explored with a file
c. Dentin shavings obtained are clean and white
d. Irrigant runs clear with no visible debris
Ans. b

2. **The degree of canal enlargement during shaping is dictated by which of the following?**
a. Method of obturation
b. Anatomy of the root
c. Plan for post placement
d. All of the above
Ans. d

3. **The apical termination point for cleaning and shaping the root canal should be which of the following?**
a. The radiographic apex
b. At the major diameter of the apical foramen
c. Within 0 to 2 mm of the radiographic apex
d. 0.5 mm beyond the radiographic apex
Ans. c

4. **To prevent extrusion of obturating material, cleaning and shaping procedures must be confined to the radicular space. Canals filled to the radiographic apex would be considered to be the perfect result.**
a. Both statements are true
b. The first statement is true; the second statement is false
c. The first statement is false; the second statement is true
d. Both statements are false
Ans. b

5. **For the irrigating solution to effectively reach the apical third of the canal, the apical canal should be enlarged to at least a No._________file.**
a. 25 or 30
b. 20 or 25
c. 35 or 40
d. 45 or 50
Ans. c

6. **Which of the following is the most widely used irrigant solution?**
a. Sodium hypochlorite
b. Ethylenediaminetetraacetic acid (EDTA)
c. MTAD
d. Saline
Ans. a

7. **The best description of a difference between nickel- titanium and stainless steel instruments is which of the following?**
a. Nickel-titanium tends to result in better shaping (less transportation) in curved canals
b. Nickel-titanium usually results in better debridement

c. Nickel-titanium can usually be reused many more times than stainless steel
d. Nickel-titanium has sharper cutting edges
Ans. a

8. **What is the primary purpose of an irrigant such as sodium hypochlorite (NaOCl)?**
a. Kill bacteria
b. Dissolve tissue remnants
c. Flush out debris
d. Lubricate instruments
Ans. c

9. **A major advantage to using a lubricant during cleaning and shaping is:**
a. It ensures that canal transportation will not occur
b. It reduces torsional force on the instrument, decreasing the possibility of fracture
c. It minimizes debris production
d. It reduces operator fatigue
Ans. b

10. **Removal of the smear layer after cleaning and shaping does which of the following?**
a. Promotes coronal leakage
b. Decreases dentin permeability
c. Allows better adaptation of obturating materials to canal walls
d. Forces bacteria into dentinal tubules
Ans. c

11. **EDTA is most effective for which of the following uses?**
a. Decalcifying small canals to allow instruments to negotiate to length
b. Lubricating canals to facilitate instrumentation
c. Bacterial elimination in canals
d. Removing smear layer after cleaning and shaping
Ans. d

12. **How does the 'crown-down' technique differ from the 'step-back' technique?**
a. It creates a funnel-shaped preparation.
b. It facilitates tissue removal.
c. It requires fewer instruments.
d. It creates coronal flare early, reducing torsional stress on the instruments.
Ans. d

13. **Recapitulation is defined as:**
a. The removal of accumulated debris using a small file at the corrected working length
b. Confirmation of working length after completing cleaning and shaping
c. The last irrigation before drying the canal
d. Verifying the master apical file after cleaning and shaping
Ans. a

14. **Of the following, which is the most important consideration of a temporary restoration?**
a. Antimicrobial
b. Placed over a cotton pellet
c. Resistant to acids
d. At least 4 mm thick
Ans. d

PREPARATION FOR RESTORATION

1. **What is the leading cause for loss of endodontically treated teeth?**
a. Inadequate cleaning and shaping of the canals
b. Inadequate obturation of the root canal system

c. Restorative factors
d. Vertical root fracture

Ans. c

2. **How does the survival rate for a tooth restored with cusp protection compare to a tooth without cusp protection?**
   a. About the same
   b. A tooth with protected cusps has an enhanced survival rate
   c. A tooth without protected cusps has an enhanced survival rate
   d. Restorations have no effect on tooth survival rates

   Ans. b
3. **Dentin becomes more brittle following the endodontic treatment due to loss of moisture content.**
   a. True
   b. False

   Ans. b
4. **The greatest contributing factor to reduced cuspal stiffness (strength) that predisposes to fracture is which of the following?**
   a. Occlusal access opening
   b. Loss of one or both marginal ridges
   c. An amalgam restoration placed after root canal treatment
   d. A bonded composite restoration placed after root canal treatment

   Ans. b
5. **Which of the following describes a definitive restoration after root canal treatment?**
   a. It should be placed at the time of obturation
   b. It should allow cuspal flexure to absorb occlusal forces
   c. It should provide a coronal seal
   d. It should always be a full-coverage crown on posterior teeth

   Ans. c
6. **Exposure of obturating materials to oral fluids can be described by which of the following?**
   a. It is not a factor if a sealer is properly used during obturation
   b. It is a major cause of failure
   c. It leads to rapid failure
   d. It may cause pain to thermal changes

   Ans. b
7. **Which of the following describes a definitive restoration?**
   a. It should be placed as soon as practical
   b. It should be placed at the 6-month recall visit to assure symptoms do not recur
   c. It should be placed when radiographic evidence of healing becomes evident
   d. It should be delayed if there is a questionable prognosis

   Ans. a
8. **What is the only reason to delay the definitive restoration?**
   a. To maximize the patient's insurance benefit
   b. If the patient is unable to pay for the restoration
   c. To allow radiographic healing to become evident
   d. If there is a questionable prognosis and failure would lead to extraction

   Ans. d
9. **The practical principles for function and durability when designing a definitive restoration include the following except which of the following?**
   a. Conservation of tooth structure
   b. Retention

c. Placement of a post
d. Protection of the remaining tooth structure
Ans. c

10. **What is an indication for use of a direct (amalgam or composite) restoration?**
a. Excessive tooth structure has not been lost
b. The opposing arch has been restored with full coverage crowns
c. Esthetics is not a concern
d. Only one of the marginal ridges has been lost
Ans. a

11. **Fewer root fractures have been recorded in laboratory studies when what type of post has been used?**
a. Cobalt chromium alloy post
b. Stainless steel post
c. Titanium post
d. Carbon fiber post
Ans. d

12. **Which of the following describes removal of gutta- percha for post space preparation?**
a. Immediately after obturation
b. After the sealer has completely set
c. To a depth that allows 2 to 3 mm of remaining gutta-percha
d. Completed using solvents
Ans. a

13. **When using a prefabricated post system to restore a posterior tooth, the most desirable post design is:**
a. Tapered, passively cemented
b. Tapered, threaded screw type
c. Parallel sided, passively cemented
d. Parallel sided, threaded screw type
Ans. c

14. **Which of the following describes retentive pins?**
a. Retentive pins help strengthen the restoration
b. Retentive pins minimize stresses to dentin
c. Retentive pins are the most effective antirotation method for post and cores
d. Retentive pins should not be used because the risks outweigh any potential gain
Ans. d

15. **Placement of a dowel or post through a crown or an existing restoration is described by which of the following?**
a. It adds support for the existing restoration
b. It helps maintain integrity of the existing restoration
c. It improves the seal of the root canal
d. It is rarely indicated
Ans. d

OBTURATION

1. **What is a possible outcome when there is an overfill of the obturation materials?**
a. Decreased periapical inflammation
b. Improved and rapid healing of periapical lesions
c. Inadequate apical seal
d. Decreased post obturation discomfort
Ans. c

2. **What is the optimal preparation/obturation length relative to the radiographic apex with pulp necrosis?**
a. Flush
b. 0.5 to 1.0 mm short

c. Slight extrusion of sealer but not gutta-percha
d. 1.0 to 3.0 mm short
Ans. b

3. **Prognosis and histologic studies show that if there is a length error, there are less problems resulting with which of the following?**
a. Overfills
b. Underfills
Ans. b

4. **Which of the following describes lateral canals?**
a. They connect adjacent canals within the same root
b. They may allow bacterial and necrotic debris to leak into the periodontium
c. They are débrided with copious irrigation
d. They are significant in the outcome of most root canal treatments
Ans. b

5. **What factors should be considered when deciding the timing for obturation?**
a. Signs and symptoms present
b. Pulp and periapical status
c. Difficulty of the procedure
d. All of the above
Ans. d

6. **What pulp and periapical diagnosis may have completed treatment in a single visit?**
a. Symptomatic (acute) apical periodontitis
b. Asymptomatic apical periodontitis (chronic apical periodontitis)
c. Acute apical abscess
d. Painful irreversible pulpitis
Ans. d

7. **What material is currently the only universally accepted solid core obturation material?**
a. Gutta-percha
b. Synthetic polyester resin-based polymers
c. Silver points
d. Solid core (carrier) gutta-percha
Ans. a

8. **Which of the following is a disadvantage of gutta-percha?**
a. Poor adaptation to canal irregularities with compaction
b. Shrinkage if altered by heat or solvents
c. Not easily managed and manipulated
d. Difficult to partially remove from a canal
Ans. b

9. **Which of the following is an advantage of gutta-percha?**
a. Adhesiveness to dentin
b. Slight elasticity and rebound effect
c. Expansion on cooling of warmed gutta-percha
d. Adaptation to canal irregularities with compaction
Ans. d

10. **What have recent studies shown synthetic polyester resin-based polymers to be?**
a. Adhesive to canal walls throughout their length
b. Inflammatory to tissues
c. Mutagenic
d. No difference in leakage when compared to gutta-percha
Ans. d

11. Which of the following have semisolid obturation materials (pastes or cements) been shown to do?
   a. They provide easy control of obturation length.
   b. They exhibit no shrinkage upon setting.
   c. They provide an unpredictable and inconsistent apical seal.
   d. They are bio compatible and nonirritating to periapical tissues.
   Ans. c

12. Which of the following describes the complete setting of zinc oxide–eugenol (ZnOE)-based sealers?
   a. The setting occurs at approximately 1 hour if left exposed to air
   b. The setting depends on contact with dentin
   c. The setting usually requires weeks or months
   d. The setting usually is approximately 24 hours
   Ans. c

13. What type of sealer may have a problem with long-term solubility?
   a. ZnOE-based sealers
   b. Plastic sealers
   c. Glass ionomer sealers
   d. Calcium hydroxide sealers
   Ans. d

14. Which of the following describes lateral compaction of gutta-percha?
   a. It is indicated for cases with internal resorption.
   b. It involves multiple steps and special armamentarium.
   c. It manages length control well.
   d. It is difficult to retreat.
   Ans. c

15. What is a disadvantage of finger spreaders as compared to standard long-handled spreaders?
   a. Tactile sensation
   b. Instrument length control
   c. Fracture potential in curved canals
   d. Dentin stress during obturation
   Ans. c

PROCEDURAL ACCIDENTS

1. What should a patient not be told when there has been a procedural accident?
   a. The incident did occur
   b. The possible procedures that may be necessary for correction
   c. How this might affect the outcome
   d. The root canal treatment will be completed free of charge
   Ans. d

2. Which of the following is not a common cause of a perforation during access preparation?
   a. Mandibular molar with a lingual axial inclination of the tooth
   b. Searching for canals through an under-prepared access opening
   c. Directing the bur parallel to the long axis of the tooth
   d. Presence of a misaligned cast restoration
   Ans. c

3. What measures are used to prevent perforation during access preparation?
   a. Relating tooth angulations independent of the adjacent tooth
   b. Using only straight-on radiographs
   c. Always having a rubber dam in place before beginning access preparation
   d. Having a thorough knowledge of both surface and internal tooth anatomy
   Ans. d

4. **Which of the following is not an early sign or indication of a perforation?**
   a. Pain during access preparation
   b. Sudden appearance of hemorrhage
   c. Burning pain and bad taste during irrigation with NaOCl
   d. Radiographically mal positioned file
   Ans. a
5. **If a lateral root perforation does occur, what is the most favorable location for perforation repair?**
   a. At or above the height of crestal bone
   b. Below the crestal bone in the coronal third of the root
   c. On the furcal side of the coronal root surface
   d. A zipping perforation at the apex of the root
   Ans. a
6. **What is the ideal time and material for a nonsurgical repair of a furcation perforation?**
   a. Immediate repair with amalgam
   b. Immediate repair with mineral trioxide aggregate (MTA)
   c. Delayed repair with amalgam
   d. Delayed repair with MTA
   Ans. b
7. **What is a common cause of ledge formation?**
   a. Straight-line access into the canal
   b. Excess irrigating solution
   c. Over enlargement of a curved canal with files
   d. Constant recapitulation and irrigation into the apical portion of the canal
   Ans. c
8. **What type of canal is most prone to ledge formation?**
   a. Long, small, and curved
   b. Incomplete apex formation, curved
   c. Large, long
   d. Short, straight
   Ans. a
9. **What is a possible etiology for an apical (zipping) root perforation?**
   a. Inability to negotiate canals with ledges
   b. Working length determination with radiographs only
   c. Trying to locate canals in a small chamber
   d. Failure to adjust working length after curved canals are straightened during cleaning and shaping
   Ans. d
10. **What type of perforation has the poorest long-term prognosis?**
   a. Zipping (apical third) root perforation
   b. Stripping perforation in the apical third of the root
   c. Stripping perforation in the coronal third of the root below the crest of bone
   d. Direct floor to furcation perforation in a multi- rooted tooth
   Ans. c
11. **Which of the following is not a common cause of file separation?**
   a. Limited flexibility
   b. Manufacturing defects
   c. Amount of use
   d. Amount of force applied
   Ans. b

12. What approaches may be used to treat a case with a separated instrument?
a. Attempt to remove
b. Attempt to bypass
c. Prepare and obturate to the level of the segment
d. All of the above
Ans. d

13. Which of the following scenarios yields the most favorable prognosis in cases with a separated instrument?
a. A small instrument short of the working length
b. A small instrument beyond the apical foramen
c. A large instrument at an early stage of instrumentation
d. A large instrument close to the working length
Ans. d

14. Which of the following causes extrusion of sodium hypochlorite (NaOCl) irrigating solution into periapical tissues?
a. Fitting irrigation needle loosely in the canal space
b. Wedging irrigation needle in the canal space
c. Using perforated needles during irrigation
d. Using regular needles during irrigation
Ans. b

15. Which of the following occurs after minor extrusion of obturation materials into the periapical tissue?
a. It results in significant swelling
b. It results in significant symptoms
c. It causes some tissue inflammation
d. It causes more apical leakage
Ans. c

NONSURGICAL RETREATMENT

1. Nonsurgical retreatment should be the first treatment option for correction when?
a. A large well-fitting post and core is present
b. There is a separated instrument present that cannot be retrieved
c. External resorptive root defects are present
d. A negotiable canal was not initially treated
Ans. d

2. Which of the following is not a potential contraindication for nonsurgical root canal retreatment?
a. Post and core restorations
b. Ledges in the root canal walls
c. Amalgam core restorations into the chamber
d. Separated root canal instruments
Ans. c

3. Which of the following is not a potential risk associated with nonsurgical root canal retreatment?
a. Thinning and weakening of the root canal walls
b. Inability to remove the initial root canal obturation material
c. Creating a compromised crown-root ratio
d. Loosening of a well-fitting fabricated crown
Ans. c

4. Which of the following describes removal of coronal restorations before nonsurgical retreatment?
a. Removal may prolong retreatment procedures
b. Removal complicates removal of post and core restorations
c. Removal may be necessary to assess restorability
d. Removal should never be done if the previous restoration is a full-coverage crown.
Ans. c

5. **What steps are involved in retrieval of a prefabricated post during retreatment?**
   a. Section and remove the core material and the post at the level of the chamber floor.
   b. An ultrasonic activated tip is used for 3 to 5 minutes each at several locations circumferentially around the post, without water for visibility.
   c. Grasp the post with a hemostat or Steiglitz pliers to rock it back and forth to break the cement seal.
   d. Use ultrasonics, then grasp a threaded screw type post with a hemostat or small-tipped forceps to unscrew it from the canal.
   Ans. d
6. **The following steps are used to attempt removal of a canal ledge during nonsurgical retreatment except which one?**
   a. Remove all obstructions coronal to the ledge
   b. Bypass the ledge with a flexible nickel-titanium hand file
   c. File in a circumferential motion after bypassing the ledge
   d. Proceed from small-size files to larger size files
   Ans. b
7. **Which of the following is not a factor that may affect the successful removal of a separated instrument fragment?**
   a. Size of the instrument separated
   b. Length of the separated fragment
   c. Location of the fragment within the canal
   d. Length of time the fragment has been in place
   Ans. d
8. **What method or methods have been used to successfully remove gutta-percha from root canals?**
   a. Heat
   b. Ultrasonics
   c. Rotary instruments
   d. All of the above
   Ans. d
9. **When should Hedstrom hand files or regular hand reamers be the instruments of choice for gutta-percha removal, without the addition of solvents?**
   a. The root canal is well sealed with gutta-percha.
   b. The gutta-percha is well adapted to canal walls.
   c. A space can be created between the gutta-percha and the root canal.
   d. Gutta-percha fills the root canal chamber.
   Ans. c
10. **What solvent has been shown to be the most efficient (fastest) in softening gutta-percha?**
    a. Chloroform
    b. Halothane
    c. Methylchloroform
    d. Xylene
    Ans. a
11. **During the removal of a carrier-based gutta-percha obturator which of the following should occur?**
    a. The first step is to remove the solid core material.
    b. A combination of techniques for removal of gutta-percha, silver cones, and posts is employed.
    c. A small rotary file may be used to engage and remove the plastic carrier.
    d. Different solvents are used that would routinely be used to remove gutta-percha alone.
    Ans. b

12. **What is the key to success in the retrieval of silver points?**
    a. The key is to engage the silver point with the ultrasonic tip
    b. The key is to remove the silver point and core material simultaneously
    c. The key is to retain as much of the coronal extent of the point as possible
    d. The key is to remove the core material and silver point to the level of canal orifices first
    Ans. c
13. **Which of the following is not true regarding the removal and retreatment of hard-setting pastes?**
    a. They are more difficult to remove than a soft paste
    b. They may be impossible to remove
    c. Solvents have been shown to soften hard-setting pastes
    d. Use of ultrasonics is the most predictable method
    Ans. c
14. **Which of the following is true regarding inter appointment flare-ups with nonsurgical root canal retreatments?**
    a. Flare-ups occur less frequently when compared to initial root canal treatments
    b. Flare-ups occur frequently, even when debris and microorganisms are confined to the canals
    c. Flare-ups occur less frequently if irrigation is kept to a minimum
    d. High incidence dictates that retreatment should generally be treated in two visits rather than one visit
    Ans. d
15. **The prognosis for nonsurgical root canal retreatment is which of the following?**
    a. It is increased with periapical lesions
    b. It has the lowest rate of success without a periapical lesion
    c. It is similar to initial root canal treatment success rates
    d. It is best if the etiology of failure can be identified
    Ans. d

ENDODONTIC SURGERY

1. **What is the purpose of incision for drainage?**
    a. To evacuate exudates from a soft tissue swelling
    b. To obtain a biopsy specimen
    c. To prevent a postoperative swelling
    d. To avoid emergency cleaning and shaping
    Ans. a
2. **Profound anesthesia is difficult to attain before incision for drainage. What is a preferred approach for a maxillary cuspid with extensive swelling?**
    a. Start with an infraorbital block and then infiltrate at the margins of the swelling
    b. Start with posterior superior alveolar block and then use refrigerant spray
    c. Inject buffer and anesthetic directly into the swelling
    d. Use topical anesthetic and then refrigerant spray. No anesthetic is needed
    Ans. a
3. **Which of the following is not an indication for periapical surgery?**
    a. A nonnegotiable or blocked canal associated with symptomatic periradicularpathosis
    b. Gross overextension of obturating material
    c. Obtain a biopsy
    d. To resolve any endodontic treatment failure
    Ans. d
4. **Which of the following would contraindicate periapical surgery? 1. anatomical structures in the area 2. medical complications 3. lipparesthesia 4. previous malignancies 5. unidentified cause of treatment failure.**
    a. 1, 2, and 3
    b. 1, 3, and 5

c. 1, 2, and 5
d. 2, 3, and 4
e. All of the above

Ans. c

5. **Which of the following is true regarding an incision over a bony defect?**
   a. It should be avoided
   b. It may cause a postsurgical fenestration
   c. It may prevent healing of the incision
   d. All of the above

   Ans. d

6. **Which of the following describes a submarginal flap design?**
   a. It is ideal for mandibular posterior teeth
   b. It causes less scarring
   c. It is associated with less gingival recession
   d. It causes less intraoperative hemorrhage

   Ans. c

7. **What is the purpose of root end resection?**
   a. Removes irritants encased in the apical portion of the root
   b. To examine the root
   c. Exposes additional canals or fractures
   d. All of the above

   Ans. d

8. **Which of the following is true regarding a root-end cavity preparation?**
   a. It should be as shallow as possible to preserve tooth structure
   b. It should be made to a minimum depth of 3 mm
   c. It should only encompass the main portion of the canal
   d. It should be made with a very small bur

   Ans. b

9. **An ideal root-end filling material should satisfy all of the following except which one?**
   a. The material should be well tolerated by periradicular tissues
   b. The material should be easily placed
   c. The material should be absorbable
   d. The material should be visible radiographically

   Ans. c

10. **Which of the following cell types are important in the healing process after periapical surgery? 1. epithelial cells 2. macrophages 3. dendritic cells 4. fibroblasts 5. osteocytes.**
    a. 1, 2, 4, and 5 only
    b. 1 and 2 only
    c. 1, 2, and 5 only
    d. 1, 2, 3, 4, and 5
    e. 1, 3, and 4 only

    Ans. a

11. **With root amputation, the factor that most affects success is which of the following?**
    a. Occlusal force patterns
    b. The type of restoration
    c. The length of the root
    d. The patient's oral hygiene

    Ans. d

12. **All of the following procedures should be referred to a specialist with specific training in endodontic surgery except which one?**
    a. Root-end resection/root-end filling
    b. Incision for drainage
    c. Root amputation
    d. Perforation repair
    Ans. b

EVALUATION OF ENDODONTIC OUTCOMES

1. **What is the primary determinant for successful endodontic treatment?**
    a. Selecting the proper obturation technique
    b. Effective elimination of microorganisms from the pulp space
    c. Using rotary instruments to shape the canals
    d. Using an effective irrigation regimen
    Ans. b
2. **What are the major indicators of successful endodontic treatment?**
    a. Lack of discoloration, no tenderness to biting
    b. No swelling or redness of the gingival area
    c. Absence of symptoms and apical radiolucency
    d. A happy patient who has paid the bill
    Ans. c
3. **A patient presents for a posttreatment examination with no complaint of symptoms except the apical radiolucency that was present before treatment, although it appears smaller. Treatment for this patient would be classified as which of the following?**
    a. A failure
    b. A success
    c. A clinical success but radiographic failure
    d. A functional tooth with uncertain prognosis
    Ans. d
4. **Which of the following is not a clinical criterion to evaluate treatment outcome?**
    a. Absence of a radiolucency
    b. No evidence of a sinus tract
    c. No swelling present
    d. No response to percussion or palpation
    Ans. a
5. **To make valid comparisons between radiographs to assess healing, which of the following describes how films should be made?**
    a. In a reproducible manner
    b. 6 months apart
    c. At different angles
    d. By the same person to ensure consistency
    Ans. a
6. **Which of the following criteria is not considered to be a predictor of success or failure?**
    a. The patient's medical history
    b. Apical pathosis
    c. Quality of the coronal restoration
    d. Extent and quality of obturation
    Ans. a

7. **The most common preoperative cause of endodontic treatment failure includes all of the following except which one?**
   a. Misdiagnosis
   b. Leaking coronal restoration
   c. Poor case selection
   d. Error in treatment planning
   Ans. b
8. **The most common postoperative cause of endodontic treatment failure is which of the following?**
   a. Overextension of obturating material
   b. A separated instrument
   c. Coronal leakage
   d. Placement of a post unnecessarily
   Ans. c
9. **The prognosis for nonsurgical retreatment depends primarily on which of the following?**
   a. Identification and correction of the cause of failure
   b. Using a different obturation technique
   c. Placing the definitive restoration at the obturation appointment
   d. All of the above
   Ans. a

BLEACHING DISCOLORED TEETH: INTERNAL AND EXTERNAL

1. **Which of the following is not considered a natural or acquired discoloration source?**
   a. Tetracycline stain
   b. Intrapulpal hemorrhage
   c. Stain from amalgam
   d. Calcific metamorphosis
   Ans. c
2. **Which of the following is not part of the mechanism of staining caused by fluorosis?**
   a. Hypoplastic defects are produced in enamel by excess fluoride
   b. Stain is acquired from chemicals in the oral cavity
   c. Stain is present in the enamel
   d. Stain is solely caused by fluoride deposits in the enamel
   Ans. d
3. **Which of the following describes tetracycline stain?**
   a. It is classified into three groups based on severity
   b. It is often associated with a 'banding' pattern
   c. It is located in the dentin
   d. All of the above
   Ans. d
4. **What is the most common iatrogenic etiology related to tooth discoloration?**
   a. Incomplete removal of pulp tissue
   b. Incomplete removal of obturating material from the chamber
   c. The use of intracanal medicaments
   d. Intracanalirrigants
   Ans. b
5. **Which of the following restorative materials can contribute to staining?**
   a. Amalgam
   b. Pins and posts

c. Composite
d. All of the above
Ans. d

6. **What is the most common agent used for internal bleaching?**
   a. Carbamide peroxide
   b. Sodium perborate
   c. Hydrogen peroxide
   d. Sodium peroxyborate monohydrate
   Ans. b
7. **Which of the following is not an indication for internal bleaching?**
   a. Defective enamel formation
   b. Intrapulpal hemorrhage-induced stain
   c. Tetracycline-induced stain
   d. Sealer stain
   Ans. a
8. **One potential complication of internal bleaching is external root resorption, which has been associated with which of the following?**
   a. High concentration of hydrogen peroxide
   b. Heat
   c. Damage to cementum and periodontal tissues
   d. All of the above
   Ans. d
9. **What is the most common agent employed in external bleaching?**
   a. Sodium perborate
   b. Hydrochloric acid
   c. Carbamide peroxide
   d. Sodium hypochlorite
   Ans. c
10. **Which of the following describes the microabrasion technique?**
    a. It is not a true bleaching technique
    b. It uses hydrochloric acid
    c. It requires meticulous soft tissue isolation
    d. All of the above
    Ans. d

GERIATRIC ENDODONTICS

1. **Which of the following are changes that occur in the pulp with age? 1. decreased vascular elements 2. decreased amount of collagen 3.increase in numbers of fibroblasts 4. decrease in numbers of odontoblasts 5. increase in occurrence of calcifications:**
   a. 1, 2, and 3 only
   b. 1, 3, and 5 only
   c. 1, 4, and 5 only
   d. 2, 3, and 5 only
   e. 1, 2, 3, 4, and 5
   Ans. c
2. **Which of the following statements are true regarding calcifications in the pulp space?**
   a. Pulp stones are usually found in the radicular pulp
   b. Pulp stones can increase the incidence of odontogenic pain
   c. Calcifications increase with both age and irritation
   d. Diffuse calcifications are most commonly found in the pulp chamber
   e. All of the above.
   Ans. c

3. **With age, which of the following describes the pulp chamber in molars?**
   a. Decreases primarily in a mesiodistal dimension
   b. Decreases primarily in an occlusal apical dimension
   c. Remains the same in volume
   d. Increases in size in response to irritation
   Ans. b
4. **The healing capacity of older patients is significantly less than younger patients because of a decrease in periradicular vascularity. The vascularity of the periradicular tissues is a critical determinant in healing.**
   a. The first statement is false, and the second statement is true
   b. The first statement is true, and the second statement is false
   c. Both statements are true
   d. Both statements are false
   Ans. a
5. **Which of the following medical conditions may influence healing in geriatric patients?**
   a. Osteoporosis
   b. Hypertension
   c. Immunosuppression
   d. Diabetes
   Ans. d
6. **Which of the following describes bisphosphonates?**
   a. They are used in treatment of osteoporosis
   b. They are used in treatment of malignancies
   c. They are linked to idiopathic osteonecrosis of the jaws
   d. They interfere with osteoclast function
   e. All of the above.
   Ans. e
7. **Which of the following is a common finding on examination in geriatric patients?**
   a. Extensive restorative experience with multiple large restorations and crowns
   b. Lower incidence of periodontal disease
   c. Exaggerated symptoms associated with pulp pathosis
   d. Excessive salivation
   Ans. a
8. **Which of the following is a consideration between geriatric and younger patients that may affect the ability to make a diagnosis?**
   a. Older patients are more stoic
   b. Decreased response to pulp testing is common
   c. Symptoms of pulpitis are not as acute in older patients
   d. All of the above
   Ans. d
9. **A common modification in performing root canal treatment for older patients is which of the following?**
   a. Treatment planning for a shorter life span
   b. Access cavity without a rubber dam to locate a smaller chamber
   c. Greater need for anesthetic
   d. Larger restorations make isolation easier
   Ans. b
10. **Working length determination in elderly patients may be more difficult because of which of the following?**
    a. Increased bone density, making radiographs harder to interpret
    b. Increased cementum deposition, modifying the apical anatomy
    c. Differences in tissue electrical resistance, making apex locators less accurate
    d. Patients unable to sit still for radiographs
    Ans. b

AIIMS Perio Question Bank

ANATOMY OF GINGIVA AND DENTOGINGIVAL JUNCTION

1. **The part (s) of oral mucosa referred to as specialized mucosa is/are:**
   a. Gingiva
   b. Covering of the hard palate
   c. Both of the above
   d. Dorsum of the tongue
   Ans. d
2. **The normal width of the marginal gingiva is:**
   a. 1 mm
   b. 2 mm
   c. 0.5 mm
   d. 3 mm
   Ans. a
3. **All of the following are true about mucogingival junction except:**
   a. It separates the gingiva from movable mucosa
   b. It makes the apical extent of attached gingiva
   c. It is stable and remains stationary throughout the life
   d. Its position may change in a pathological condition of gingiva
   Ans. d
4. **The incorrect statement about width of attached gingiva is:**
   a. It is the distance between mucogingival junction and projection of base of sulcus on outer surface
   b. It increases with age and supraeruption of teeth
   c. It increases with pathological enlargement of gingiva
   d. It decreases with loss of epithelial attachment
   Ans. c
5. **Col is:**
   a. A pathological enlargement of gingiva
   b. Keratinized portion of interdental gingiva
   c. Valley like depression of interdental gingiva
   d. An abnormal overgrowth of interdental bony septum
   Ans. c
6. **Which of the followings is not true about interdental papilla:**
   a. It is part of interdental gingiva
   b. Its tip and lateral borders are formed by continuation of marginal gingiva
   c. It is absent in diastema
   d. It is keratinized and less prone to infection
   Ans. d
7. **Probing depth of clinically healthy gingiva is:**
   a. 0–1 mm
   b. 1–2 mm
   c. 2–3 mm
   d. More than 4 mm
   Ans. c

8. **The principal cells of gingival epithelium are:**
   a. Keratinocytes
   b. Langerhans' cells
   c. Merkel cells
   d. Melanocytes
   Ans. a
9. **The main function(s) of gingival epithelium is/are:**
   a. Protection of underlying structures
   b. Nutrition of underlying structures
   c. To allow selective interchange with oral environment
   d. Both (A) and (C)
   Ans. d
10. **The width of attached gingiva:**
    a. Increases with age and supraeruption of the teeth
    b. Decreases with pocket formation
    c. Both of the above
    d. None of the above
    Ans. c
11. **Which of the following is incorrect about Langerhans' cells:**
    a. These are dendritic cells
    b. These are modified monocytes
    c. These are absent in junctional epithelium
    d. These are present in basal cell layer of oral epithelium
    Ans. d
12. **The nuclei are absent in stratum corneum of:**
    a. Orthokeratinized gingival epithelium
    b. Parakeratinized gingival epithelium
    c. None of the above
    d. Both of the above
    Ans. a
13. **The stratum granulosum is absent in:**
    a. Orthokeratinized epithelium
    b. Parakeratinized epithelium
    c. Both of the above
    d. None of the above
    Ans. b
14. **Merkel cells are:**
    a. Present in superficial layers of gingival epithelium
    b. Antigen presenting cells for lymphocytes
    c. Tactile preceptors
    d. All of the above
    Ans. c
15. **Sulcular epithelium is:**
    a. Semipermeable in nature
    b. Non keratinized
    c. Can be keratinized when exposed to oral cavity
    d. All of the above
    Ans. d

16. **The length of junctional epithelium is:**
    a. 0.1 to 0.2 mm
    b. 0.25 to 1.35 mm
    c. 1.35 to 2.00mm
    d. 2 to 2.5 mm
    Ans. b
17. **Which of the followings is not the function of sulcular fluid:**
    a. It helps in removing harmful materials from the sulcus
    b. It provides plasma proteins that help in adhesion of junctional epithelium of the tooth
    c. It carries antibodies to help in defence mechanism of gingiva
    d. It helps in plaque formation by providing glycoproteins which are an important component of dental pellicle
    Ans. d
18. **The gingival fibers are arranged into following groups except:**
    a. Dentogingival group
    b. Dentoalveolar group
    c. Circular group
    d. Trans-septal group
    Ans. b
19. **The cells present in connective tissue of gingiva include:**
    a. Mast cells, macrophages, adipose cells
    b. Histocytes, eosinophils, mast cells
    c. Macrophages, histocytes, melanocytes
    d. Both (A) and (B)
    Ans. d
20. **Blood supply to the gingiva is provided by:**
    a. Supraperiosteal arterioles
    b. Vessels of periodontal ligament
    c. Vessels emerging from the crest of the interdental septa
    d. All of the above
    Ans. d
21. **The coral pink color of the normal gingiva is produced due to:**
    i. Vascular supply of gingiva
    ii. Thickness of gingival epithelium
    iii. Degree of keratinization of gingival epithelium
    iv. Presence of pigment containing cells
    a. (i) and (iv)
    b. (i), (ii) and (iii)
    c. (i) and (iii)
    d. (i), (ii), (iii) and (iv)
    Ans. d
22. **Choose the incorrect statement:**
    a. Stippling is absent in marginal gingiva
    b. Stippling is absent in infants and appears at about 5 years of age
    c. Stippling is more prominent on facial surface than on lingual surface
    d. Stippling is lost permanently in gingivitis
    Ans. d
23. **The earliest sign of gingival inflammation is:**
    a. Increased gingival fluid production rate
    b. Change in color of gingiva
    c. Loss of stippling of gingiva
    d. Bleeding on gentle probing
    Ans. d

24. **Passive eruption is divided into:**
    a. Two stages
    b. Three stages
    c. Four stages
    d. Not divided into stages
    Ans. c
25. **Mark the wrong statement(s):**
    a. Active eruption is a physiological process
    b. Passive eruption is a physiological process
    c. Passive eruption is divided into four stages
    d. Both (B) and (C)
    Ans. b
26. **The attachment apparatus of the tooth is composed of:**
    a. Periodontal ligament and cementum
    b. Periodontal ligament and alveolar bone
    c. Periodontal ligament alone
    d. Periodontal ligament, cementum and alveolar bone
    Ans. d
27. **The group of periodontal fibers not attached to the bone include(s):**
    a. Transseptal group
    b. Horizontal group
    c. Interradicular group
    d. Both (A) and (C)
    Ans. a
28. **The principal fiber group that gets reconstructed even after the destruction of alveolar bone is:**
    a. Transseptal group
    b. Horizontal group
    c. Tnterradicular group
    d. Oblique group
    Ans. a
29. **The largest group of principal fibers is:**
    a. Transseptal group
    b. Horizontal group
    c. Oblique group
    d. Apical group
    Ans. c
30. **The principal fiber group that prevents extrusion of the tooth and resists lateral tooth movements is:**
    a. Transseptal group
    b. Apical group
    c. Alveolar crest group
    d. Oblique group
    Ans. c
31. **The principal connective tissue cells present in periodontal ligament are:**
    a. Fibroblasts
    b. Cementoblasts
    c. Osteoblasts
    d. All of the above
    Ans. a
32. **All of the followings are true about fibroblasts except:**
    a. Fibroblasts are principal connective tissue cells of periodontal ligament
    b. Fibroblasts synthesize collagen

c. Fibroblasts have pseudopodia like processes
d. Fibroblasts are not capable of phagocytosis for collagen destruction
Ans. d

33. **Epithelial rests:**
a. Are remnants of Hertwig's root sheath
b. May calcify to form cementicles
c. May proliferate under stimulation to form a periapical cyst
d. All of the above
Ans. d

34. **Myelinated fibers of nerve bundles entering the periodontal ligament ultimately terminate into:**
a. Free endings with treelike configuration
b. Ruffini-like corpuscles
c. Coiled forms
d. Any of above structures
Ans. d

INFLAMMATION OF PERIODONTIUM AND HOST RESPONSE

1. **Cytoplasmic granules of mast cells contain:**
a. Histamine
b. Slow releasing substances of anaphylaxis
c. Heparin
d. All of the above
Ans. d

2. **Principal cells of defense against injury and infection are:**
a. Plasma cells
c. Lymphocytes
b. Mast cells
d. Neutrophils
Ans. d

3. **Antibodies are produced mainly by:**
a. Helper T-cells
b. Suppressor T-cells
c. B-cells
d. Plasma cells
Ans. d

4. **Suppressor T-cells:**
a. Release interleukin-4 and interleukins
b. Stimulate cytotoxic and microbicidal activity of immune cells
c. Are CDS positive
d. All of the above
Ans. d

5. **Macrophages are formed by differentiation of:**
a. Monocytes
b. Plasma cells
c. Lymphocytes
d. Basophils
Ans. a

6. **Plasma cells are formed by differentiation of:**
a. Monocytes
b. Neutrophils
c. B Lymphocytes
d. T lymphocytes
Ans. c

7. **Effector cell for local and systemic humoral immunity is produced by:**
   a. Plasma cells
   b. Macrophages
   c. Neutrophils
   d. All of the above
   Ans. a
8. **Antibodies are:**
   a. Mucopolysaccharides
   b. Proteins
   c. Glycoproteins
   d. None of the above
   Ans. c
9. **Specificity of every antibody with a particular antigen is due to:**
   a. Its unique ammo acid sequence
   b. Tertiary structure of its antigen combining sites
   c. Both of the above
   d. None of the above
   Ans. c
10. **The number of antibody binding sites in the immunoglobulin molecule is referred to as:**
   a. Potency of immunoglobulin molecule
   b. Valence of immunoglobulin molecule
   c. Both of the above
   d. None of the above
   Ans. b
11. **Most abundant immunoglobulin in the serum is:**
   a. IgG
   b. IgA
   c. IgM
   d. IgE
   Ans. a
12. **Which of the followings is wrong about IgG:**
   a. It is most abundant of serum immunoglobulins
   b. It is distributed equally between blood and extracel lular fluids
   c. It enhances phagocytosis by binding to microorgan isms
   d. It does not cross placental barrier
   Ans. d
13. **Antibodies responsible for acute allergic reactions belong to the class:**
   a. IgG
   b. IgE
   c. IgA
   d. IgM
   Ans. b
14. **The principal immunoglobulin in exocrine secretions is:**
   a. IgA
   b. IgD
   c. IgE
   d. IgM
   Ans. a
15. **Immunoglobulin first to be formed in response to initial attack of infections is:**
   a. IgA
   b. IgE

c. IgG
d. IgM
Ans. d

16. The basis for complement fixation assay (an important laboratory procedure) is:
a. Increased permeability of small blood vessels
b. Phagocytic activity by leucocytes and macrophages
c. Hemolysis
d. All of the above
Ans. c

17. Type III hypersensitivity reactions are also known as:
a. Cytotoxic reactions
b. Arthus reactions
c. Immune complex reactions
d. Both B and C
Ans. d

18. Which of the followings is cell mediated hypersensitivity reaction:
a. Type I
b. Type II
c. Type III
d. Type IV
Ans. d

19. Type I hypersensitivity is also known as:
a. Anaphylaxis
b. Cytotoxic reactions
c. Arthus reactions
d. Delayed hypersensitivity
Ans. a

20. Pharmacological actions of histamine include following except:
a. Increased capillary permeability
b. Contraction of striated muscles
c. Stimulation of exocrine glands
d. Increased venule dilation permeability
Ans. b

21. Examples of cytotoxic reactions include:
a. Hemolytic transfusion reaction
b. Hemolytic disease of newborn
c. Autoallergic hemolytic anemia
d. All of the above
Ans. d

22. Which of the followings is not a cytokine:
a. Interleukin 1
b. Tumor necrosis factor
c. Transforming growth factor
d. None of the above
Ans. d

ANATOMY OF CEMENTUM

1. A cellular cementum is mainly found in:
a. Cervical third of the root
b. Apical third of the root
c. Middle third of root
d. None of the above
Ans. a

2. **Thickness of a cellular cementum is:**
   a. 10 μ
   b. 2 μ
   c. 100 μ
   d. It varies from 30 to 230 μ
   Ans. d
3. **Increased function of tooth causes:**
   a. Increase is number of Sharpey's fibers
   b. Increase in size of Sharpey's fibers
   c. Both of the above
   d. None of the above
   Ans. c
4. **An cementum, cementocytes are contained in the individual spaces known as:**
   a. Lamellae
   b. Canaliculi
   c. Lacunae
   d. None of the above
   Ans. c
5. **All of the following are true about cellular cementum except:**
   a. It contains cementocytes
   b. It is formed before the tooth reaches its occlusal plane
   c. It is less calcified than a cellular cementum
   d. It has smaller amount of Sharpey's fibers as compared to a cellular cementum
   Ans. b
6. **The hyper calcified lines that separate lamellae of cellular cementum from that of a cellular cementum are known as:**
   a. Incremental lines
   b. Lines of Ritzius
   c. Both of the above
   d. None of the above
   Ans. a
7. **The incremental lines of cementum represent:**
   a. Active periods of cementum formation
   b. Rest periods of cementum formation
   c. Both of the above
   d. None of the above
   Ans. b
8. **Total inorganic content of cementum is:**
   a. 90 to 95 percent
   b. 70 to 80 percent
   c. 60 to 65 percent
   d. 45 to 50 percent
   Ans. d
9. **Cementum is thickest at:**
   a. Cervical third of the roots
   b. Middle third of the roots
   c. Apical third and furcation areas of roots
   d. Uniform all over the root
   Ans. c

10. Cementum overlaps the enamel at cementoenamel junction in about:
   a. 60 to 65 percent of cases
   b. 30 percent of cases
   c. 5 to 10 percent of cases
   d. None of the above
   Ans. a

11. The prominent thickening of cementum on root is termed as:
   a. Hypercementosis
   b. Cementum hyperplasia
   c. Both of the above
   d. None of the above
   Ans. c

12. Fusion of Cementum with alveolar bone resulting into obliteration of periodontal ligament is known as:
   a. Both of the above
   b. A true pocket never forms in ankylosed tooth
   Ans. b

13. Resorption of cementum may occur in:
   a. Erupted tooth
   b. Partially erupted tooth
   c. Unerupted tooth
   d. All of the above
   Ans. d

14. Newly formed cementum during the period of cemental repair is demarcated from rest of the cementum by a line known as:
   a. Incremental line
   b. Reversal line
   c. Both of the above
   d. None of the above
   Ans. d

ANATOMY OF ALVEOLAR BONE

1. Which of the following parts of alveolar bone gives attachment to principal fibers of periodontal ligament:
   a. Inner cortical plates
   b. Alveolar bone proper
   c. Both of the above
   d. None of the above
   Ans. b

2. Inner wall of the tooth socket is formed by:
   a. Cancelloustrabeculae
   b. Inner cortical plates
   c. Alveolar bone proper
   d. All of the above
   Ans. c

3. Alveolar bone proper is formed of:
   a. Haversian bone
   b. Compact bone lamellae
   c. Bundle bone
   d. Partly of lamellated and partly of bundle bone
   Ans. d

4. **Lamina dura is:**
   a. Thin lamella of bone that forms the inner wall of the socket
   b. Dense radiopaque line around the roots seen in radiographs
   c. Both of the above
   d. None of the above
   Ans. b
5. **Alveolar process is formed:**
   a. Before the eruption of the tooth
   b. At the time of tooth eruption
   c. After the eruption of the tooth
   d. None of the above
   Ans. b
6. **Lacunae of the alveolar bone communicate with each other through:**
   a. Cytoplasmic cell processes of osteocytes
   b. Intercellular matrix
   c. Canaliculi
   d. All of the above
   Ans. c
7. **Inorganic matter of alveolar bone consists of:**
   a. ½ of the bone
   b. 2/3rd of the bone
   c. 3/4th of the bone
   d. 1/4th of the bone
   Ans. b
8. **Type I collagen forms:**
   a. 60 to 65 percent of organic matrix of alveolar bone
   b. 65 to 70 percent of organic matrix of alveolar bone
   c. 76 to 82 percent of organic matrix of alveolar bone
   d. 88 to 89 percent of organic matrix of alveolar bone
   Ans. d
9. **Which of the followings is wrong about interdental septum:**
   a. Cancellous bone is bounded from facial and lingual sides by alveolar bone proper
   b. Cancellous bone may be absent in case of narrow interdental space
   c. Bone may be absent in some area of interdental septum in case the roots are too close to each other
   d. Cancellous bone is bounded from mesial and distal sides by alveolar bone proper
   Ans. a
10. **The outer layer of periosteum of alveolar bone:**
    a. Has cells that have potential to differentiate into osteoblasts
    b. Consists of fibroblasts and collagen fibers and is rich in nerves and blood vessels
    c. Both of the above
    d. None of the above
    Ans. b
11. **Osteoid is:**
    a. Freshly secreted bone matrix
    b. Freshly mineralized bone matrix
    c. Both of the above
    d. None of the above
    Ans. a
12. **Mineralization:**
    a. Always precedes bone matrix formation
    b. Always lags behind bone matrix formation
    c. Occurs simultaneously with bone matrix formation
    d. None of the above
    Ans. b

13. **The ruffled border is the characteristic structural feature of:**
    a. Osteocytes
    b. Osteoblasts
    c. Osteoclasts
    d. All of the above
    Ans. c
14. **Acid/acids secreted by osteoclasts at the ruffle border is/are:**
    a. Citric acid
    b. Lactic acid
    c. Hydrochloric acid
    d. Both (A) and (B)
    Ans. d
15. **Osteoclasts:**
    a. Are formed by fusion of circulating monocytes
    b. May differentiate from mesenchymal cells in sites
    c. Are irregularly oval or club shaped with many branching processes
    d. All of the above
    Ans. d
16. **Choose the correct statement:**
    a. In fenestrations the denuded area extends through the marginal bone
    b. In dehiscence the marginal bone is intact
    c. Both of the above
    d. None of the above
    Ans. d
17. **Most common cause(s) of physiologic mesial migration is/are:**
    a. Failure to replace extracted 1st permanent molar
    b. Flattening of proximal contact area due to proximal wear of teeth
    c. Both of the above
    d. None of the above
    Ans. a
18. **In response to increased occlusal demands:**
    a. Bony trabeculae realign perpendicular to root surface
    b. Width of periodontal ligament increases
    c. There is increased diameter and number of Sharpey's fibers
    d. All of the above
    Ans. d
19. **In response to reduced occlusal demand:**
    a. Thickness and number of trabeculae reduce
    b. Periodontal ligament becomes thin and atrophied
    c. Periodontal fibers get disoriented and ultimately arranged parallel to the root surface
    d. All of the above
    Ans. d
20. **Source (s) of blood supply to periodontal ligament is (are):**
    a. Branches given off by apical vessels before entering the dental pulp
    b. Transalveolar vessels that enter periodontal ligament after perforating the lamina dura.
    c. Gingival vessels anastomosing with periodontal ligament vessels of cervical region
    d. All of the above
    Ans. d

SULCULAR FLUID AND SALIVA DEFENSE MECHANISMS OF GINGIVA

1. **Sulcular epithelium can be penetrated by substances with a molecular weight of up to:**
   a. One million
   b. Two million
   c. Three million
   d. Ten million
   Ans. a
2. **Sulcular fluid is:**
   a. An inflammatory exudate
   b. A normal transudate
   c. Derived from saliva
   d. None of the above
   Ans. a
3. **The amount of fluid collected on a paper strip can be evaluated by:**
   a. Measuring the wetted area
   b. The help of an electronic device
   c. Both of the above
   d. None of the above
   Ans. c
4. **The concentration of carbohydrates in the sulcular fluid is:**
   a. Less than that in the blood
   b. 3 to 4 times more than that in the blood
   c. Same as in the blood
   d. None of the above
   Ans. b
5. **Concentration of proteins in the sulcular fluid is:**
   a. Less than that in the blood
   b. More than that in the blood
   c. Same as in the blood
   d. None of the above
   Ans. a
6. **The amount of gingival fluid usually increases with:**
   a. Severity of the inflammation
   b. Vigorous tooth brushing
   c. Mastication of coarse food
   d. All of the above
   Ans. d
7. **Smoking:**
   a. Increases the flow of sulcular fluid
   b. Decreases the flow of sulcular fluid
   c. First increases then decreases the flow of sulcular fluid
   d. Does not have any effect on the flow of sulcular fluid
   Ans. a
8. **During ovulation, pregnancy and use of hormonal contraceptives, the production of gingival fluid:**
   a. Increases
   b. Decreases
   c. Remains unchanged
   d. None of the above
   Ans. a

9. **Saliva helps in maintaining the oral tissues in physiological state by:**
   a. Mechanically cleaning the exposed oral surface by its flushing action
   b. By buffering the acids produced by bacteria
   c. By controlling the bacterial activity
   d. All of the above
   Ans. d
10. **The most dominant immunoglobulin found in saliva is:**
   a. IgA
   b. IgG
   c. IgM
   d. IgD
   Ans. a
11. **Proteolytic enzymes found in saliva are produced by:**
   a. Oral bacteria
   b. Host tissue cells
   c. Both (A) and (B)
   d. None of the above
   Ans. c
12. **Antiprotease (s) found in saliva is/are:**
   a. Cathepsins
   b. Tissue inhibitor of matrix metalloproteinase (TIMP)
   c. Antileucoproteases
   d. All of the above
   Ans. d
13. **The activity of collagen degrading enzymes in the saliva is inhibited by:**
   a. Cathepsins
   b. TIMP
   c. Antileucoproteases
   d. All of the above
   Ans. b
14. **Concentration of which of the following enzyme (s) increases in saliva in periodontal disease:**
   a. Hyaluronidase
   b. Chondroitin sulphatase
   c. Peroxidase
   d. All of the above
   Ans. d
15. **Orogranulocytic migratory rate refers to:**
   a. The rate of migration of monocytes into oral cavity
   b. The rate of migration of polymorphonuclear leucocytes into the oral cavity
   c. The rate of immigration of lymphocytes into the oral cavity
   d. All of the above
   Ans. b
16. **The most important buffer system in the saliva is:**
   a. Bicarbonate-carbonic acid buffers
   b. Protein buffers
   c. Phosphate buffers
   d. All of the above
   Ans. a
17. **The important coagulation factors present in saliva include:**
   a. Factors VIII, IX, and X
   b. Hageman factor
   c. Plasma thromboplastin antecedent (PTA)
   d. All of the above
   Ans. d

18. Besides its defensive role, the saliva also helps in the production of periodontal diseases due to its:
   a. High molecular weight glycoproteins
   b. Proteolytic enzymes
   c. Both (A) and (B)
   d. None of the above
   Ans. c

AGING OF PERIODONTIUM

1. Which of the following changes in gingiva is not identified with aging:
   a. Decreased connective tissue cellularity
   b. Diminished keratinization
   c. Reduced or unchanged amount of stippling
   d. Decreased width of attached gingiva
   Ans. d

2. The keratinizing potential of which of the following does not change with age:
   a. Lip
   b. Cheek
   c. Hard palate
   d. Attached gingiva
   Ans. c

3. In the periodontal ligament, aging results in:
   a. Increase in the number of elastic fibers
   b. Decrease in the number of collagen fibers
   c. Both of the above
   d. None of the above
   Ans. c

4. A reduction in the width of periodontal ligament with Caging is due to:
   a. Lower functional demand owing to decrease in strength of the masticatory musculature
   b. Increased functional demand owing to decrease in strength of the masticatory musculature
   c. Lower functional demand owing to increase in strength of the masticatory musculature
   d. Increased functional demand owing to increase in strength of the masticatory musculature
   Ans. a

5. Change (s) in alveolar bone with aging is/are:
   a. Osteoporosis
   b. Decreased vascularity
   c. Decreased healing capacity
   d. All of the above
   Ans. d

6. Occlusal wear results in all, except:
   a. Reduction in cusp height
   b. Reduction in cusp inclination
   c. Loss of sluiceways
   d. Decrease in food table area
   Ans. d

7. With age the anteroposterior length of the dental arch:
   a. Reduces by approximately 0.5 cm by age 40
   b. Increases by approximately 0.5 cm by age 40
   c. Remains the same by age 40
   d. Remains the same by age 60
   Ans. a

MICROBIOLOGY OF PERIODONTAL DISEASES

1. **One gram of plaque (wet weight) contains approximately:**
   a. 1 × 1010 bacteria
   b. 2 × 10″ bacteria
   c. 1 × 10″ bacteria
   d. 2 × 10′ bacteria
   Ans. b
2. **The initial bacteria colonizing the pellicle coated tooth surface are predominantly:**
   a. Gram-positive facultative microorganisms
   b. Gram-negative facultative microorganisms
   c. Both gram-positive facultative microorganisms and gram-negative facultative microorganisms
   d. Gram-positive aerobic microorganisms
   Ans. a
3. **Secondary colonizers of the dental plaque are all of the following, except:**
   a. Prevotellaintermedia
   b. Streptococcus sanguis
   c. Porphyromonasgingivalis
   d. Fusobacteriumnucleatum
   Ans. b
4. **Which of the following microorganisms is identified as predominant pathogen in localized juvenile periodontitis:**
   a. Prevotellagingivalis
   b. Actinobacillusactinomycetemcomitans
   c. Streptococcus sanguis
   d. Actinomycesviscosus
   Ans. b
5. **The change in periodontal microbiology from a healthy periodontium to a diseased periodontium includes:**
   a. Increase in gram-positive facultative rods and cocci and gram-negative rods
   b. Decrease in gram-positive facultative rods and cocci and increase in gram-negative rods
   c. Decrease in gram-positive facultative rods and cocci and gram-negative rods
   d. Increase in gram-positive facultative rods and cocci and decrease in gram-negative rods
   Ans. b
6. **Pregnancy gingivitis is associated with increase in the levels of:**
   a. Prevotellaintermedia
   b. Streptococcus mitis
   c. Campylobacter species
   d. Actinomycesnaeslundii
   Ans. a
7. **Mjeroorganisms predominantly found in ANUG lesions are:**
   a. Prevotella gingivalis and Prevotella inter media
   b. Prevotella intermedia and Spirochetes
   c. Porphyromonas gingivalis and Prevotella intermedia
   d. Porphyromonas gingivalis and capnocytophaga
   Ans. b
8. **In chronic adult periodontitis the microorganisms often cultivated at high levels include:**
   a. Porphyromonasgingivalis
   b. Prevotellaintermedia
   c. Actinobacillusactinomycetemcomitans
   d. All of the above
   Ans. d

9. **The microorganisms significantly associated with rapidly progressive periodontitis are:**
   a. P. gingivcilis and A.actinomyceteiuconiitans
   b. P. gingivalis and capnocytophaga
   c. A. actinomycetemcomitansand capnocytophaga
   d. P. gingivalisonly
   Ans. a
10. **According to Koch's postulates, the causative agent in human infections must:**
    a. Be routinely isolated from diseased individuals
    b. Be grown in pure culture in the laboratory
    c. Produce a similar disease when inoculated into susceptible laboratory animals
    d. All of the above
    Ans. d
11. **Actinomycesviscosus that initially colonizes the periodontal environment most likely attaches to the pellicle or saliva coated tooth surface through:**
    a. Membrane protein
    b. Heat sensitive protein
    c. Fimbriae
    d. Outer membrane protein
    Ans. c
12. **Bacteria may enter host tissues through:**
    a. Ulcerations in the epithelium of the gingival sulcus or pocket
    b. Direct penetration of bacteria into host epithelial or connective tissue cells
    c. Both of the above
    d. None of the above
    Ans. c
13. **Selected bacterial properties involved in evasion of host defense mechanisms include:**
    a. Immunoglobulin degrading proteases
    b. Inhibition of superoxide production
    c. Production of leukotoxin
    d. All of the above
    Ans. d
14. **The virulence factors of periodontal pathogens work in which of the following ways:**
    a. Bacterial adherence in the periodontal environment
       → Bacterial evasion of host defense mechanisms
       → Host tissue invasion
    b. Bacterial evasion of host defense mechanisms—Host tissue Invasion— Bacterial adherence in the periodontal environment
    c. Host tissue Invasion—Bacterial adherence in the periodontal environment—Bacterial evasion of host defense mechanisms
    d. Bacterial Adherence in the Periodontal environment—Host tissue Invasion—Bacterial evasion of host defense mechanisms
    Ans. d
15. **The bacterial products that inhibit the growth or alter the metabolism of host tissue cells include:**
    a. Ammonia
    b. Volatile sulfur compounds
    c. Fatty acids, peptides and indole
    d. All of the above
    Ans. d
16. **Trypsin like enzyme capable of degrading host tissues is produced by all, except:**
    a. P. gingivalis
    b. Campylobacter rectus
    c. A. actinomycetemcomitans
    d. Treponemadenticola
    Ans. b

17. Bacterial enzymes may facilitate:
   a. Tissue destruction
   b. Invasion of the bacteria into host tissues
   c. Both of the above
   d. None of the above
   Ans. c

18. The microorganisms colonizing the gingival pockets utilize which of the following as energy source:
   a. Saliva and sugars
   b. Saliva and amino acids
   c. Amino acids and sugars
   d. Amino acids and simple peptides
   Ans. d

19. Host defense mechanisms in the dentogingival area include all of the following, except:
   a. Host parasite inter-relations
   b. Defense by saliva
   c. Microbial perturbation of the local humoral defense
   d. 'Defence by RBCs'
   Ans. d

CALCULUS AND PERIODONTAL DISEASES

1. A hard deposit that forms by mineralization of dental plaque is:
   a. Marginal plaque
   b. Calculus
   c. Materiaalba
   d. All of the above
   Ans. b

2. Calculus is generally covered by a layer of:
   a. Mineralized plaque
   b. Unmineralized plaque
   c. Materiaalba
   d. None of the above
   Ans. b

3. Supragingival calculus occurs most frequently and in greatest quantity on the:
   a. Buccal surfaces of the maxillary molars and lingual surfaces of the mandibular anterior teeth
   b. Lingual surfaces of the maxillary molars and lingual surfaces of the mandibular anterior teeth
   c. Buccal surfaces of the mandibular molar and lingual surfaces of the maxillary molars
   d. Lingual surfaces of the maxillary anterior teeth and buccal surfaces of maxillary molars
   Ans. a

4. Which of the followings is not a property of subgingival calculus:
   a. It is usually dark brown or greenish black in color
   b. It is not visible on routine clinical examination
   c. It can be easily detached from the tooth surface
   d. It is hard or flintlike in consistency
   Ans. c

5. Which of the followings is the main mineral source for subgingival calculus:
   a. Saliva
   b. Gingival fluid which resembles
   c. Gingival fluid which resembles plasma
   d. None of the above
   Ans. b

6. Which of the following crystal forms occur in greater amounts in supragingival calculus:
   a. Hydroxyapatite and magnesium whitlockite
   b. Octacalcium phosphate and Brushite
   c. Hydroxyapatite and octacalcium phosphate
   d. Brushite and Magnesium whitlockite
   Ans. c

7. **Which of the following crystal forms is more in subgingival calculus compared to supragingival calculus:**
   a. Hydroxyapatite
   b. Magnesium whitlockite
   c. Octacalcium phosphate
   d. Brushite
   Ans. b
8. **The content of the following increases with the depth of periodontal pockets:**
   a. Calcium
   b. Phosphate
   c. Sodium
   d. Potassium
   Ans. c
9. **The mode(s) of attachment of dental calculus to the tooth surface is/are:**
   a. By means of an organic pellicle
   b. By penetration of calculus bacteria into cementum
   c. Mechanical locking into surface irregularities such as resorption lacunae and caries
   d. All of the above
   Ans. d
10. **Which of the following chromogenic bacteria is most commonly responsible for black stains:**
   a. Flavobacterium
   b. Actinomyces
   c. Prevotellamelaninogenicus
   d. Aspergillus
   Ans. b
11. **Calcifying plaques may become 50 percent mineralized in:**
   a. 1 day
   b. 2 days
   c. 12 days
   d. 21 days
   Ans. b
12. **In the supragingival plaque calcification begins along the:**
   a. Outer surface of the supragingival plaque
   b. Inner surface of the supragingival plaque adjacent to the tooth
   c. Equally on both the outer and inner surfaces to the supragingival plaque
   d. It never calcifies
   Ans. b
13. **The primary effect of calculus in periodontal disease seems to be:**
   a. Its irritating nature
   b. By initiating gingivitis
   c. Its retention site role for plaque
   d. Disruption of the attachment of junctional epithelium with tooth
   Ans. c

PUBLIC HEALTH ASPECT OF PERIODONTAL DISEASES

1. **The following gingival score of the gingival index is associated with moderate degree of gingivitis:**
   a. 0.1 to 1.0
   b. 1.1 to 2.0
   c. 2.1 to 3.0
   d. 3.1 to 4.0
   Ans. b

2. **All are indices of gingival bleeding, except:**
   a. Sulcus bleeding index
   b. Papillary bleeding index
   c. Gingival bleeding index
   d. Periodontal bleeding index
   Ans. d
3. **The highest prevalence of gingivitis occurs during:**
   a. Age of 5 years
   b. Puberty
   c. Adulthood
   d. Old age
   Ans. b
4. **The prevalence and severity of periodontal disease in males as compared to females is:**
   a. Higher
   b. Lower
   c. Equal
   d. Cannot be estimated
   Ans. a
5. **The primary etiologic agent of the gingival and periodontal disease is:**
   a. Poor oral hygiene
   b. Malnutrition
   c. Adverse habits
   d. Lack of fluorides in diet
   Ans. a
6. **Which of the following area of mouth is most severely affected by gingivitis:**
   a. Buccal surfaces of gingiva
   b. Lingual surfaces of gingiva
   c. Interproximal areas
   d. Both (A) and (B)
   Ans. c
7. **Which of the following parts of mouth has a slightly higher tendency towards gingivitis:**
   a. Right half of the arch
   b. Left half of the arch
   c. Complete upper arch
   d. Complete lower arch
   Ans. a
8. **The subgingival calculus is found in greater amount in association with:**
   a. Lower first molars
   b. Lower second molars
   c. Lower centrals and laterals
   d. Upper centrals and laterals
   Ans. c
9. **The teeth that are most severely affected by periodontal disease are the:**
   a. Lower centrals and laterals
   b. Lower premolars
   c. Upper centrals and laterals
   d. Upper premolars
   Ans. a

10. **In the gingivitis index, mild to moderately severe gingivitis extending all around the tooth is given the gingival status of:**
    a. 0
    b. 1
    c. 2
    d. 3
    Ans. c
11. **If the periodontal index score is between 0.7 and 1.9, it means that the periodontal disease is:**
    a. Absent
    b. Reversible
    c. Irreversible
    d. Treated
    Ans. b
12. **In the PMA index, P, M and A stand for:**
    a. P-periodontium, M-mobility, A-attrition
    b. P-dental papilla, M-migration of teeth, A-attrition
    c. P-dental papilla, M-gingival margin, A-attached gingiva
    d. P-plaque, M-gingival margin, A-attached gingiva
    Ans. c

TREATMENT OF HIV INFECTED PATIENTS

1. **The percentage of AIDS patients having oral lesions is:**
    a. 20 percent
    b. 35 percent
    c. 55 percent
    d. 95 percent
    Ans. c
2. **HIV infection is strongly correlated with:**
    a. Oral candidiasis
    b. Oral hairy leukoplakia
    c. Oral Kaposi's sarcoma
    d. All of the above
    Ans. d
3. **In HIV infected patients oral hairy leukoplakia is found almost exclusively on the:**
    a. Buccal mucosa
    b. Soft palate
    c. Hard palate
    d. Lateral borders of the tongue
    Ans. d
4. **The Kaposi's sarcoma that occurs in HIV ini'ectedpatients presents different clinical features in that it is:**
    a. Very slowly growing lesion
    b. Much more aggressive lesion
    c. Frequently involves the oral mucosa, particularly the palate and the gingiva
    d. Both (B) and (C)
    Ans. d
5. **Which of the following statements is wrong about oralhairy leukoplakia and AIDS:**
    a. Oral hairy leukoplakia in AIDS patients is found almost exclusively on the lateral borders of the tongue
    b. Oral hairy leukoplakia is caused by human papilloma
    c. The number of HIV infected patients with hairy leukoplakia who eventually develop AIDS approaches 100 percent
    d. Small lesions are as diagnostically significant as extensive lesions
    Ans. b

6. **The most common oral lesion in HIV infected patients is:**
   a. Oral hairy leukoplakia
   b. Oral candidiasis
   c. Oral Kaposi's sarcoma
   d. Oral hyperpigmentation
   Ans. b
7. **The percentage of AIDS patients suffering from candidiasis is approximately:**
   a. 50 percent
   b. 60 percent
   c. 90 percent
   d. 100 percent
   Ans. c
8. **HIV associated gingivitis is best described by the term:**
   a. Juvenile gingivitis
   b. Acute necrotizing gingivitis
   c. Linear gingival erythema
   d. Necrotizing ulcerative gingivitis
   Ans. c
9. **HIV positive individuals can anticipate reasonably good periodontal health throughout the course of their disease by:**
   a. Periodontal surgery
   b. Antibiotic treatment
   c. Proper home care and appropriate periodontal treatment and maintenance
   d. Proper scaling and root planing
   Ans. c
10. **HIV infected patients are more susceptible to periodontal infections as their immune system becomes more compromised. HIV infected patients are not the potential candidates for procedures such as periodontal surgery and implant placement:**
   a. Both the statements are wrong
   b. Only first statement is wrong
   c. Only second statement is wrong
   d. Both the statements are correct
   Ans. c

BACTERIAL INTERACTION IN PERIODONTAL DISEASES

1. **The cell constituent (s) of various bacteria that play a in periodontal disease is/are:**
   a. Endotoxins
   b. Bacterial surface complements
   c. Capsular components
   d. All of the above
   Ans. d
2. **Endotoxins are highly toxic substances, affecting periodontal tissues:**
   a. Directly
   b. Through activation of host responses
   c. Both of the above
   d. None of the above
   Ans. c
3. **A central characteristic of periodontal destruction is the degradation of:**
   a. Collagen
   b. Elastin
   c. Fibroblasts
   d. Mucopolysaccharides
   Ans. a

4. **A significant immune finding in pregnancy gingivitisis:**
   a. PMN chemotactic defect
   b. Occurrence of immune complexes in tissues
   c. No significant findings reported
   d. Elevated antibody levels to Prevotellagingivalis
   Ans. c
5. **The primary source of collagenase in the periodontal pocket is probably:**
   a. Host tissue cells
   b. Bacteria
   c. Diet
   d. Blood
   Ans. a
6. **Secreting immune system affects the periodontal disease by:**
   a. Decreasing bacterial colonization on surfaces exposed to saliva
   b. Causing tissue destruction
   c. Controlling immune responses to bacteria
   d. All of the above
   Ans. a
7. **Which of the following neutrophil disorder(s) is/are associated with periodontal disease:**
   a. Diabetes mellitus
   b. Down's syndrome
   c. Papillon-Lefevre syndrome
   d. All of the above
   Ans. d
8. **Which of the following periodontal disease (s) is/are associated with neutrophil disorders:**
   a. Acute necrotizing ulcerative gingivitis
   b. Prepubertal periodontitis
   c. Rapidly progressing periodontitis
   d. All of the above
   Ans. d
9. **Immunoglobulins are inactivated or destroyed by bacterial:**
   a. Collagenase
   b. Hyaluronidase
   c. Catalase
   d. Protease
   Ans. d
10. **The immunologic findings in adult periodontitis include all of the following except:**
    a. Elevated antibody titer to Prevotella gingivalis and other periodonto pathogens
    b. Cell mediated immunity to gingival bacteria
    c. Occurrence of immune complexes in tissue
    d. PMN and monocytic chemotactic defects
    Ans. d
11. **The host factor (s) which is/are responsible for tissue destruction in periodontal disease is/are:**
    a. Anti body mediated hypersensitivity
    b. Cell mediated hypersensitivity
    c. Activation of tissue factor such as collagenase
    d. All of the above
    Ans. d

FUNCTIONS OF LEUKOCYTES IN PERIODONTAL DISEASES

1. **The three primary leukocytes participating in the immune response to periodontal diseases are:**
   a. Neutrophils, Monocytes and Eosinophils
   b. Basophils, Neutrophils and Eosinophils
   c. Neutrophils, Monocytes and Lymphocytes
   d. Neutrophils, Basophils and Lymphocytes
   Ans. c
2. **Neutrophils virtually derive all their energy from:**
   a. Fermentation of stored glycogen
   b. Oxidative phosphorylation
   c. Both of the above
   d. None of the above
   Ans. a
3. **The chemoattractant for the neutrophils produced bybacteria is:**
   a. Leukotriene B4
   b. Interleukin 1
   c. FMet peptides
   d. Endothelial IL8
   Ans. c
4. **Neutrophils with megabodies is a characteristic feature of:**
   a. Neutropenia
   b. Agranulocytosis
   c. Leukocyte adhesion deficiency
   d. Chediak-Higashi syndrome
   Ans. d
5. **Presence of hyperproliferation of peripheral blood lymphocytes indicative of:**
   a. Less gingival inflammation
   b. Normal gingiva
   c. Less periodontal disease
   d. Severe periodontitis
   Ans. d
6. **Chronic inflammation begins with the infiltration of:**
   a. Neutrophils and Monocytes
   b. Monocytes and Lymphocytes
   c. Lymphocytes and Plasma cells
   d. Plasma cells and Neutrophils
   Ans. b
7. **Monocytes and Lymphocytes primarily infiltrate:**
   a. Connective tissue
   b. Junctional epithelium
   c. Gingival crevice
   d. None of the above
   Ans. a
8. **Which of the following serves as opsonin helping binding of phagocytes to target cells:**
   a. Complement metabolite C3b
   b. Complement metabolite C3a
   c. Complement metabolite C5b
   d. Complement metabolite C5a
   Ans. a

EFFECT OF LOCAL AND LATROGENIC FACTORS

1. **Subgingivally located margins of restorations are associated with:**
   a. Increased plaque accumulation
   b. Increased gingival inflammation
   c. Increased rate of gingival fluid flow
   d. All of the above
   Ans. d
2. **Overhanging margins contribute to periodontal disease by:**
   a. Providing ideal locations for the accumulation of plaque
   b. Changing the etiologic balance of the gingival sulcus area to one that favors the growth of disease associated organisms
   c. Both of the above
   d. None of the above
   Ans. c
3. **In general, restorative materials are not themselves injurious to periodontal tissues, except:**
   a. Glass ionomer cement
   b. Self curing acrylic
   c. Light curingcomposites
   d. Amalgam
   Ans. b
4. **Normally, the forceful wedging of food is prevented by:**
   a. Integrity and location of the proximal contacts
   b. The contour of marginal ridges
   c. The contour of facial and lingual surfaces
   d. All of the above
   Ans. d
5. **Cusps that tend to forcibly wedge food interproximally are known as:**
   a. Wedging cusps
   b. Trauma cusps
   c. Plunger cusps
   d. Sharp cusps
   Ans. c
6. **The common site of gingivitis associated with mouth breathing is:**
   a. Maxillary anterior region
   b. Mandibular anterior region
   c. Maxillary posterior region
   d. Mandibular posterior region
   Ans. a
7. **Smoking causes gingival fluid flow to:**
   a. Decrease
   b. Increase
   c. First decrease then increase
   d. No impact on gingival fluid flow
   Ans. b
8. **When compared with non-smokers of similar age and oral hygiene status, the bone height in smokers is:**
   a. Reduced
   b. Remains same
   c. Increased
   d. First reduces then increase
   Ans. a

9. **Chronic toothbrush trauma results in:**
   a. Gingival recession
   b. Denudation of the root surface
   c. Linear grooves extending from the marginal to the attached gingiva
   d. All of the above
   Ans. d
10. **Which of the following is/are the causative factor (s) for the development of periodontal diseases:**
   a. Orthodontic therapy
   b. Tongue thrusting habit
   c. Radiation
   d. All of the above
   Ans. d

EFFECT OF SYSTEMIC DISEASES ON THE PERIODONTIUM

1. **Which of the following statement (s) is/are correct:**
   a. Nutritional deficiencies initiate gingivitis and periodontal pockets
   b. Nutritional deficiencies aggravate the injurious effects of local irritants on gingiva and periodontium
   c. Both of the above
   d. None of the above
   Ans. b
2. **Which of the following types of diet leads to accumulation of plaque and development of gingivitis:**
   a. Soft diet
   b. Hard diet
   c. Fibrous diet
   d. All of the above
   Ans. a
3. **Glossitis, angular cheilitis, seborrheic dermatitis and superficial vascularizing keratitis are due to deficiency of:**
   a. Vitamin A
   b. Vitamin B
   c. Vitamin C
   d. Vitamin D
   Ans. b
4. **Bleeding, swollen gingiva and loosened teeth are the common features of:**
   a. Beri-beri
   b. Ariboflavinosis
   c. Scurvy
   d. Pellagra
   Ans. c
5. **Hormonal disturbances may affect the periodontal tissues:**
   a. Directly, as periodontal manifestations of endocrine disease
   b. By modifying the tissue response to plaque in gingival and periodontal disease
   c. By producing anatomic changes in the oral cavity that favor plaque accumulation
   d. All of the above
   Ans. d
6. **Decreased skeletal growth leading to crowding and malposition of teeth is due to:**
   a. Hypothyroidism
   b. Hypopituitarism
   c. Hyperpituitarism
   d. Hyperthyroidism
   Ans. b

7. **Insulin dependent diabetic children tend to have more destruction around the:**
   a. Anteriors
   b. First molars and incisors
   c. Premolars and canines
   d. First molars and canines
   Ans. b
8. **Frequent periodontal abscesses is an important feature of periodontal disease in:**
   a. Hypothyroidism
   b. Hypopituitarism
   c. Diabetes
   d. Starvation
   Ans. c
9. **The gingival fluid level of cyclic adenosine monophosphate (CAMP) in diabetics when compared with that of nondiabetics is:**
   a. Lower
   b. Higher
   c. Same
   d. No correlation of CAMP level and diabetes
   Ans. a
10. **Which of the following statement (s) is/are correct:**
   a. Pregnancy itself does not cause gingivitis
   b. Pregnancy accentuates the gingival response to plaque
   c. No notable changes occur in the gingiva
   d. All of the above
   Ans. d
11. **The highest incidence of leukemic gingival proliferative lesions is in:**
   a. Acute monocytic leukemia
   b. Chronic monocytic leukemia
   c. Acute lymphocytic leukemia
   d. Chronic lymphocytic leukemia
   Ans. a
12. **Leukemic gingival enlargement is not found in:**
   a. Children
   b. Edentulous patients
   c. Patients with chronic leukemia
   d. Both (B) and (C)
   Ans. d
13. **Which of the following is the early oral sign of leukemia:**
   a. Oral ulcerations
   b. Gingival enlargement
   c. Bleeding gingiva
   d. Pain
   Ans. c
14. **A syndrome consisting of glossitis and ulcerations of the oral mucosa and oropharynx, including dysphagia, has been described in patients with:**
   a. Pernicious anemia
   b. Megaloblastic anemia
   c. Sickle cell anemia
   d. Iron deficiency anemia
   Ans. d

15. **Bluish-black discoloration of the gingival margin in areas of pre-existing gingival inflammation is due to:**
    a. Bismuth intoxication
    b. Lead intoxication
    c. Mercury intoxication
    d. Arsenic intoxication
    Ans. a
16. **The absence of a notable gingival inflammatory reaction to the local irritants is a striking feature of:**
    a. Chediak-Higashi syndrome
    b. Arteriosclerosis
    c. Agranulocytosis
    d. Thrombocytopenic purpura
    Ans. c

OCCLUSION AND PERIODONTIUM

1. **In the physiologic rest position, the masticatory muscles are in:**
   a. Mild state of relaxation
   b. Mild state of contraction
   c. Strong state of relaxation
   d. Strong state of contraction
   Ans. c
2. **The space between the mandibular and maxillary teeth when the mandible is in postural position is called the:**
   a. Vertical dimension of rest
   b. Free way space
   c. Both of the above
   d. None of the above
   Ans. c
3. **Gradual physiologic attrition is characterized by:**
   a. Lack of inflammatory changes on the alveolar bone surfaces
   b. Severe inflammatory changes on the alveolar bone surfaces
   c. Resorption of the alveolar bone
   d. None of the above
   Ans. d
4. **Wear of the non-occluding tooth surfaces with sharply defined, wedge shaped depression in the facial cervical areas of the tooth is termed as:**
   a. Attrition
   b. Wear facets
   c. Erosion
   d. Abrasion
   Ans. c
5. **Frictional ablation is considered to be caused by:**
   a. The action of brush used against the dentition
   b. The action of dentifrices used against the dentition
   c. The action of hard food eaten
   d. The action of soft tissue and saliva against the dentition
   Ans. d
6. **The vertical dimension of occlusion is naturally maintained by:**
   a. Compensatory rate of both occlusal wear and proximal wear
   b. Compensatory rate of both proximal wear and mesial drifting
   c. Compensatory rate of both occlusal wear and continuous tooth eruption
   d. Compensatory rate of both continuous tooth eruption and mesial drifting
   Ans. c

7. **No signs of traumatic occlusion in healthy dentalarches appear if vertical dimension of occlusion is increased to a maximum up to:**
   a. 5 mm
   b. 0.5 mm
   c. .05 mm
   d. 3 mm
   Ans. d
8. **Occlusal or incisal surfaces worn by attrition are called:**
   a. Worn surfaces
   b. Erosion
   c. Facets
   d. Ablation
   Ans. c
9. **Bruxism and periodontal condition:**
   a. Appear to be independent phenomena
   b. Appear to be dependent phenomena
   c. Are proved to be independent phenomena
   d. Arc proved to be dependent phenomena
   Ans. a
10. **Facets generally represent:**
   a. Only functional wear
   b. Only parafunctional wear
   c. Both functional and parafunctional wear
   d. Neither functional nor parafuctional wear
   Ans. c

DIET AND NUTRITION IN PERIODONTIUM

1. **The dietary effect on plaque is mostly due to:**
   a. Carbohydrates
   b. Fats
   c. Proteins
   d. Nucleic acids
   Ans. a
2. **Large numbers of lactobacilli in saliva are related to a high consumption of:**
   a. Nonfermentable carbohydrates
   b. Fermentable carbohydrates
   c. Fermentable fats
   d. Nonfermentable fats
   Ans. b
3. **The plaque dry weight constituted by carbohydrates is about:**
   a. 0.1 percent
   b. 10 percent
   c. 20 percent
   d. 50 percent
   Ans. c
4. **The extracellular polysaccharides synthesized in plaque from dietary sucrose are:**
   a. Fructans and levans
   b. Glycogen amyiopectin and glucose amylopectin
   c. Dextran and glucan
   d. Fructans and glucans
   Ans. d

5. **Which of the following functions primarily as structural stabilizer of intermicrobial matrix:**
   a. Levans
   b. Fructans
   c. Dextrans
   d. Mutans
   Ans. d

GINGIVITIS

1. **The stage I gingivitis is termed as:**
   a. The early lesion
   b. The initial lesion
   c. The established lesion
   d. The advanced lesion
   Ans. b
2. **Clinically in subclinical gingivitis, the initial response of the gingiva to bacterial plaque is:**
   a. Not apparent
   b. Manifested by reddened gingiva
   c. Manifested by spontaneous bleeding of gingiva
   d. Manifested by bleeding of gingiva on probing
   Ans. a
3. **The predominant immune cells infiltrating the connective tissue and gingival sulcus in the initial lesions of gingivitis are:**
   a. Eosinophils
   b. Neutrophils
   c. Lymphocytes
   d. Plasma cells
   Ans. b
4. **The percentage of collagen destroyed around the cellular infiltrate in the stage II gingivitis is:**
   a. 10 percent
   b. 25 percent
   c. 50 percent
   d. 70 percent
   Ans. d
5. **The changes in color, size and texture of gingiva are seen in:**
   a. Stage I gingivitis
   b. Stage II gingivitis
   c. Stage III gingivitis
   d. Stage IV gingivitis
   Ans. c
6. **The term chronic gingivitis is refers to the following stage of gingivitis:**
   a. Stage I gingivitis
   b. Stage II gingivitis
   c. Stage III gingivitis
   d. Stage IV gingivitis
   Ans. c
7. **All of the following enzyme levels are found to be elevated in chronically inflamed gingiva except:**
   a. Acid phosphatase
   b. Alkaline phosphatase
   c. Lactic dehydrogenase
   d. Neutral mucopolysaccharide
   Ans. d

8. **Advanced lesion is also termed as:**
   a. Chronic gingivitis
   b. Phase of intensive inflammatory infiltration
   c. Phase of periodontal breakdown
   d. Phase of collagenolytic activity
   Ans. c
9. **The sequence of developing gingivitis is as follows:**
   a. The early lesion — The initial lesion — The advanced lesion — The established lesion
   b. The initial lesion — The early lesion — The established lesion — The advanced lesion
   c. The early lesion — The initial lesion — The established lesion — The advanced lesion
   d. The initial lesion — The early lesion — The advanced lesion — The established lesion
   Ans. b
10. **Erythema and bleeding on probing are initially evident in:**
    a. The initial lesion
    b. The early lesion
    c. The established lesion
    d. The advanced lesion
    Ans. b
11. **The main fiber groups affected in early gingivitis appear to be:**
    a. The circular and horizontal fibers
    b. The circular and dentogingival fibers
    c. The horizontal and alveolar crest fibers
    d. The dentogingival and alveolar crest fibers
    Ans. b

CLINICAL FINDINGS OF GINGIVITIS

1. **The earliest symptom of gingival inflammation which precedes established gingivitis is:**
   a. Change in color of gingiva
   b. Change in texture of gingiva
   c. Bleeding from the gingival sulcus on gentle probing
   d. Change in position of gingiva
   Ans. c
2. **In most cases the cellular infiltrate of sites that bleed on probing is predominantly:**
   a. Neutrophilic
   b. Lymphocytic
   c. Eosinophilic
   d. Plasma cells
   Ans. b
3. **The gingiva becomes more red than its normal color when there is:**
   a. An increase in vascularization and decrease in degree of epithelial keratinization
   b. An increase in vascularization and degree of epithelial keratinization
   c. A decrease in vascularization and degree of epithelial keratinization
   d. A decrease in vascularization and increase in degree of epithelial keratinization
   Ans. a
4. **Bluish red or deep blue linear pigmentation of the gingival margin is due to:**
   a. Bismuth
   b. Arsenic
   c. Mercury
   d. Lead
   Ans. d

5. **Leathery texture of the gingiva is due to:**
   a. Acute gingivitis
   b. Chronic gingivitis
   c. Hyperkeratosis
   d. Non-inflammatory gingival hyperplasia
   Ans. c
6. **The severity of recession is determined by:**
   a. The actual position of the gingiva
   b. The apparent position of the gingiva
   c. Both of the above
   d. None of the above
   Ans. a
7. **Gingival recession may be caused by:**
   a. Faulty toothbrushing technique
   b. Tooth malposition
   c. High frenum attachment
   d. All of the above
   Ans. d
8. **Me Call's festoons occur most frequently in:**
   a. Incisor areas on the facial surface
   b. Canine and premolar areas on the facial surface
   c. Premolar and molar areas on the facial surface
   d. Incisor and canine areas on the facial surface
   Ans. b
9. **The severity of the bleeding and the ease with which it is provoked depend on the:**
   a. Duration of the inflammation
   b. Position of the inflammation
   c. Intensity of the inflammation
   d. All of the above
   Ans. c
10. **Acute bleeding can occur:**
    a. Only in the absence of gingival disease
    b. Only in the presence of gingival disease
    c. Both in the presence and absence of gingival disease
    d. Neither in the presence nor in the absence of gingival disease
    Ans. b

GINGIVAL ENLARGEMENT

1. **Chronic inflammatory gingival enlargement originates as a slight ballooning of the:**
   a. Attached gingiva
   b. Free gingiva
   c. Interdental papilla and/or marginal gingiva
   d. Interdental papilla and attached gingiva
   Ans. c
2. **Gingival enlargement lesions that are relatively firm, resilient and pink have greater:**
   a. Vascular component
   b. Inflammatory cells
   c. Degenerative changes
   d. Fibrotic component
   Ans. d

3. **Chronic inflammatory gingival enlargement is caused by:**
   a. Dental calculus
   b. Genetic influences
   c. Prolonged exposures to dental plaque
   d. External physical trauma
   Ans. c
4. **The following is the most common site of gingival enlargement due to mouth breathing:**
   a. Maxillary posterior region
   b. Maxillary anterior region
   c. Mundinular posterior region
   d. Mandibular anterior region
   Ans. b
5. **A localized, painful, rapidly expanding lesion that is usually of sudden onset is termed as:**
   a. Gingival hyperplasia
   b. Gingival hypertrophy
   c. Gingival abscess
   d. Gingival ulceration
   Ans. c
6. **Gingival abscess is generally limited to:**
   a. Gingival sulcus
   b. Attached gingiva
   c. Marginal gingiva and interdental papilla
   d. Marginal gingiva and attached gingiva
   Ans. c
7. **Phenytoin induced gingival hyperplasia is absent in:**
   a. Presence of profuse local irritants
   b. Absence of local irritants
   c. Region where teeth are present
   d. Edentulous spaces
   Ans. d
8. **Which of the following drugs induces gingival hyperplasia:**
   a. Phenytoin
   b. Cyclosporine
   c. Nifedipine
   d. All of the above
   Ans. d
9. **In combined gingival enlargement the primary component is:**
   a. Hyperplasia of connective tissue and epithelium
   b. Inflammation of connective tissue
   c. Both of the above
   d. None of the above
   Ans. a
10. **In pregnancy the gingival enlargement tends to be more prominent:**
   a. In interproximal areas
   b. On facial surfaces
   c. On lingual surfaces
   d. Equal enlargement on all surfaces
   Ans. a

11. Tumor like gingival enlargement in pregnancy usually appears after the:
a. First month of pregnancy
b. Third month of pregnancy
c. Second trimester of pregnancy
d. First trimester of pregnancy
Ans. b

12. An exaggerated conditioned response to minor trauma resulting in tumor like gingival enlargement is termed as:
a. Atypical gingivitis
b. Gingivostomatitis
c. Granuloma pyogenicum
d. Granulomatosis
Ans. c

13. True leukemic gingival enlargement occurs commonly in:
a. Acute leukemia
b. Chronic leukemia
c. Both of the above
d. None of the above
Ans. a

14. Most lesions referred to as epulis are:
a. Neoplastic gingival enlargements
b. Malignant gingival enlargements
c. Inflammatory gingival enlargements
d. False gingival enlargements
Ans. c

15. Which of the following is the most common malignant tumor of the gingiva:
a. Malignant melanoma
b. Fibrosarcoma
c. Squamous cell carcinoma
d. Lymphosarcoma
Ans. c

16. Peripheral giant cell granuloma occurs most frequently on the:
a. Interproximal areas
b. Labial surface
c. Lingual surface
d. Col area
Ans. b

ACUTE NECROTIZING ULCERATIVE GINGIVITIS

1. Punched out, crater like depressions at the crest of interdental papillae are found in:
a. Acute necrotizing ulcerative gingivitis
b. Trench mouth
c. Vincent's infection
d. All of the above
Ans. d

2. Which of the following is/are the oral symptoms of acute necrotizing ulcerative gingivitis:
a. Metallic foul taste
b. Crater like depression at interdental papillae
c. Pasty saliva
d. Both (A) and (C)
Ans. d

3. **Systemic signs and symptoms in severe case of acute necrotizing ulcerative gingivitis are:**
   a. Local lymphadenopathy
   b. Slight elevation in temperature
   c. Loss of appetite
   d. Increased salivation
   Ans. c
4. **Which of the following statements is/are not true acute necrotizing ulcerative gingivitis (ANUG).**
   a. ANUG may result in destruction of periodontium
   b. ANUG may result in pulmonary infections
   c. ANUG may lead to periodontal pocket formation
   d. ANUG can be superimposed on periodontal pocket
   Ans. c
5. **Numerous leukocytes with bacteria including spirochetes are found in which of the following zones of necrotic lesion of ANUG:**
   a. ZONE 1
   b. ZONE 2
   c. ZONE 3
   d. ZONE 4
   Ans. b
6. **Diffuse erythema of the posterior areas of the oral mucosa including the gingiva is the clinical feature of:**
   a. Streptococcus gingivostomatitis
   b. Agranulocytosis
   c. ANUG
   d. Gonococcal stomatitis
   Ans. b
7. **The disease common in newborns characterized by oral mucosa covered with grayish membrane that sloughs off exposing bleeding surface is:**
   a. Acute herpetic gingivostomatitis
   b. Gonococcal stomatitis
   c. Vincent's angina
   d. ANUG
   Ans. d
8. **Painful membranous ulceration of the throat with edema and hyperemic patches is found in:**
   a. Vincent's infection
   b. Vincent's stomatitis
   c. Vincent's angina
   d. All of the above
   Ans. c
9. **Loss of soft tissue and bone and formation of sequestra is found in:**
   a. ANUG in leukemia
   b. ANUG in AIDS
   c. Necrotizing ulcerative periodontitis
   d. Chronic destructive periodontal disease
   Ans. b
10. **Which of the following clinical features is not observed in agranulocytosis, that distinguish it from ANUG:**
    a. Ulceration of the gingiva
    b. Necrosis of the gingiva
    c. Severe inflammatory reaction
    d. All of the above
    Ans. c

ACUTE HERPETIC GINGIVOSTOMATITIS

1. **Acute herpetic gingivostomatitis is caused by:**
   a. Herpes simplex virus type 1
   b. Herpes simplex virus type 2
   c. Herpes simplex virus type 6
   d. Cytomegalovirus
   Ans. c
2. **Which of the following oral signs is/are found in acute herpetic gingivostomatitis:**
   a. Edema and gingival bleeding
   b. Erythematous and shiny gingiva
   c. "Soreness" of the oral cavity
   d. Both (A) and (B)
   Ans. c
3. **Painful small ulcers with red, elevated margin and depressed yellowish central portion on the gingiva and the adjacent oral mucosa are found in:**
   a. Chronic desquamative gingivitis
   b. Acute necrotizing ulcerative gingivitis
   c. Streptococcai gingivostomatitis
   d. Acute herpetic gingivostomatitis
   Ans. c
4. **The oral symptom of acute herpetic gingivostomatitis in infants is:**
   a. Soreness of the oral cavity
   b. Pain and sensitivity in ruptured vesicles
   c. Refusal to take food
   d. None of the above
   Ans. c
5. **Diffuse involvement of the gingiva with 'peeling' the epithelial surface is characteristic feature of:**
   a. Erythema multiforme
   b. Desquamative gingivitis
   c. ANUG
   d. Acute herpetic gingivostomatitis
   Ans. b

PERICORONITIS

1. **Pericoronitis occurs most frequently in the:**
   a. Maxillary third molar area
   b. Mandibular third molar area
   c. Maxillary first molar area
   d. Mandibular second molar area
   Ans. b
2. **Red, swollen, suppurating lesion in third molar area with radiating pain to ear, throat and floor of mouth is found in:**
   a. Periodontal abscess
   b. Desquamative gingivitis
   c. Pericoronitis
   d. None of the above
   Ans. c
3. **Abscess spreading posteriorly into the oropharyngeal area and medially to the base of the tongue is:**
   a. Periodontal abscess
   b. Peritonsillar abscess
   c. Pericoronal abscess
   d. Gingival abscess
   Ans. c

4. **Which of the following is/are the clinical features of pericoronitis:**
   a. Swelling of the cheek
   b. Lymphadenitis
   c. Fever and malaise
   d. All of the above
   Ans. d
5. **Primary incubation zone in acute necrotizing ulcerative gingivitis is:**
   a. Periodontal pockets
   b. Pericoronal flaps
   c. Chronic gingival disease
   d. Both (A) and (B)
   Ans. d

CHRONIC DESQUAMATIVE GINGIVITIS AND DERMATOSES

1. **Which of the following is the clinical feature of the moderate form of desquamative gingivitis:**
   a. Diffuse erythema of the gingiva
   b. Bright red and grey patches on the gingiva
   c. Denuded and strikingly red gingiva
   d. Burning sensation in the mouth
   Ans. b
2. **Speckled gingiva with dry and burning sensation throughout the mouth is found in desquamative gingivitis of:**
   a. Mild form
   b. Moderate form
   c. Severe form
   d. None of the above
   Ans. c
3. **Recommended dose of prednisone for the treatment of desquamative gingivitis is:**
   a. Daily dose of 40 mg to 50 mg reduced to daily maintenance dose of 5 to 10 mg
   b. Daily dose of 30 to 40 ma reduced to daily maintenance dose of 5 to 10 mg
   c. Daily dose of 30 to 40 mg reduced to daily maintenance dose of 10 to 20 mg
   d. Daily dose of 50 to 60 mg reduced to daily maintenance dose of 10 to 20 mg
   Ans. b
4. **Grayish white, linear, lace like elevations on the oral mucosa in lichen planus are known as:**
   a. Vesicular lesions
   b. Bullous lesions
   c. Dendritic lesions
   d. None of the above
   Ans. c
5. **Atrophic involvement of gingiva in lichen planus is characterized by:**
   a. Raised white lesion
   b. Thinning of epithelium
   c. Erosive gingivitis
   d. Both (B) and (C)
   Ans. d
6. **Chronic desquamative gingivitis is the oral manifestation of which of the following disease:**
   a. Lichen planus
   b. Bullous pemphigoid
   c. Mucous membrane pemphigoid
   d. All the above
   Ans. d

7. **Purplish red macules or papules with interspersed bullous lesions on oral mucosa are found in:**
   a. Lupus erythematous
   b. Pemphigus
   c. Erythema multiforme
   d. Bullous pemphigoid
   Ans. c
8. **Swollen, bluish red and everted lips with adherent scales and crusts are the clinical feature of:**
   a. Erythema multiforme
   b. Chronic discoid type lupus erythematosus
   c. Acute systemic type lupus erythematosus
   d. Scleroderma
   Ans. b
9. **The oral manifestations of the scleroderma are characterized by:**
   a. Impaired mobility of tongue
   b. Thin and rigid lips
   c. Restricted mouth opening
   d. All the above
   Ans. d
10. **Local reaction from the use of a medicament in the oral cavity is termed as:**
    a. Contact stomatitis
    b. Stomatitis venenata
    c. Stomatitis medicamentosa
    d. Both (A) and (B)
    Ans. d
11. **The most common mycotic infection of the oral mucosa is:**
    a. Acute candidiasis
    b. Chronic candidiasis
    c. Actinomycosis
    d. Histoplasmosis
    Ans. a
12. **The drug of choice for the treatment of chronic candidiasis is:**
    a. Clotrimazole
    b. Mycostatin
    c. Amphotericin B
    d. All of the above
    Ans. c
13. **Large numbers of hyphae and spores of Candida albicansare present at mucosal surface in:**
    a. Hyperplastic type oral candidiasis
    b. Pseudomembranous type candidiasis
    c. Atrophic type candidiasis
    d. Perioral type candidiasis
    Ans. b
14. **Drug of choice for the treatment of oral pemphigus is:**
    a. Diphenhydramine hydrochloride
    b. Methyl prednisolone
    c. Acyclovir
    d. Foscarnet
    Ans. b
15. **Increase in the width of the periodontal space, more often in posterior teeth is found in:**
    a. Diffuse scleroderma

b. Acrosclerosis
c. Circumscribed scleroderma
d. Both (A) and (B)
Ans. d

16. **The interdental gingiva of the deciduous dentition is:**
a. Broad mesiodistally and narrow faciolingually
b. Broad faciolingually and narrow mesiodistally
c. Same as in permanent dentition
d. None of the above
Ans. b

17. **The mean gingival sulcus depth for the primary dentition is:**
a. 2.1 mm ± 0.2 mm
b. 2.5 mm ±0.2 mm
c. 2.1 mm ± 0.4 mm
d. 2.5 mm ± 0.4 mm
Ans. a

PERIODONTAL POCKET

1. **Which of the following is/are the symptoms of periodontal pocket:**
a. Gingival bleeding
b. Tooth mobility
c. Localized pain
d. Diastema formation
Ans. c

2. **Periodontal pocket is generally painful, when explored with a probe because of:**
a. Degeneration of epithelium
b. Ulceration on the inner aspect of the pocket wall
c. Suppurative inflammation of the inner wall
d. None of the above
Ans. b

3. **The soft tissue wall of the periodontal pocket showing flat surface with minor depressions and shedding of cells is seen in:**
a. Areas of ulceration
b. Areas of hemorrhage
c. Areas of relative quiescence
d. Areas of leukocytic bacterial interaction
Ans. c

4. **Excessive pus formation occurs in:**
a. Deep periodontal pockets
b. Shallow periodontal pockets
c. Both (A) and (B)
d. None of the above
Ans. c

5. **The most dominant microorganisms in root surface caries is:**
a. Streptococcus sanguis
b. Fusobacterium nucleates
c. Staphylococcus
d. Actinomycesviscosus
Ans. d

6. **The distance between the bottom of the calculus and the alveolar crest in periodontal pockets is constant, having a mean length of:**
   a. 2 mm ±33.6 percent
   b. 1.97 mm ±43.16 percent
   c. 1.97 mm ±33.16 percent
   d. 2 mm ±43.16 percent
   Ans. c
7. **Localized purulent inflammation in the periodontal tissues is known as:**
   a. Lateral abscess
   b. Periodontal abscess
   c. Parietal abscess
   d. All the above
   Ans. d
8. **The bone destructive pattern is angular in:**
   a. Infrabony pocket
   b. Suprabony pocket
   c. Both of the above
   d. None of the above
   Ans. a
9. **The periodontal cyst occurs most often in:**
   a. Maxillary canine - premolar area
   b. Maxillary incisor canine area
   c. Mandibular canine —premolar area
   d. Maxillary molar area
   Ans. c
10. **In periodontal pocket, bone and connective tissue attachments are lost and pocket deepens during:**
    a. Period of quiescence
    b. Period of exacerbation
    c. Period of inactivity
    d. None of the above
    Ans. b

BONE LOSS IN PERIODONTAL DISEASES

1. **The most common cause of bone destruction in periodontal disease is:**
   a. Bone necrosis
   b. Chronic inflammation
   c. Trauma from occlusion
   d. All the above
   Ans. b
2. **The three wall bone destruction pattern appearing most frequently on second and third maxillary and mandibular molars is known as:**
   a. Hemiseptum
   b. Combined osseous defect
   c. Angular defect
   d. Intrabony defect
   Ans. d
3. **Defects produced by loss of interdental bone, including facial and/or lingual plates without concomitant loss of radieular bone are known as:**
   a. Bulbous bone contours
   b. Ledges
   c. Reversed architecture
   d. Osseous craters
   Ans. c

4. **The most common site of furcation involvement is:**
   a. Mandibular first molars
   b. Maxillary second molars
   c. Mandibular premolar
   d. Maxillary first molar
   Ans. a
5. **The 'cul-de-sac' feature appears in which of the following grades of furcation involvement:**
   a. Grade I
   b. Grade II
   c. Grade III
   d. Grade IV
   Ans. b
6. **Trauma from occlusion resulting from reduced ability of the tissues to resist the occiusal forces is known as:**
   a. Primary trauma from occlusion
   b. Secondary trauma from occlusion
   c. Acute trauma from occlusion
   d. Chronic trauma from occlusion
   Ans. b
7. **Thinning of periodontal ligament, atrophy of fibers and osteoporosis of alveolar bone occur in:**
   a. Trauma from occlusion
   b. Excessive occiusal forces
   c. Insufficient occiusal forces
   d. None of the above
   Ans. c
8. **During pathologic migration, premolars frequently drift:**
   a. Mesially
   b. Distally
   c. Labially
   d. Lingually
   Ans. b
9. **A shift in the position of the tooth may occur due to:**
   a. Pathologic migration
   b. Trauma from occlusion
   c. Pressure from the tongue
   d. All the above
   Ans. d
10. **Plateau like bone margins caused by resorption of thickened bone plates are called:**
    a. Osseous craters
    b. Exostoses
    c. Ledges
    d. Reversed architecture
    Ans. c
11. **The cells responsible for degradation of organic matrix during bone resorption are:**
    a. Osteoclasts
    b. Fibroblasts
    c. Mononuclear cells
    d. All the above
    Ans. c

12. The most common pattern of bone loss in periodontal disease is:
   a. Vertical bone loss
   b. Horizontal bone loss
   c. Osseous defects
   d. Osseous craters
   Ans. b

13. The area of the periodontium most susceptible to injury from excessive occlusal forces is:
   a. Cementum
   b. Inter-radicular bone
   c. Alveolar bone
   d. Furcation
   Ans. d

14. Which of the following statements is not true about trauma from occlusion:
   a. Trauma from occlusion is reversible
   b. Trauma from occlusion doesn't cause pockets or gingivitis
   c. Marginal gingiva is affected by trauma from occlusion
   d. Trauma from occlusion changes the shape of alveolar crest
   Ans. c

15. The most common clinical sign of trauma to the periodontium from occlusion is:
   a. Tooth pain
   b. Increased tooth mobility
   c. Sensitivity to percussion
   d. Tooth wear
   Ans. b

16. "Thickened periodontal ligament, which is funnel shaped at the crest with angular defects in the bone" is observed in which of the following stages of tissue response to occlusal forces:
   a. Stage I
   b. Stage II
   c. Stage HI
   d. Stage IV
   Ans. c

PERIODONTITIS

1. Deep, crater like osseous lesions, mostly located in interdental areas are found in:
   a. Acute necrotizing ulcerative gingivitis
   b. Necrotizing ulcerative periodontitis
   c. Refractory periodontitis
   d. Localized juvenile periodontitis
   Ans. b

2. Periodontitis that does not respond to therapy and recurs soon after adequate treatment is referred to as:
   a. Juvenile periodontitis
   b. Necrotizing ulcerative periodontitis
   c. Rapidly progressive periodontitis
   d. Refractory periodontitis
   Ans. d

3. Which of the following diseases is/are associated with prepubertal periodontitis:
   a. Blood dyscrasias
   b. Papillon-Lefevre syndrome
   c. Hypophosphatasia
   d. All the above
   Ans. d

4. Hyperkeratotic skin lesions, severe destruction of the periodontium with calcification of dura are the characteristic features of:
a. Blood dyscrasias
b. Papillon-Lefevre syndrome
c. Hypophosphatasia
d. All the above
Ans. b

5. Periodontal disease in Down's syndrome is most severe in:
a. Lower anterior region
b. Upper anterior region
c. Lower posterior region
d. Upper posterior region
Ans. a

6. The lesions of localized juvenile periodontitis are mostly found in:
a. Canines and first premolars
b. Second molars and incisors
c. First molars and incisors
d. Second molars and canines
Ans. c

7. The most common initial clinical symptom of early juvenile periodontitis are mostly found in:
a. Canines and first premolars
b. Second molars and incisors
c. First molars and incisors
d. Second molars and canines
Ans. c

8. The most common initial clinical symptom of early juvenile periodontitis is:
a. Deep, dull radiating pain in teeth
b. Deep periodontal pockets
c. Denuded root surface sensitive to thermal and tactile stimuli
d. Migration of first molar and incisor
Ans. d

9. Bacteria considered to be pathogenic in juvenile periodontitis is/are:
a. A. actinomycetemcomitans
b. Capnocytophaga
c. Peptostreptococcus micros
d. Both (A) and (B)
Ans. d

10. Whitish-yellowish soft material that covers the areas of ulceration and necrosis of the gingival margin in ANUG is referred to as:
a. Pyogenic membrane
b. Pseudomembrane
c. Materiaalba
d. None of the above
Ans. b

11. Periodontal destruction associated with Down's syndrome is due to:
a. Defect in T-cell maturation
b. Defect in polymorphonuclear leukocyte chemotaxis
c. Reduced resistance to infection
d. All the above
Ans. d

GENERAL CONSIDERATIONS IN THE MANAGEMENT OF PERIODONTAL DISEASES

1. **Curved Nabers probe is mainly used to:**
   a. Locate subgingival deposits
   b. Measure depth of periodontal pockets
   c. Evaluate horizontal component of furcation areas
   d. None of the above
   Ans. c
2. **Which of the following sickle sealers is used in mandibular anterior area if there is little interproximal space:**
   a. Jaquette sealer
   b. U 15/30 sealer
   c. Ball sealer
   d. Morse sealer
   Ans. d
3. **Gracey curettes number 11–12 are used for:**
   a. Anterior teeth
   b. Posterior teeth facial surface
   c. Posterior teeth distal surface
   d. Posterior teeth mesial surface
   Ans. d
4. **The tip action of piezoelectric ultrasonic unit is:**
   a. Orbital
   b. Linear
   c. Elliptical
   d. None of the above
   Ans. b
5. **The proximal surfaces of the tooth can be polished by:**
   a. Rubber cups
   b. Bristle brushes
   c. Dental tape
   d. Airpowder polishing
   Ans. c
6. **Knife/ves used for interdental areas during gingivectomy is/are:**
   a. Merrifield knife
   b. Kirkland knife
   c. Both (A) and (B)
   d. None of the above
   Ans. c
7. **The finger rest established on tooth surfaces adjacent to the working areas is known as:**
   a. Finger on finger
   b. Cross arch finger
   c. Onventional finger rest
   d. Palm up finger rest
   Ans. c
8. **Stroke used for the removal of both supragingival and subgingival calculus should be:**
   a. Light to moderate pull stroke
   b. Short, powerful pull stroke
   c. Short, moderate push stroke
   d. Powerful push stroke
   Ans. b

9. **The distance between the apical edge of the calculus and the bottom of pocket usually ranges from:**
   a. 0.5 to 1.0 mm
   b. 0.2 to 0.5 mm
   c. 0.2 to 1.0 mm
   d. 0.4 to 0.8 mm
   Ans. c
10. **Sharply defined wedge shaped depression in the cervical area of the facial tooth surface is known as:**
   a. Abrasion
   b. Erosion
   c. Cuneiform defect
   d. None of the above
   Ans. c
11. **Less than adequate remaining bone support, some tooth mobility, and grade I furcation involvement establish one of the following prognosis:**
   a. Excellent prognosis
   b. Good prognosis
   c. Fair prognosis
   d. Poor prognosis
   Ans. c
12. **Periodontal surgery, including placement of implants, is carried out in:**
   a. Phase I therapy
   b. Phase II therapy
   c. Phase III therapy
   d. Phase IV therapy
   Ans. b
13. **Embedding of new periodontal ligament fibers into new cementum and attachment of gingival epithelium to tooth surface is referred to as:**
   a. Epithelial adaptation
   b. Repair
   c. Reattachment
   d. New attachment
   Ans. d
14. **Recommended prophylactic dose of amoxicillin for periodontal procedure in patients at risk for infective endocarditis is:**
   a. 2 to 3 gm orally 1 hour before procedure
   b. 1 gm orally 1 hour before procedure
   c. 3 gm IV 30 minutes before procedure
   d. 2 gm IM 30 minutes before procedure
   Ans. a
15. **Drug of choice for antibiotic prophylaxis for the prevention of infection during periodontal therapy in diabetic patient is:**
   a. Amoxicillin
   b. Erylhromycin
   c. Penicillin
   d. Ampicillin
   Ans. c
16. **Which of the following drugs shows development of loss of alveolar bone in periodontitis:**
   a. Alendronate
   b. Flurbiprofen
   c. Ibuprofen
   d. All the above
   Ans. d

17. A sinus opening onto the gingival mucosa along the length of root and covered by small, pink, bead like mass of granulation tissue is known as:
   a. Acute periodontal abscess
   b. Chronic periodontal abscess
   c. Periapical abscess
   d. Gingival abscess
   Ans. b

NONSURGICAL MANAGEMENT

1. Diameters of bristles of commonly used soft tooth brushes is:
   a. 0.007 inch
   b. 0.010 inch
   c. 0.012 inch
   d. 0.014 inch
   Ans. a

2. Which of the following statements is not true about abrasion of teeth:
   a. Abrasion is more prevalent on maxillary teeth
   b. Abrasion results in saucer shaped indentations with smooth shiny surface
   c. Abrasion is more frequent on left half of the dental arch
   d. Abrasion also occurs on incisal edges
   Ans. d

3. Which of the following brushing techniques is recommended for cleaning in areas with progressive gingival recession:
   a. Bass method
   b. Stillman method
   c. Modified Stillman method
   d. Charters method
   Ans. c

4 The step 4 during the preparation of tooth surface in the initial phase of periodontal therapy is:
   a. Supragingivai removal of calculus
   b. Subgingival root treated
   c. Plaque control instructions
   d. Obturation of carious lesions
   Ans. d

5. Which of the following drugs is most frequently used in treating refractory periodontitis, including localized juvenile periodontitis:
   a. Metronidazole +Amoxicillin
   b. Tetracycline
   c. Ciprofloxacin
   d. Penicillin
   Ans. a

6. The recommended dose of amoxicillin for the treatment of refractory or juvenile periodontitis is:
   a. 250 mg tid
   b. 500 mg bid
   c. 500 mg tid
   d. 250 mg qid
   Ans. a

7. 'Keyes technique' refers to:
   a. Application of various medicaments to root surfaces
   b. Application of slurryof sodium bicarbonate and hydrogen peroxide to tooth surface
   c. Subgingival irrigation by oral mouthwashes
   d. None of the above
   Ans. b

8. **The recommended dose of doxycycline applied to root surface for root bio modification is:**
   a. 100 mg/ml
   b. 50 mg/ml
   c. 150 mg/ml
   d. 25 mg/ml
   Ans. a
9. **The minimal daily dose of chlorhexidine gluconate required to be effective as a rinse in reducing gingivitis may be as low as:**
   a. 10 ml of a 0.1 percent solution
   b. 20 ml of a 0.16 percent solution
   c. 50 ml of a 0.1 percent solution
   d. 50 ml of a 0.2 percent solution
   Ans. c
10. **Concentration of stannous fluoride required for direct pocket iiivage in advanced periodontitis is:**
   a. 0.64 percent
   b. 1.64 percent
   c. 2 percent
   d. 2.64 percent
   Ans. b
11. **The drug (s) of choice for the treatment of acute necrotizing ulcerative gingivitis is/are:**
   a. Amoxicillin 250 or 500 mg every 6 hours
   b. Erythromycin 250 or 500 mg every 6 hours
   c. Metronidazole 250 to 500 mg every 8 hours
   d. All of the above
   Ans. d
12. **Which of the following are referred to as primary in cubation zones in acute necrotizing ulcerative?**
   a. Pre-existing chronic gingival disease
   b. Periodontal pockets
   c. Pericoronal flaps
   d. All the above
   Ans. c
13. **The drug of choice for the treatment of refractory periodontitis in which associated microflora primarily consists of black pigmented bacteria and spirochetes is:**
   a. Tetracycline
   b. Metronidazole
   c. Azithromycin
   d. Ciprofloxacin
   Ans. b
14. **Oral Kaposi's sarcoma is treated by:**
   a. Laser excision
   b. Radiation therapy
   c. Intralesional injection with vinblastine
   d. All of the above
   Ans. d
15. **Reducing the supracontact while restoring the original tooth contour during occlusal adjustment is referred to as:**
   a. Coronoplasty
   b. Grooving
   c. Spheroiding
   d. Pointing
   Ans. c

16. **The flap technique involving an internal bevel incision about 0.5 to 1 mm from the gingival margin for surgical treatment of periodontitis is known as:**
    a. Papilla preservation flap
    b. Modified widman flap
    c. Apically displaced flap
    d. None of the above
    Ans. b
17. **The recommended dose of ibuprofen for pre surgical medication in periodontal patients is:**
    a. 400 mg 1 hour before the procedure
    b. 200 mg 1/2 hour before the procedure
    c. 800 mg 1 hour before the procedure
    d. 400 mg 2 hour before the procedure
    Ans. c
18. **Restoration and epithelialization of sulcus after curettage, takes place in:**
    a. 1 day
    b. 2 to 7 days
    c. 7 to 14 days
    d. 21 days
    Ans. b
19. **Removal of inflamed soft tissue lateral to the gingival pocket wall is known as:**
    a. Coronoplasty
    b. Gingivectomy
    c. Gingival curettage
    d. Subgingival curettage
    Ans. c
20. **Gingivectomy is contraindicated in which of the following conditions?**
    a. Elimination of suprabony periodontal abscesses
    b. Elimination of gingival enlargements
    c. Elimination of suprabony pockets
    d. Elimination of pocket located apical to mucogingival junction
    Ans. d
21. **Complete repair of connective tissue after surgical gingivectomy takes about:**
    a. 5 to 14 days
    b. 4 weeks
    c. 7 weeks
    d. 10 weeks
    Ans. c
22. **The incision made from base to the pocket to the crest of the bone is known as:**
    a. Internal bevel incision
    b. Reverse bevel incision
    c. Crevicular incision
    d. Interdental incision
    Ans. c
23. **Furcation involvement in which interradicular bone is completely absent but the furcation involvement can not be seen clinically, is classified under:**
    a. Grade I involvement
    b. Grade II involvement
    c. Grade III involvement
    d. Grade IV involvement
    Ans. c

24. Which of the following teeth have the most favourable anatomic features for respective therapy?
a. Mandibular first molar
b. Maxillary first molar
c. Maxillary second molar
d. Mandibular second molar
Ans. b

25. Marginal tissue recession that extends beyond the mucogingival junction with no loss of bone or soft tissue in the interdental area is classified under:
a. Class I
b. Class II
c. Class III
d. Class IV
Ans. c

26. Guided tissue regeneration technique for root coverage is indicated when the recession is more than:
a. 3.98 mm apicocoronally
b. 2.98 mm apicocoronally
c. 4.98 mm apicocoronally
d. 4.08 mm apicocoronally
Ans. c

27. The most widely used metal in the manufacturing of the implants is:
a. Gold
b. Platinum
c. Chromium
d. Titanium
Ans. d

28. Screws shaped dental implant, made of commercially pure titanium and applied in two stage surgical procedure is known as:
a. Nobel pharma system
b. ITI system
c. IMZ system
d. Integral system
Ans. d

29. The pontic design with the least affect on the periodontium is the:
a. Ovate pontic
b. Modified ridge lap pontic
c. Sanitary pontic
d. Ridge lap pontic
Ans. c

30. Technique using mixture of bone dust and blood for autogenous bone grafts is known as:
a. Bone blend
b. Osseous coagulum
c. Bone blending
d. None of the above
Ans. b

31. The suturing technique appropriate for the maxillary arch is:
a. Horizontal suture
b. Anchor suture
c. Closed anchor suture
d. Continuous, independent sling suture
Ans. d

32. **Which of the following removable appliances is more hygienic and can be used for patients with less than ideal plaque control?**
 a. The Hawley appliance
 b. The Crozat appliance
 c. Both of the above
 d. None of the above
 Ans. b
33. **The suture-needle and sutures most commonly used in periodontal surgery are:**
 a. Circle curved needle and 50 cotton sutures
 b. 3/8 circle reverse cutting needle and 30 black braided silk
 c. Circle curved needle and 60 absorbable suture
 d. Straight needle and nylon suture
 Ans. b

MISCELLANEOUS

1. **In a healthy gingival, the distance between gingival margin and free gingiva groove is:**
 a. 0.1–0.5 mm
 b. 0.5–1 mm
 c. 0.5–1.5 mm
 d. 1–2 mm
 Ans. d
2. **What is the difference between gingivitis and periodontitis?**
 a. Gingival sulcus
 b. Periodontal pocket
 c. Loss of epithelial attachment
 d. Mobility of tooth
 Ans. c
3. **Which of the following is true is case of AIDS patient?**
 a. Acute pain
 b. Diffuse red lesion of the attached gingiva
 c. Gingiva covered with pseudomembrane
 d. Gingival itching
 Ans. b
4. **Which of the following step should be most preferably taken in root planing procedure?**
 a. Removal of root caries
 b. Removal of necrosed cementum and calculus
 c. Removal of calculus
 d. Removal of dentine
 Ans. b
5. **If periodontal surgery in necessary in case of horizontal bone loss in upper anterior region. Which of the following procedure is the most appropriate?**
 a. Papilla preservation flap
 b. Widman flap
 c. Coronary displaced flap
 d. Gingivectomy
 Ans. a
6. **A young adult shows non-fluctuant, tender and redness swelling in the marginal gingival lesion:**
 a. Periodontal abscess
 b. Periapical abscess
 c. Gingival abscess
 d. Periapical sinus
 Ans. a

7. **Which of the following periodontal diseases does not have calculus:**
   a. ANUG
   b. Chronic adult periodontitis
   c. Juvenile periodontitis
   d. Periodontal abscess
   Ans. c
8. **In which of the following conditions gingivectomy is contraindicated:**
   a. Gingival sulcus beyond mucogingival junction
   b. Enlargement due to acute systemic disease
   c. Papillary enlargement
   d. Enlargement due to chromic systemic disease
   Ans. a
9. **What is the normal average distance between the crest of the alveolar bone and the cementoenamel junction in young adult?**
   a. 1.0 mm
   b. 1.08 mm
   c. 2.08 mm
   d. 2.80 mm
   Ans. b
10. **In which percentage chlorhexidine is used as a mouthwash?**
    a. 2 percent
    b. 0.02 percent
    c. 0.2 percent
    d. 1.0 percent
    Ans. c
11. **Which probe is used to detect the furcation involvement:**
    a. Periodontal probe
    b. Nabers probe
    c. Florida probe
    d. Probe No. 11
    Ans. b
12. **Which of the following areas of the oral cavity are affected by inflammatory papillary hyperplasia?**
    a. Lips
    b. Tongue
    c. Palate
    d. Gingiva
    Ans. d

E-Course MCQs

ENDODONTICS : APICAL FLARE PREPARATION

1. **The file used to explore the apical third of a canal is called a:**
   a. Spreader
   b. Seeker
   c. Endodontic explorer
   d. Endodontics probe
   Ans. b

2. **The file used to explore the apical is normally:**
   a. Size 3 or 5
   b. Size 8 or 10
   c. size 15 or 20
   d. Size 25 or 30
   Ans. b

3. **Which are you NOT looking for when exploring the apical third of a canal?**
   a. Hypercementosis
   b. Branches
   c. Lateral canal opening
   d. Internal root resorption
   Ans. a

4. **You have discovered a canal is curved and have precurved your file accordingly. How can you best tell which direction the file is pointing when inside the tooth?**
   a. By mentally noting which direction the file is curved when inserting it
   b. By looking at the position of the number on the side of the file
   c. By cutting a notch in the rubber stop
   d. By taking a diagnostic radiograph
   Ans. c

5. **If a canal is very narrow, which of the following can be used to make exploration easier?**
   a. Water
   b. Bleach
   c. EDTA
   d. Calcium hydroxide
   Ans. c

6. **In a straight canal, how large should the apical 1mm be prepared to?**
   a. The size of the first file that binds
   b. Two or three sizes larger than this
   c. Size 30
   d. It depends on which tooth is being treated
   Ans. b

7. **Approximately how many canals are curved in the apical third?**
   a. 5%
   b. 30 %

c. 60%
d. 90%
Ans. d

8. **What is the largest size you would normally use in a slightly curved canal?**
   a. 20
   b. 25
   c. 30
   d. 35
   Ans. c

9. **What is the largest size you would normally use in a more curved canal (>20°)?**
   a. 20
   b. 25
   c. 30
   d. 35
   Ans. b

10. **A canal is prepared apically to size 40, It is found that sizes 20 to 35 can pass beyond working length, but size 40 won't, what kind of apical prep is this?**
    a. Apical stop
    b. Apical seat
    c. Open apex
    d. Closed apex
    Ans. a

11. **A canal is prepared apically to size40, It is no found no files between 20 and 40 can pass beyond working length. What kind of apical prep is this?**
    a. Apical stop
    b. apical seat
    c. Open apex
    d. Closed apex
    Ans. a

12. **Which of these instruments would you NOT use to create an apical flare?**
    a. K-flex files
    b. NiTi rotary files
    c. GT files
    d. X files
    Ans. d

13. **What is recapitulation?**
    a. Syringing bleach into a canal to irrigate it and wash out debris
    b. Using a small hand file to loosen dentine shavings
    c. Using a small hand file to smooth the steps on the canal wall
    d. Using a series of hand files to create a tapered preparation
    Ans. b

14. **When creating an apical flare with hand files. What is the technique normally used?**
    a. Crown down
    b. Step down
    c. Tug back
    d. Step back
    Ans. d

15. **To create the flare, large files are used at decreasing lengths. How much is the difference in each length?**
    a. 0.5 mm
    b. 1 mm
    c. 1.5 mm
    d. 2 mm
    Ans. b

16. **When creating the flare by using files of decreasing length, what size file do you normally finish with?**
    a. 40–45
    b. 50–55
    c. 60–70
    d. 80–90
    Ans. c

17. **What is the MAF (Master Apical File)?**
    a. The file used to measure the length of the tooth
    b. The file used to clear debris from the apical region with recapitulating
    c. The first file to bind at working length
    d. The file used to set the final diameter of the apical region preperation
    Ans. d.

18. **When a canal is properly prepared apically to size 30 and adequate circumstance filling is completed, the canal diameter will be:**
    a. A little less than size 30
    b. Same as that of size 30
    c. A little more than size 30
    d. A lot more than size 30
    Ans. c

19. **What is patency filling?**
    a. A small file is pushed through the apex to keep it clear of debris
    b. A small file is used circumferentially on the canal walls to prevent lateral canals from getting blocked
    c. A nickel-titanium rotary file is used as an Archimedes Screw to remove debris from the canal
    d. A small file is used, together with bleach, to recapitulate
    Ans. a

20. **What is 'Resistance Form' in endodontics?**
    a. A shape which resists extrusion of filling through the apex
    b. A shape which resists fracture of the root tip during condensation
    c. A shape which insertion of a plugger for vertical condensation
    d. A shape which allows insertion of a spreader for lateral condensation
    Ans. a

21. **What feature is most important to give a canal resistance form?**
    a. An apical stop
    b. An apical seat
    c. An open apex
    d. The canal walls are tapered
    Ans. d

22. **What taper is created by preparing the apical third with successively larger hand files at decreasing lengths?**
    a. 1 %
    b. 2%
    c. 5%
    d. 10%
    Ans. c

MCQs : AMALGAM

1. **What is an Amalgam?**
   a. A mercury alloy
   b. A silver alloy
   c. An alloy of mercury and silver
   d. An alloy of mercury, silver, tin, zinc, and may be copper
   Ans. a

2. **What is a dental amalgam alloy?**
   a. A mercury alloy
   b. A silver Alloy
   c. An alloy of mercury and silver
   d. An alloy of mercury,silver,tin,zinc and may be copper
   Ans. b

3. **How much copper is in a high-copper dental amalgam alloy?**
   a. 2–12%
   b. 12–32 %
   c. 32–52%
   d. Above
   Ans. b

4. **What is another name for a high-copper dental amalgam alloy?**
   a. Gamma 2
   b. Non gamma 2
   Ans. b

5. **Zinc is often added to improved dental amalgam properties. What happens to a zinc containing low-copper alloy if it gets moisture in it?**
   a. It corrodes
   b. It contracts
   c. It expands
   d. It creeps
   Ans. c

6. **What happens to a zinc containing high-copper alloy if it gets moisture in it?**
   a. It corrodes
   b. It contracts
   c. It expands
   d. It creeps
   e. None of these
   Ans. e.

7. **Which of these is a mixture of lathe-cut and spherical alloy particles?**
   a. Hybrid
   b. Admixed
   c. Gamma 2
   d. Non gamma 2
   Ans. b

8. **When amalgam is polished, the metal crystals at the surface get flattened. This layer is called the:**
   a. Dalby layer
   b. Beelby layer
   c. Triby layer
   d. Whitby layer
   Ans. b

9. Why is there tin in dental amalgam?
- a. To slow down the reaction rate and give adequate working time
- b. To reduce corrosion
- c. To scavenge water molecules
- d. To give the filling strength

Ans. a

10. Which is the gamma 1 phase?
- a. Ag_3Sn
- b. Ag_2Hg_3
- c. AgCu
- d. Cu_6Sn_5
- e. Sn_7Hg

Ans. b

11. Which is the gamma 2 phase?
- a. Ag_3Sn
- b. Ag_2Hg_3
- c. AgCu
- d. Cu_6Sn5
- e. Sn_7Hg

Ans. e

12. What is the most serious problem with restoring posterior teeth with amalgam?
- a. Mercury toxicity
- b. Unaesthetic
- c. Lots of sound tooth needs to be removed
- d. Expansion can cause cusp fracture
- e. Short lifetime compare to many other restorative materials

Ans. c

13. Which is more important when comparing dental amalgam?
- a. Low creep
- b. High compressive strength
- c. High shear strength

Ans. a

14. What is the ration of mercury to alloy?
- a. 0.5:1
- b. 0.75:1
- c. 1:1
- d. 1.25:1
- e. 1.5:1
- f. 2:1

Ans. c

15. What is Trituration?
- a. Mixing
- b. Packing
- c. Carving
- d. Polishing

Ans. a

16. How long before amalgam forms a seal with the tooth?
   a. 1 hour
   b. 24 hour
   c. 1 week
   d. 1 month
   e. 3 months
   Ans. e

MCQs HANDLING MATERIALS : CHEMFILL (GIC)

1. What type of material is ChemFill?
   a. Composite
   b. Compomer
   c. Glass lonomer
   d. Resin Modified Glass Ionomer
   e. Synthetic Porcelain
   Ans. c

2. ChemFill's elasticity (elastic modules) matches that of?
   a. Cementum
   b. Dentine
   c. Enamel
   d. None of these
   Ans. b

3. What is the consistency of chemFill, when used as an restoration?
   a. Very thick
   b. Medium thick
   c. Thin
   d. Runny
   e. Watery
   Ans. a

4. What is the mixing time for ChemFill?
   a. 20 Sec
   b. 40 Sec
   c. 60 Sec
   d. 90 Sec
   Ans. a

5. How does ChemFill set?
   a. Light cured
   b. Chemical cured
   c. Dual cured (i.e. sets quickly with light, slowly without light)
   Ans. b

6. When newly placed, it is essential to protect ChemFill from moisture. How?
   a. Cover with petroleum jelly (Vaseline)
   b. 1 coat of ChemFill Varnish
   c. 2 coats of CehmFil Varnish
   d. Use rubber dam
   Ans. c

7. **How is ChemFill placed into a cavity?**
   a. Place and pack with a flat plastic instrument, then allow to set
   b. Use a matrix or strip to hold it in place
   c. Either way is satisfactory
   Ans. b

8. **Ideally how long must a ChemFill restoration be left before finishing and polishing it?**
   a. 3 minutes
   b. 7 minutes
   c. 1 hour
   d. 24 hours
   Ans. d

9. **What is the minimum time before it can be finished?**
   a. 3 minutes
   b. 7 minutes
   c. 1 hour
   d. 24 hours
   Ans. a

10. **If you have to finish a ChemFill restoration on the same visit, how would prevent heat from polishing?**
   a. Use water spray from the polishing handpiece
   b. Use Vaseline on the restoration
   c. Both of these
   Ans. b

11. **What is the working time for ChemFil?**
   a. 20 Sec
   b. 40 Sec
   c. 60 Sec
   d. 90 Sec
   Ans. a

12. **What liquid is ChemFil powder4 mixed with?**
   a. Polycrylic acid
   b. Phosphoric acid
   c. Unfilled resin
   d. Water
   e. Acetone
   Ans. d

13. **What is the bond strength of ChemFil to dentine? (1 MegaPascal = 1 kg/mm^2)**
   a. 0.1 Mpa
   b. 1 Mpa
   c. 5 Mpa
   d. 10 Mpa
   e. 25 Mpa
   Ans. c

14. **Ideally, what type of margin should be prepared on a cavity before a ChemFil restoration?**
   a. Feather edge
   b. 1 mm bevel
   c. Butt joint
   Ans. c

15. **Which of these would you Not use to finish a ChemFil restoration?**
    a. Steel finishing burs
    b. High speed diamond burs
    c. 3 M 'Enhance' polishing cup and disc
    d. Tungsten Carbide finishing burs
    e. Impregnated rubber points
    f. Abrasive polishing paste
    Ans. a

ENDODONTICS : INFECTION CONTROL AND CORONAL SEAL

1. **What is an amalcore?**
   a. An amalgam restoration that enters and plugs the canal orifice(s)
   b. A cast post with an amalgam on top of it
   c. A pinned amlgam core for a crown
   d. A amalgam that covers the entire occulsal surface of the tooth.
   Ans. c

2. **Why is infection control so expecially important in endodontics?**
   a. To prevent cross infection of the operator and nurse
   b. To allow healing of the per-radicular tissues
   c. To prevent the patient picking up infection from previous patients
   d. To reduce New Variant CJD transmission
   Ans. b

3. **What is meant by aseptic technique?**
   a. Working in a field as near sterile as possible
   b. Limiting infection to the patients own oral bacteria
   c. Ensuring all micro-organisms are removed or killed as part of the procedure
   d. Not introducing any micro organism to the canal that weren't already there before you
   Ans. d

4. **Which is NOT a function of Rubber Dam?**
   a. Preventing saliva contamination
   b. Improving visibility
   c. Confining excess irrigants
   d. Making access to the pulp chamber easier
   e. Improving patient comfort
   f. Reducing mediolegal liability
   Ans. d

5. **What strength of Sodium Hypochlorite (bleach) is used for canal irrigation?**
   a. 1%
   b. 2%
   c. 5%
   d. 10%
   e. 20%
   f. 50%
   Ans. c

6. **About how long does it take bacteria contacting the coronal end of a very well condensed root filling to penetrate through it to apex?**
   a. 1 day max
   b. 1 week max
   c. 6 weeks max
   d. 6 months max
   e. Many years
   Ans. c

7. **If you can't get dam onto a tooth for root treatment, which solution is unacceptable?**
   a. Rstoration tooth first to enable dam placement, them drill access through the new restoration
   b. Crwon lengthening by electrocurgery
   c. Working without dam
   d. Restoring with a copper band
   e. Placing the dam clamp beaks directly onto the gintival
   Ans. c

8. **Which of these is NOT true when Vitrebond is used as a canal orifice sealant?**
   a. Hard to identify if re-treatment is needed
   b. May not be fully set all the way through
   c. Does not bond well to dentine
   Ans. c

9. **What is a hermetic seal as applied to endodontics?**
   a. Airtight
   b. Waterproof
   c. Saliva can't pass
   d. Micro-organisms can't pass
   e. All of these
   Ans. e

10. **If a patient has gingival recession, how far should the guttapercha be trimmed back before sealing the coronal?**
    a. 1 mm below the level of the recession
    b. 1 mm below the ACJ
    c. 1 mm below the canal opening
    d. 1 mm below the roof of the pulp
    Ans. a

11. **What intra-canal medication should normally be placed in the canal between visits?**
    a. Ledermix (combined anti-biotic and anti inflammatory)
    b. Hypocal
    c. Dycal of Life
    d. Para-chloro-mono-phenol (PCMP)
    e. Paper point
    Ans. b

12. **When irrigating with bleach, how far should the needle inserted?**
    a. Into the pulp chamber only
    b. 7 mm from the apex
    c. To the point before it just binds on the canal walls, but must be short of the working length.
    d. To the working length
    Ans. c

13. **Which of these does bleach NOT do?**
    a. Lubricate the canal
    b. Dissolve organic debris
    c. Kill bacteria
    d. Wash out debris
    e. Dissolve sclerosed dentine
    Ans. e.

14. **What needle is used for deliyering bleach when irrigating a canal?**
    a. Side venting wide bore
    b. Side venting narrow bore
    c. End venting wide bore
    d. End venting narrow bore
    Ans. b

15. If a patient has No gingival recession, how far should the gutta-percha be trimmed back before sealing the coronal?
   a. 1 mm below the level of the recession
   b. 1 mm below the ACJ
   c. 1 mm below the canal opening
   d. 1 mm below the roof of the pulp chamber
   Ans. b

16. If you choose to temporarily seal the access cavity of a tooth with Kalzinol, how thick should it be?
   a. 1 mm
   b. 2 mm
   c. 3 mm
   d. 4 mm
   Ans. c

17. Which of these is the material as a temporary dressing for an access cavity after endo is completed?
   a. Life or Dycal
   b. Chemfil
   c. Kalzinol
   d. Poly-F
   Ans. d

18. Which of these pulp locations can be removed mechanically?
   a. Lateral canals
   b. Pulp horns
   c. Cul-de-sacs (dead ends)
   d. Apical Ramifications
   e. Isthmi
   f. Concavities
   Ans. b

19. To control infection during endo, the files must be cleaned between uses. How?
   a. Dry guaze in a ring holder
   b. Gauze dampened with water
   c. Guaze dampened with bleach
   d. Guaze dampened with chlorhexine
   Ans. c

HANDLING MATERIALS : RUBBER DAM

1. You notice during an endo that saliva is creeping through your rubber dam hole. What should you do:
   a. Put on a new piece with a smaller hole
   b. Put in a new piece using thicker dam
   c. Use caulking paste to seal the leak
   d. Use a curved saliva elector in the mouth under the dam
   Ans. c

2. When doing an MO restoration under dam on an upper first premolar, you should apply the dam clamp to the:
   a. Canine
   b. First premolar
   c. Second premolar
   d. Any of these
   e. None of these you must be wedges
   Ans. c

3. **It is essential to lubricate dam before applying it. Which of these is NOT a suitable lubricant?**
   a. Shaving cream
   b. Liquid soap
   c. Hibiscrub
   d. Vaseline
   Ans. d

4. **When doing an endo, how many teeth would you normally have coming through the dam?**
   a. just the one being root treated
   b. 2
   c. 3
   d. As many as possible and practical
   Ans. a

5. **You have problem with dam tearing. What might you consider?**
   a. Using thinner dam
   b. Using thicker dam
   c. Making the holes closer together
   d. Making the holes further apart
   Ans. b

6. **Which of these will make the dam most likely to tear?**
   a. A large tooth
   b. A large clamp
   c. A small hole
   d. A rusty dam puch
   Ans. a

7. **You care having trouble getting the dam between the contact points for four anterior teeth. what might you NOT do?**
   a. Punch the holes closer together
   b. Oush it through with floss
   c. Use lubricant
   d. Use wooden wedges for a short while to separate the teeth
   e. Use an abrasive finishing strip to reduce the contact points
   f. Use an abrasive finishing strip to smooth off rough interproximal fillings
   Ans. e

8. **Where does the metal dam frame go?**
   a. Under the dam
   b. Over the dam
   Ans. b

9. **Which is true?**
   a. The curved parts of the clamp beaks should rest on the tooth
   b. The pointed parts of the clamp beaks should rest on the tooth
   Ans. b

10. **Which of these medical conditions is not relevant when considering use of dam?**
   a. Latex allergy
   b. Sleep apnoea
   c. Claustrophobia
   d. Sinusitis
   e. Emphysema
   Ans. b

11. **You are unable to apply dam to an upper molar that require endodontic treatment. What should you do?**
    a. Advise extraction
    b. Dress the pulp with a mummifying paste and provide a good coronal seal
    c. Continue without dam
    d. Refer the patient to an endodontics specialist
    Ans. d

12. **Which is NOT a function of dam in endodontics?**
    a. Preventing saliva contamination
    b. Improving visibility
    c. Confining excess irrigants
    d. Making access to the pulp chamber easier
    e. Improving patient comfort
    f. Reducing medicolegal liability
    Ans. d

13. **If you can't get dam onto a tooth for root treatment, which solution is unacceptable?**
    a. Restore the tooth first to enable dam placement, then drill access through the new restoration
    b. Crown lengthening by electrosurgery
    c. Working without dam
    d. Restoring with a copper band
    e. Placing the dam clamp beaks directly onto the gingival
    Ans. c

14. **You are providing anterior composite tip restoration, but the dam clamp is in the way. What is the best option?**
    a. Proceed without dam
    b. Use rubber or wooden wedges instead to hold the dam in place
    c. Use adhesive to fix the dam to the gingival
    Ans. b

15. **Which is WRONG way to apply dam using a winglesclamp?**
    a. Put the clamp on the tooth, then pull the dam over it
    b. Place the dam on the tooth with fingers, then position the clamp over it
    c. Attach the dam to the clamp and frame outside the mouth, then put the assembly over the tooth using clamp holders over the dam
    d. Attach the dam to the clamp and frame outside the mouth, then put the assembly over the tooth using clamp holdes under the dam
    Ans. c

16. **When the dam is in place, which of these will further improve the seal to the tooth?**
    a. Placing Vaseline round the tooth margins
    b. Inverting the edge of the dam around the tooth with a small plastic instrument
    c. Leaving strips of floss interproximally
    d. Coating the assembly with cavity varnish
    Ans. b

HANDLING MATERIALS : PARAPOST

1. **What is the minimum acceptable length for a post?**
    a. 5 mm
    b. 7 mm
    c. 9 mm
    d. 5 mm from apical constriction

e. 3 mm from apical constriction
f. The same length as the crown it supports
Ans. b

2. **Parapost drills are:**
a. Side cutting
b. End cutting
Ans. b

3. **A black Parapost drill has the same diameter as which size Gates Glidden drill?**
a. No. 3
b. No. 4
c. No. 5
d. No. 6
Ans. d

4. **Approximately how many roots are curved in the apical third?**
a. 5%
b. 25 %
c. 50%
d. 75 %
e. 95 %
Ans. e

5. **Why is it important to retain as much coronol dentine as possible when preparing a post crown?**
a. To resist post roation
b. To increase post retention
c. To reduce the crowbar effect
d. All of these
Ans. d

6. **Which parapost is used for the impression?**
a. The metal one
b. The smooth plastic one
c. The serrated plastic one
Ans. c

7. **Which parapost is used for the temporary crown?**
a. The metal one
b. The smooth plastic one
c. The serrated plastic one
Ans. a

8. **Which parapost is used for the burn-out post?**
a. The metal one
b. The smooth plasltic one
c. The serrated plastic one
Ans. a

8. **Which post hole design provides the most acceptable antirotation effect?**
a. An antirotation notch
b. An oval cross section in the coronal third
Ans. a

9. **What is the minimum thickness (width) of coronal dentine that can be left?**
a. 0.1 mm
b. 0.5 mm

c. 1 mm
d. 21.5 mm
e. 2 mm
Ans. b

10. **What type of impression should be used in conjunction with the parapost technique?**
    a. One state
    b. Two stage
    Ans. a

11. **How should the impression be removed from the mouth with the parapost technique?**
    a. Snap action
    b. Slowly, in line with the post
    c. By tilting it to break the seal posteriorly
    Ans. b

12. **How should the inside of the post hole be cleared of residual sealer paste and Gutta-Percha strands?**
    a. With a high speed handpiece
    b. With a finishing bur on a speed (RA) handpiece
    c. With a sonic scaler
    d. With hand files and Gates Glidden drills
    Ans. d

ENDODONTIC: THE CORONAL FLARE

1. **What is the point of coronal flare preparation?**
   a. To allow straight line across to the apical third
   b. To remove infected dentine from the walls of the canal
   c. To crease space for a tapered post
   Ans. a

2. **You notice the opening to a canal is very narrow, what should you do?**
   a. Prepare the flare using Gates Gliddens, stepping back from a size 2
   b. Prepare the flare with a NiTI orifice shaper
   c. Pre-enlarge the canal with hand files to size 35 before preparing the flare
   d. Prepare the flare using Gates Gliddens, stepping down from a size 4
   Ans. c

3. **How big is the tip of a size 4 Gates Glidden?**
   a. Size 50
   b. Size 70
   c. Size 90
   d. Size 110
   Ans. d

4. **How big is the tip of a size 2 Gates Glidden?**
   a. Size 50
   b. Size 70
   c. Size 90
   d. Size 110
   Ans. b

5. **Which of these is NOT true about Gates Glidden drills?**
   a. If they fracture, they are easier to retrieve than Rotary NiTi flies
   b. They can be 'swept away' fro danger areas like furcations, unlike most rotary NiTis
   c. They leave a smooth step-free surface on the canal wall
   d. They are cheaper than NiTis
   Ans. c

6. **Which part of an instrument is used to cut dentine when preparing a canal?**
   a. The tip region
   b. The side
   Ans. b

7. **Which statement is false?**
   a. The crown down approach to NiTi orifice shapers reduced transportation of bacterial applicably
   b. Orifice shapers remove shavings with an Archimedes Screw action, aiding debris removal
   c. Orifice shapers are long (25 mm), making them harder to use them on back teeth
   Ans. b

8. **Which of these is NOT likely to occur in the absence of a good coronal flare?**
   a. Zip perforation
   b. Dentine ledge
   c. Elbow
   d. Wall grooving
   e. Through-the-foramen Apical over-instrumentation
   Ans. e

9. **What is a zip perforation?**
   a. A perforation caused by the side of a file going round a curve
   b. A perforation caused by the tip of a file that was used too heavily
   c. A perforation of the pulp chamber floor, often caused by using an over-large. Gates Glidden
   d. A perforation of the pulp chamber floor, often caused by making the access cavity too deep
   Ans. a

10. **What can cause a ledge?**
   a. Using a file that is too thick
   b. Failure to create a proper coronal flare before exploring the apical region
   c. Using a file that is inflexible
   d. Failure to irrigate and recapitulate between every instrument
   e. All of these
   Ans. b

HANDLING MATERIALS: ACID ETCH

1. **What acid is normally used to etch teeth in restorative dentistry?**
   a. Using a file that is too thick
   b. Acetic acid
   c. Phosphoric acid
   d. Hydrochloric acid
   e. Poly-acrylic acid
   Ans. c

2. **What strength of this acid a normally used to etch teeth is restorative dentistry?**
   a. 1%
   b. 5%
   c. 10%
   d. 20%
   e. 35%
   f. 50%
   Ans. b

3. **When etching enamel, approximately how long should the acid be in place?**
   a. 10 sec
   b. 25 sec
   c. 40 sec
   d. 60 sec
   e. 90 sec
   Ans. b

4. **What is 'conditioner'?**
   a. Acid
   b. Alcohol
   c. Dentine priming agent
   d. Dentine bonding agent
   e. Acetone
   Ans. a

5. **When etching dentine, approximately how long should the acid be in place?**
   a. 10 sec
   b. 25 sec
   c. 40 sec
   d. 60 sec
   e. 90 sec
   Ans. a

6. **When washing the acid off a tooth, approximately how long should you spray water?**
   a. 5 sec
   b. 10 sec
   c. 30 sec
   d. 60 sec
   e. 90 sec
   Ans. c

7. **What is the point of the water spraying?**
   a. T ensure all the acid is washed off
   b. To ensure the calcium phosphate precipitates caused by the etching are washed away
   c. Both of these
   Ans. c

8. **How deep is the minor-porous layer created by etching the enamel (in micrometers)?**
   a. 0.5–5
   b. 5–50
   c. 50–500
   d. 500–5000
   Ans. b

9. **How much general surface enamel is removed by etching (in micrometers)?**
   a. 0.1
   b. 1
   c. 10
   d. 100
   Ans. c

10. **How dry should enamel be after etching and before placement of a bonding resin?**
   a. Absolutely
   b. Almost dry

c. Slightly moist
d. Wet
Ans. a

11. **What is the appearance of correctly etched enamel?**
a. Frosted
b. Blotchy
c. Speckled
d. Translucent
Ans. a

12. **Why is etch usually presented as a gel instead of a solution:**
a. To make identification easier
b. To allow better control over placement
c. To entrance and concentrate the action of the acid
d. To make it easier to wash off
Ans. b

13. **Why is the etch gel colored?**
a. To make identification easier
b. Legal requirement
c. The color changes when etching is completed
Ans. a

14. **How should you protect adjacent teeth from being etched?**
a. Rubber dam
b. Vaseline
c. Mylar matrix strip
d. Cavity varnish
Ans. c

15. **How should the patient he protected from the acid when it is being washed off?**
a. Excess should be wiped off with cotton wool first
b. Rubber dam should be used
c. Protective glasses
d. Full size bib
e. High speed aspiration
Ans. e

16. **How should the pulp be protected from etch in a very deep cavity?**
a. Line it with Life or Dycal (Calcium hydroxide liner)
b. Line it with Life or Dycal, covered with Vitrebond (a light curred resin modified glass ionomer)
c. Line it with Kalzino (Zinc, oxide/eugenol)
d. Protect it with Copalite (cavity varnish)
e. Protect it with Vitrebond
Ans. b

17. **What type of enamel (restoration bond is created when an acid-etch technique is used?**
a. Chemical (Ionic)
b. Chemical (Hydrogen)
c. Chemical (Covalent)
d. Micro-mechanical
Ans. d

HANDLING MATERIALS: BONDING COMPOSITE TO TEETH

1. **What does Enamel Bonding Agent (EEA) consist of?**
   a. Unfilled resin
   b. A mixture of resin in an acetone or ethanol solvent
   c. A wetting agent and resins
   d. A mixture of printing and bonding agents
   Ans. a

2. **Which of these products in an EEA?**
   a. Prime and Bond
   b. Durafill
   c. One step
   d. Liner bond
   e. Gluma
   Ans. b

3. **Etched enamel does not 'wetting' before the Enamel Agent in applied. Why not?**
   a. It has a high surface free energy
   b. It has a low surface free energy
   c. Enamel Bonding Agent has low surface tension
   d. The negative charge in EEA is attracted to the positive Calcium irons in etched enamel
   Ans. a

4. **What is the bond strength achievable using EEA on etched enamel? (1 MPa =1 kg/mm^2)**
   a. 1 MPa
   b. 5 MPa
   c. 15 MPa
   d. 30 MPa
   Ans. d

5. **What is the approximate stress caused by polymerization contraction of composite?**
   a. 1 MPa
   b. 5 MPa
   c. 15 MPa
   d. 30 MPa
   Ans. b

6. **Does the bond strength of EEA to enamel exceed the contraction stress of polymerized composite?**
   a. No
   b. About equal
   c. Yes, slightly
   d. Yes, greatly
   Ans. d

7. **Can a dentine bonding system be used on etched enamel?**
   a. Yes
   b. No
   Ans. a

8. **Which of these is NOT an advantage of EEA over dentine bonding systems?**
   a. Less marginal leakage
   b. Better color stability

c. Higher bond strength
d. Easier to apply
e. Cheaper
f. Less moisture sensitive
Ans. f

9. **A dentine 'Primer'**
a. Etches the dentine
b. Raises the surface free energy of (i.e. 'wets) the dentine
c. Removes the smear layer
d. Bonds the composite
e. Conditions the dentine
Ans. b

10. **A dentine 'Conditioner' in:**
a. Removes the smear layer
b. Raises the surface free energy of the dentine
c. Bonds the composite
d. Thinly coats the collagen fibrils with resin
Ans. a

11. **The resin in EEA is usually:**
a. HEMA
b. Bis-GMA
c. PENTA
d. Di-Methyl Methacrylate
e. Methyl Methacrylate
Ans. b

12. **The resins in a Dentine Bonding system Primer:**
a. Have a high molecular weight
b. Are viscous
c. Have high surface tension
d. Are hydrophilic
Ans. d

13. **The solvent that helps dentine 'wetting' in DBS's in often:**
a. Water
b. Acetone or Ethanol
c. Carbon Tetrachloride
d. Ethylamine
e. Low molecular weight resin
Ans. b

14. **Including etching, how many stages are involved in dentine bending?**
a. 2
b. 3
c. 4
d. Varies with different systems
Ans. d

HANDLING MATERIALS: CALCIUM HYDROXIDE

1. **Which of these is NOT a form of Calcium Hydroxide?**
a. Life
b. Dycal

c. Hypocal
d. Caitosol
e. Apexit
Ans. d

2. **Calcium hydroxide causes production of tertiary dentine – How?**
a. By direct stimulation of odonotiblasts
b. By killing bacteria, allowing natural healing processes to occur
c. By sealing dentinal tubules
Ans. b

3. **Why is calcium hydroxide anti-bacterial?**
a. Calcium irons disrupt bacterial metabolism
b. It has a high pH
c. It is acidic
Ans. b

4. **Approximately how long does the antibacterial effect of a calcium hydroxide lining last?**
a. 2 days
b. 2 weeks
c. 2 months
d. 2 years
e. Permanently
Ans. c

5. **Which these is NOT a good use for calcium hydroxide?**
a. Lining under an amalgam restoration
b. Dressing inside a root canal in between visits
c. Promoting apical closure in a young non vital tooth
d. Pulp capping
e. Lining under a composite restoration
Ans. a

6. **Which of close is NOT essential for a successful direct pulp cap?**
a. There should be no spontaneous pain from the tooth
b. When stimulated by hot or cold, the pain should disappear as soon as the stimulus is removed.
c. Bleeding from the pulp should be minimal and easily controlled
d. The exposure must be traumatic, i.e. no infected dentine present
e. Hard leathery infected dentine should be present
Ans. e

ENDODONTICS : PREPARING THE MASTER CONE

1. **What is meant by 'Friction Fit'?**
a. A gentle resistance to withdrawal of the master cone
b. A firm resistance to withdraw of the master cone
c. A good fit of the master cone in the apical third of the canal
Ans. a

2. **What is meant by 'Tug Back'?**
a. A gentle resistance to withdrawal of the master cone
b. A firm resistance to withdrawal of the master cone
c. A good fit of the master cone in the apical third of the canal
Ans. b

3. **What is the taper of a standard GP cone?**
   a. 0%
   b. 1%
   c. 2%
   d. 5%
   e. 10%
   Ans. c

4. **You have prepared the apical 1mm of a canal with a size 30 Master File. What size master cone, would you expect to fit?**
   a. Size 25
   b. Slightly less than size 30
   c. Size 30
   d. Slightly more than size 30
   Ans. d

5. **What is the ISO color code for size 25?**
   a. White
   b. Yellow
   c. Red
   d. Blue
   e. Green
   f. Black
   Ans. c

6. **You have trimmed 1mm off a standard size 30 cone and found it is now a friction fit region of a canal you prepared. What is the diameter of your apical region preparation?**
   a. 0.28 mm (size 29)
   b. 0.29 mm (size 29)
   c. 0.30 mm (size 30)
   d. 0.31 mm (size 31)
   e. 0.32 mm (size 32)
   Ans. e

7. **How wide is the tip of a size 20 Mater cone?**
   a. 0.02 mm
   b. 0.2 mm
   c. 2 mm
   d. 20 mm
   Ans. b

8. **You have prepared an apical region to size 25. What is the first cone you would try in?**
   a. Size 20
   b. Size 25
   c. Size 30
   d. Size 35
   Ans. c

9. **If a canal is prepared to a 5% taper, why not use a 5% master cone instead of the Standard when obturating by cold lateral condensation?**
   a. Cold lateral condensation would be very difficult
   b. Sealant would be expressed through the apex
   c. It would be too rigid to negotiate curved canals
   d. They are very expensive
   Ans. a

10. Recommended master cone sizes for upper central incisor fall in the range of:
   a. Size 8 to 15
   b. Size 20 to 30
   c. Size 35 to 60
   d. Size 65 to 90
   Ans. c

11. Which statement is true about an apical seat?
   a. The master cone will go further than the working length
   b. The master cone stops at working length, but smaller ones go further
   c. The master cone, and smaller ones, all stop at the working length
   d. The master cone will not reach the working length
   Ans. b

12. Standard files have a 2% taper. What is the percentage taper you create when you step back by 1 mm per file?
   a. 1%
   b. 2%
   c. 4%
   d. 5%
   e. 10%
   Ans. d

13. When checking the taper of a prepared canal with a finger spreader, how for would go the instrument?
   a. To the apex
   b. To working length
   c. To 1mm short of working length
   d. 2/3rds down the root
   Ans. c

14. When checking that the taper is adequate, and that lateral condensation is possible?
   a. Place the master cone, then check the spreader reaches the desired length alongside it
   b. Place the spreader into the empty canal
   Ans. b

15. Approximately how much sealer paste would you place on the Master Cone prior to its insertion.
   a. The length of the canal
   b. The length of the tooth
   c. 5 mm
   d. 2 mm
   e. 1 mm
   Ans. c

DENTAL PATHOLOGY MCQs

1. Which one of the following would normally be found in the oral cavity of a newborn baby?
   a. Actinomycesviscosus
   b. Streptococcus sanguis
   c. Streptococcus salivarius
   Ans. c

2. (i) The acquired pellicle is normally 1-3 mm thick
   (ii) The acquired pellicle attains its full thickness within approximately two hours of prophylaxis
   a. Only (i) is true
   b. Only (ii) is true

c. Both (i) and (ii) are true
d. Both (i) and (ii) are false
Ans. b

3. **Which one of the following is the normal serum fluoride concentration in the absence of a dietary fluoride supplement?**
   a. 0.1 ppm
   b. 0.1 ppm
   c. 1.0 ppm
   d. 2.0 ppm
   e. 5.0 ppm
   Ans. b

4. **Which one of the following is an histological feature of dentine caries?**
   a. Liquelaction foci
   b. Transverse clefts
   c. Cholesterol clefts
   Ans. c

5. **Flaque extracelluar polysacoharide synthesis is greatest when which one of the following sugars is present in the diet?**
   a. Glucose
   b. Manose
   c. Fructose
   d. Sucrose
   e. Sorbitol
   Ans. d

6. **Which one of the following occurs earliest in caries of dentine?**
   a. Beading of tubules
   b. Invasion of pioneer bacteria
   c. Initial dermineralization
   d. Liquefaction foci
   Ans. c

7. **Which one of the following becomes more prominent in various enamel?**
   a. Striae of Retzius
   b. Hunter Scherger band
   c. Imbrication lines of Pickerill
   d. Striae of Wickham
   e. Dead tracts of Fish
   Ans. a

8. **Which statement is true?**
   a. An apical granuloma always precedes a radicular cyst
   b. An apical granuloma may not precede a radicular cyst
   c. An apical granuloma never precedes a radicular cyst
   Ans. a

9. **Tertiary dentine:**
   a. Can be observed in routine intraoral radiographs
   b. Can be observed in demineralized histological sections
   c. Is inimically deposited as secondary dentine
   d. Starts begin deposited with the onset of early enamel carious lesions
   Ans. b

10. **Regarding pulp inflammation:**
    A. The size of the apical vessels in the pulp
    B. Rigidity of pulp chamber due to dentine walls
    a. Only A influences pulp inflammation
    b. Only B influences pulp inflammation
    c. Both A and B influence pulp inflammation
    d. Neither A nor B influence pulp inflammation
    Ans. c

MATERIALS THEORY: GLASS IONOMER CEMENTS

1. **Which of these is a more proper name for Glass Ionomer?**
   a. Glass Polyalkelete
   b. Glass Polyalkenate
   c. Glass Polyalkencate
   d. Glass Polyalkenite
   Ans. c

2. **Why is GIC called a cement?**
   a. It sticks to teeth tissues
   b. It sets with an acid base reaction in a water solvent
   c. It can be used to cement crowns, bridges etc.
   Ans. b

3. **Which of these irons it NOT released from the glass filler with GIC seta?**
   a. Aluminium
   b. Calcium
   c. Fluoride
   d. Zinc
   e. Silicate
   f. Sodium
   Ans. d

4. **What type of bond joins (cross0links) the polymer matrix together when GIC is set?**
   a. Ionic
   b. Covalent
   c. Hydrogen
   d. Micromechanical
   Ans. a

5. **Which of these are most involved in the GIC polymer cross-links?**
   a. Aluminium and Calcium
   b. Aluminium and Sodium
   c. Sodium and Calcium
   d. Fluoride and Silicate
   e. Calcium and Zinc
   f. Carboxylate
   Ans. a

6. **What is a main feature of the polymer of GIC?**
   a. Alkaline
   b. Acidic
   c. Acid soluble
   d. Neutral pH
   Ans. b

7. **What is a main feature of the glass filler in GIC?**
   a. Silane coated
   b. Acidic
   c. Acid soluble
   d. Neutral pH
   Ans. c

8. **Which is the most useful feature of GIC?**
   a. Adheres to tooth tissues
   b. Release fluoride
   c. GIC elasticity matches dentine's elasticity
   d. Good biocompatibility
   Ans. a

9. **When fluoride ions leach out of GIC, what replaces them?**
   a. Aluminium ions
   b. Hydroxyl ions
   c. Carboxylate ions
   d. Silicate ions
   Ans. b

10. **What does 'chelate' means when we say 'GIC chelates calcium atoms?**
   a. Dissolve
   b. Replace
   c. Grab
   d. Ionise
   e. Preciptate
   Ans. c

11. **Which part of a GIC bonds to dentine?**
   a. Carboxylic groups of the polymer chains
   b. Metal ions
   c. Unsaturated carbon carbon bonds
   d. Polymer Cross-links
   Ans. a

12. **Which of these is NOT true about GIC?**
   a. Brittle
   b. Lo tensile strength
   c. Law fracture toughness
   d. Poor long term aesthetics
   e. Very technique sensitive
   f. Poor marginal seal
   Ans. f

13. **Which of these is a RM-GIC?**
   a. Vitemer
   b. Dyract
   c. Gluma
   d. Chemfil
   e. Herculite
   f. Fuji IX
   Ans. a

14. **What is the typical bond strength of GIC to enamel?**
    a. 1 MPa
    b. 5 MPa
    c. 15 MPa
    d. 30 MPa
    Ans. b

15. **What is the typical bond strength of GIC to dentine?**
    a. 1 MPa
    b. 5 MPa
    c. 15 MPa
    d. 30 MPa
    Ans. b

16. **Which is the best material for treatment of non-carious class V cavities in unstable acid erosion cases?**
    a. GIC
    b. RM-GIC
    c. Compomer
    d. Composite
    Ans. d

MCQs – COMPOSITE

1. **What is the Matrix in Composite?**
   a. The resin into which the filler particles are inserted
   b. A transparent strip which holds it against the tooth
   c. The polymerization initiator
   d. An energy source for machines
   Ans. a

2. **What is the Matrix usually made of?**
   a. HEMA
   b. Mylar
   c. EDTA
   d. Bis-GMA
   e. Celluloid
   Ans. d

3. **In composites what are the filler particles made of?**
   a. Methacryclate resins
   b. Glass
   c. Glass Ionomer
   d. Titanium Dioxide
   Ans. b

4. **What is the initiator?**
   a. Light
   b. A chemical which starts the polymerization reaction
   c. Either of these
   Ans. b

5. **How are the filler particples joined to the matrix?**
   a. Micro-mechanical retention
   b. Biploar bond
   c. With a silane coupling egent
   d. The outside of the particles is dissolved and a metal ionic bond is formed
   Ans. c

6. **What is the typical particle size in microfilled composite, in micrometers?**
   a. 0.04
   b. 0.4
   c. 4
   d. 40
   Ans. a

7. **What is special about a hybrid composite?**
   a. It is a mixture of composite and compomer
   b. It contains both large and small filler particles
   c. The matrix is a mixture of Bis-GMA and TEG-GMA
   d. The filler particles are a mixture are a mixture of glass and Silicon Dioxide
   Ans. b

8. **What is special about a posterior composite?**
   a. It is dual-cured
   b. It is very heavly filled
   c. If flows easily during placement
   d. It is cured outside the mouth and cemented into the tooth
   Ans. b

9. **Which of these lining materials should not be used with composite?**
   a. Life
   b. Poly-F
   c. Vitrebond
   d. Kalzinol
   e. Zinc phosphate
   Ans. d

10. **What is the maximum thickness of composite that a curing light can polymerize?**
    a. 0.5 mm
    b. 1 mm
    c. 2 mm
    d. 3 mm
    Ans. c

11. **What is the approximate polymerization contraction stress when composite sets?**
    a. 1 MPa
    b. 5 MPa
    c. 15 MPa
    d. 30 MPa
    Ans. c

12. **What is NOT a common result microleakage at a composite margin?**
    a. Secondary caries
    b. Sensitivity
    c. Staining
    d. Enamel fracture
    Ans. d

MCQs COMPOMER

1. **Which of these is a compomer?**
   a. Herculite
   b. Gluma

c. Fuji IX
d. Dyract
e. Vitremer
Ans. c

2. **How does compomerset?**
   a. Acid-base reaction
   b. Polymer chains cross linked with metal ions
   c. Polymerization of methacrylates resins
   d. Precipitation of soluble ions
   Ans. a

3. **What is the most useful property of compomer?**
   a. Release fluroide
   b. Handles easily
   c. Bonds to enamel and dentine
   Ans. b

4. **Does the bond strength to dentine when a DBS is used exceed the contraction stress of polymerized composite?**
   a. No
   b. About equal
   c. Yes
   Ans. c

5. **Which of these does acid etch NOT do to dentine?**
   a. Remove the smear layer
   b. Open up the dentinal tubules
   c. Expose collagen fibrils
   d. Increase the surface free energy
   Ans. d

6. **Bond strength of DBS to dentine is?**
   a. 1 Mpa
   b. 5 Mpa
   c. 15 Mpa
   d. More than 15 Mpa
   Ans. d

ENDODONTICS : WORKING LENGTH

1. **How far short of the enatomical apex would one normally prepare the root canal?**
   a. 0 mm
   b. 0.5 mm
   c. 1 mm
   d. 1.5 mm
   e. 2 mm
   f. 3 mm
   Ans. c

2. **When estimating the working length of a tooth?**
   a. The estimate should be the as the true working length
   b. The estimate should err on the long side
   c. The estimate should err on the short side
   d. It doesn't matter because the canal preparation does not start until the true working length is known
   Ans. c

3. **To estimate a working length:**
   a. At undistorted pre-op radiograph is essential
   b. Knowledge of the average length of teeth is sometimes enough. If the radiograph a distorted
   Ans. b

4. **When estimating working length using a parallel technique radiograph, how much enlargement of the image is allowed for?**
   a. None
   b. 1 mm
   c. 2 mm
   d. 3 mm
   Ans. c

5. **If a canal was curved away from the lean to a pre-up radiograph how would this affect you estimated working length?**
   a. It would be on the short side
   b. It would have no effect
   c. It would be on the ling side
   Ans. a

6. **When estimating working length from your knowledge of average lengths of teeth and a blasting angle radiograph, which of these would you NOT make an allowance for?**
   a. Apical root resorbtion
   b. Incisal wear
   c. Incisal fracture
   d. Canal calcluli pulp stones
   e. Elongation or foreshortening on the radiograph
   f. Hypercementosis
   Ans. d

7. **Which of these is the canal reference point for a molar?**
   a. Level of access cavity
   b. A cusp tip
   c. A rubber stop
   d. A graduated 'seeker' file
   Ans. b

8. **To obtain the estimated working length from a Parallel technique radiograph one subtracts how much from the tooth image's length?**
   a. 0 mm
   b. 1 mm
   c. 2 mm
   d. 3 mm
   Ans. d

9. **For canines, it is usually side to introduce a file:**
   a. 15 mm
   b. 18 mm
   c. 20 mm
   d. 22 mm
   Ans. c

10. **For all other teeth (not canines), it is usually safe to introduces of file:**
   a. 16 mm
   b. 18 mm
   c. 20 mm
   d. 22 mm
   Ans. b

11. **A tooth has apical root resorption, when judging the working length, it will probably be:**
   a. When it usually is i.e. 1mm short of the apex
   b. More than this
   c. Less than this
   Ans. b

12. **The true working length is determined with an apex locator and a side 8 or 10 file:**
   a. After access to the canal orfice has been made
   b. After the coronal 2/3" has been shaped
   c. After the apical 1/3rd has been shaped
   Ans. b

13. **The true working length is condoned with a radiograph using a:**
   a. Size 8 file
   b. Size 10 file
   c. Size 15 file
   d. Size 25 file
   Ans. c

14. **The filel must be repositioned and a new working length radiograph takes if it is short of the true working length by:**
   a. 1 mm
   b. 2 mm
   c. 3 mm
   d. 4 mm
   e. 5 mm
   Ans. c

15. **A.W.L radiograph has a file inserted 17 mm. It is 2.5 mm short of the anatomical apex. What is the true working length?**
   a. 17 mm
   b. 18 mm
   c. 18.5 mm
   d. 19 mm
   e. 19.5 mm
   f. 20.5 mm
   Ans. c

16. **With a multi canal teeth:**
   a. Each root requires a separate W.I radiograph
   b. All roots should be measured an one radiograph, using their nearest cusp (If positive) as a landmark
   c. All roots should be measured on one radiograph using the some cusp if positive as a landmark
   Ans. c

17. **Which of these would NOT sometimes give a false reading on an electronic apex 'locater?**
   a. Lateral canal
   b. Root fracture

c. Contact with metal restoration
d. Fluid in canal
f. Canal calculus (pulp stones)
Ans. b

18. In endodontics, what level of accuracy is reasonably achievable with good technique?
a. ± 0.1 mm
b. ± 0.25 mm
c. ± 0.5 mm
d. ± 1 mm
e. ± 1.5 mm
Ans. b

Q1. What is the objective of coronal access?
a. To expose and unroof the pulp chamber to gain visibility, inclulding removal of pulp horns
b. To locate the canal openings
c. To enable a small file to be placed down the canal openings
Ans. a

Q2. What instrument is NOT ever needed for access preparation?
a. High speed diamond burs
b. RA Steel round burs
c. Gates Glidden Drills
d. Long shank burs
e. Swan neck burs
Ans. c

Q3. How can you identify dentine on the floor of the pulp chamber in a molar?
a. It is smooth
b. It is grey
c. It is knobbly
d. It is dark brown
e. It is hard
Ans. b

Q4. What shape is the access cavity for upper and lower incisors?
a. Triangular
b. Ovoid
c. Round
d. Oblong
Ans. a

Q5. What shape is the access cavity for upper and lower canines?
a. Triangular
b. Ovoid
c. Round
d. Oblong
Ans. b

Q6. What shape is the access cavity for upper and lower premolars?
a. Triangular
b. Ovoid
c. Round
d. Oblong
Ans. d

Q7. What shape is the access cavity for upper and lower molars?
a. Triangular
b. Ovoid
c. Round
d. Oblong
Ans. a

Q8. How many upper incisors have two canals?
a. 5%
b. 5%
c. 25%
d. 50%
e. 75%
f. 95%
Ans. a

Q9. How many lower incisors have two canals?
a. Hardly any
b. 5%
c. 25%
d. 50%
e. 75%
f. 95%
Ans. d

Q10. Where is an 'extra' canal often found in upper molars?
a. Mesiobuccal root
b. Distobuccal root
c. Palatal root
d. Mesiolingal root
Ans. a

Q11. The opening of the distal canal(s) in molars is usually directly under:
a. The distal marginal ridge
b. The centre of the tooth
c. The buccal groove
d. The palatal fissure
e. The cusp of Caribelli
Ans. b

Q12. Upper first premolars usually have:
a. One canal
b. Two canals
c. Three canals
Ans. b

Q13. Upper second premolars usually have:
a. One canal
b. Two canals
c. Three canals
Ans. a

Q14. If the canal orifice in an upper second premolar appears under the buccal cusp, one might suspect:
a. Pulpal sclerosis
b. A palatal canal
c. Internal resorbtion
Ans. b

Q15. When preparing an access cavity, you find what appears to be the canal opening much earlier than expected. What might explain this?
a. Incorrect measurement of the pre-op radiograph
b. You have hit a pulp horn
c. Internal resorbtion
Ans. b

Q16. When preparing an access cavity, you come across an orange-yellow slurry inside the pulp chamber. What is it likely to be?
a. Pus
b. Ledermix placed by a previous dentist
c. Necrotic pulp
d. Unset composite resin
Ans. b

Q17. True or false? After entering the pulp chamber, an option is to continue preparation without water spray.
a. True
b. False
Ans. a

Q18. True or false? You should not normally extend the access for anterior teeth under the cingulum.
a. True
b. False
Ans. b

Q19. Why is often advisable to remove an artificial crown from a tooth before preparing an access cavity?
a. Metal shavings may drop into the canal
b. The metal will create false readings when the electronic apex locator is used
c. The tooth may be rotated or tilted under the crown, and the crown just makes it look straight.
d. Dam clamps may loosen the crown
Ans. c

Q20. To find pulp horns, which instrument is most useful?
a. A Briault probe
b. A file with a curved tip
c. A small round bur
d. A Hedstrom file
Ans. a

COHEN's MCQs

DIAGNOSTIC PROCEDURES

1. **A cold test best localizes:**
   a. Pain of pulpal origin
   b. Periodontal pain
   c. Pulp necrosis
   d. Referred pain
   Ans. a

2. **Anesthetic testing is most effective in localizing pain:**
   a. To a specific tooth
   b. To the mandible or maxilla
   c. Across the midline of the face
   d. To a posterior tooth
   Ans. b

3. **Dental history taking:**
   a. Is less important than X-ray examination
   b. Has as its principal goal to identify the offending tooth
   c. Principally assess intensity of pain
   d. Focuses heavily on the quality of pain
   Ans. b

4. **Percussion testing:**
   a. Differentiates pain of periodontal origin
   b. Stimulates proprioceptive fibers in the periodontal ligament
   c. Indicates tooth fracture
   d. Must be performed with a blunt instrument
   Ans. b

5. **Areas of rarefaction are evident on X-ray examination when:**
   a. The tooth is responsive to cold
   b. The tooth is responsive to heat
   c. A tooth fracture has been identified
   d. The cortical layer of bone has been eroded
   Ans. d

6. **An area of rarefaction in the lower premolar areas indicates:**
   a. Definite pathology
   b. Torus mandibularis
   c. Possible mental foramen
   d. Root fracture
   Ans. c

7. **Percussion palpation, and thermal testing:**
   a. Are not to be performed on patients with pacemakers
   b. Should involve testing of contralateral teeth for comparison
   c. Are best compared when using ipsilateral teeth
   d. obviate radiographs
   Ans. b

8. **Irreversible pupitis is often defined by:**
   a. A moderate response to percussion
   b. A strong painful response to cold that lingers
   c. A strong painful response to cold
   d. A response to heat
   Ans. b

9. **Medical history of heart disease is significant:**
   a. And contraindicates endodontic treatment
   b. For referred pain to the left mandible indicating possible myocardial infarction
   c. And indicates the need for premedication with antibiotics
   d. And contraindicates local anesthetic with epinephrine
   Ans. b

10. **The best approach for diagnosis of odontogenic pain is:**
    a. X-ray examination
    b. Percussion
    c. Visual examination
    d. A step-by-step sequenced examination and testing approach following the same procedure
    Ans. d

11. **Calcification of the pulp:**
    a. Is a response to aging
    b. Does not relate to the periodontal condition
    c. Precedes internal resorption
    d. Indicates the presence of addition canals
    Ans. a

12. **Electric pup tests should be performed on patients who have a:**
    a. Hearing aid
    b. Hip implant
    c. Dental implant
    d. Pacemaker
    Ans. d

13. **A false-negative response to the pup tester may occur:**
    a. Primarily in anterior teeth
    b. In a patient heavily premedicated with analgesics, narcotics, alcohol, or transquilizers
    c. Most often in teenagers
    d. In the presence of periodontal disease
    Ans. b

14. **A test cavity:**
    a. Is the first test in diagnostic sequence
    b. Often results in a dull pain response
    c. Is employed only when all other test findings are equivocal
    d. Should be performed with local anesthetic
    Ans. c

OROFACIAL DENTAL PAIN EMERGENCIES

1. **Pulpal pain response is:**
   a. Dull and throbbing when carried by A-delta myelinated nerve fibers
   b. Dull and throbbing when carried by A-delta unmyelinated nerve fibers

c. Quick and sharp when carried by A-delta myelinated nerve fibers
d. Quick and sharp when carried by A-delta unmyelinated nerve fibers
Ans. c

2. **Pulpal pain response is:**
a. Dull and throbbing when carried by myelinated C fibers
b. Dull and throbbing when carried by unmyelinated C fibers
c. Quick and shapr when carried by myelinated C fibers
d. Quick and sharp when carried by unmyelinated C fibers
Ans. b

3. **Nonspecific biochemical mediators are:**
a. Pyruvic acid, prostaglandins, and aspartic acid
b. Arachidonic acid and the complement system
c. Histamine, bradykinin, prostaglandins and leukotrienes
d. Arachidonic acid and serotonin
Ans. c

4. **Neuropeptides such as substance P and calcitonin gene-related peptide (CGRP):**
a. Are released from capillaries
b. Are released from sensitized nerves
c. Are not part of the inflammatory cycle
d. Are found in the absence of pain and inflammation
Ans. b

5. **Trigeminal neuralgia differs from odontogenic pain by being:**
a. Continuous and dull
b. Sharp and shooting
c. Sharp, shooting, repetitive, and triggered
d. Dull and throbbing
Ans. c

6. **Maxillary sinusitis associated with acute tooth pain:**
a. Is a seasonal phenomenon
b. Can involve the entire quadrant up to the midline
c. Can involve the mandible
d. Is initiated by psychogenic factors
Ans. b

7. **Pain is most commonly referred from:**
a. Lower anterior teeth to ipsilateral upper molars
b. Lower molars to upper anteriors
c. Posterior molars to the opposing quadrant or to other teeth in same quadrant
d. Upper molars to the contralateral lower quadrant
Ans. c

8. **Odontogenicsymptons are elicited primarily by the following provoking stimuli:**
a. Thermal (heat, cold), percussion, palpation
b. Postural changes
c. Pain following exertion
d. Barometric changes
Ans. a

9. **In the presence of an intense inflammatory process, nerve block injections are rendered less effective owing to:**
a. Distance to source of irritation
b. pH changes of inflammation

c. Length of needle,
d. Prior use of analgesics
Ans. b

10. **For effective urgent care management of the routine endodontic emergency:**
a. Leave the pulp chamber open for drainage
b. Pulpotomy will suffice
c. After pulpectomy, close the pulp chamber with a temporary dressing
d. Incise with a scalpel
Ans. c

11. **Localized swelling as an extension of pulpal disease:**
a. Requires antibiotic therapy alone
b. Requires analgesics
c. Is managed using incision, drainage, and an indwelling drain
d. Resolves without treatment
Ans. c

12. **Flare-ups occur more often:**
a. In the afternoon and evening
b. In endodontic treatment of vital teeth
c. In endodontic treatment of pulpless teeth
d. In teenagers
Ans. c

13. **To assess pain intensity, the most useful measure is:**
a. How much analgesia the patient requires
b. How well he patient eats and sleeps
c. Zero to ten verbal analogue scale
d. The patient's own words
Ans. c

14. **Pain can most frequency be expected as a result of:**
a. Pulpitis
b. A nonvital tooth
c. An overinstrumented root canal system
d. After routine endodontic therapy
Ans. c

NONODONTOGENIC FACIAL PAIN AND ENDODONTICS

1. **Pain in the absence of identifiable disease is recognized as:**
a. Acute pain
b. Inflammation mediated
c. Hypersensitivity
d. Chronic pain
Ans. d

2. **Given time, diffuse pain of odontogenic origin:**
a. Will be referred
b. Will readily abate
c. Will localize to specific site
d. Can be controlled with analgesics
Ans. c

3. **Trigeminal neuralgia can be treated:**
   a. With analgesics
   b. By anesthetizing the trigger area
   c. With lysis of the terminal nerve endings
   d. With anticonvulsant drugs
   Ans. d

4. **Cluster headache differs from migraine in being:**
   a. Unilateral and involving the teeth
   b. Principally a female complaint
   c. Unilateral and involving the eye
   d. Bilateral
   Ans. c

5. **Acute maxillary sinusitis:**
   a. Results in referred pain to a single tooth
   b. Results in referred pain to the orbit and maxillary posterior teeth
   c. Is exacerbated by cold testing
   d. Is usually a noninfections process
   Ans. b

6. **Degenerative joint disease most often:**
   a. Results in posterior displacement of the meniscus
   b. Result in irreversible pulpitis
   c. Allows for wide mouth opening
   d. Can lead to adhesions and arthritic changes
   Ans. d

7. **TMJ pain can be:**
   a. sharp, lancinating and electrical
   b. exacerbated by jaw closing
   c. the result of ipsilateral maxillary odontalgia
   d. found in males
   Ans. c

8. **A typical facial pain can be treated most effectively by:**
   a. Microvascular decompression
   b. Radio frequency gangliolysis
   c. NSAIDs
   d. Tricyclic antidepressant drugs
   Ans. d

9. **Phantom tooth pain or differentiation pain:**
   a. Can occur briefly after tooth extraction
   b. Is simply a peripheral phenomenon
   c. Can occur for an extended period after pulp extirpation
   d. Is managed by analgesics
   Ans. c

10. **A definite of facial causalgia can be made:**
    a. By lidocaine infiltration
    b. By use of analgesics
    c. By use of ipsilateral stellate ganglion block
    d. By observation of symptoms
    Ans. c

CASE SELECTION AND TREATMENT PLANNING

1. **Patients with rheumatic heart disease should:**
   a. Be premeditated with antibiotics per American Heart Association guidelines
   b. Be premedicated with psychosedation
   c. Be premedicated with nonsteriodal anti-inflammatory drugs
   d. Postpone elective endodontic therapy
   Ans. a

2. **Diabetes patients in need of endodontic therapy:**
   a. A should not receive elective therapy
   b. Should maintain normal insulin and meal schedules
   c. Do well with intracanal steroid therapy
   d. Heal as well as nondiabetics
   Ans. b

3. **Patients with HIV infection, including AIDS:**
   a. Should be premedicated with analgesics
   b. Are at less risk from root canal therapy than from extraction
   c. Are at less risk from extraction than from root canal therapy
   d. Have fewer complications during and after treatment
   Ans. d

4. **Pregnant patients in the first trimester:**
   a. Should receive the normal X-ray dose for endodontic therapy
   b. Are not candidates for electronic apex locators
   c. Should delay use of X-ray until the second trimester
   d. Are not at risk from pharmacologic intervention
   Ans. c

5. **Patients taking daily steroid therapy (e.g. for systemic lupus erythematosus):**
   a. May demonstrate adrenocorticoid depression
   b. Respond well to stress
   c. Are candidates for intracanalcorticisteriod therapy
   d. Do not require antibiotic premedication
   Ans. a

6. **Extra canals:**
   a. Are rarely found in molar teeth
   b. Are often found in molar teeth
   c. If not found, have little effect on the success of endodontic therapy
   d. Are often found in upper canines
   Ans. b

7. **Treatment consideration(s) for referral are:**
   a. Poor oral hygiene
   b. A patient who breaks appointments
   c. Calcified and curved root canals
   d. A patient who does not have dental insurance
   Ans. c

8. **Differentiate between external and internal root resorption:**
   a. Internal resorption is contiguous with the canal, and external resorption is superimposed on X-ray examination

b. Internal resorption appears superimposed, and external resorption contiguous with the canal on X-ray examination
c. The apex iocator is very useful
d. Internal resorption is larger in size
Ans. a

9. **Crown and root perforations:**
a. Are not treatable by surgical intervention
b. Heal after routine root canal therapy
c. Can respond to a matrix of hydroxyapatite and seal with glass ionomer
d. Respond whether or not crown-root is sealed
Ans. c

10. **The prognosis is compromised:**
a. When patient presents with pain
b. When patient experiences interappointment pain
c. With class III mobility and loss of bone support
d. For molar teeth
Ans. c

11. **The sequence of therapy recommended for emergency treatment is:**
a. A caries control, pulp-periodontal, oral surgery
b. Oral surgery, caries, pulp/periodontal
c. Pulp/periodontal, caries control, extraction
d. Pulp/periodontal oral surgery, caries control
Ans. d

12. **Single-visit root canal therapy:**
a. Is an unacceptable procedure
b. Should be performed with apicoectomy
c. Is an acceptable and successful procedure
d. Requires antibiotic premedication
Ans. c

13. **One-appointment endodontic therapy is not indicated for:**
a. Fractured anterior teeth where aesthetics is a concern
b. Patients requiring sedation or operating room procedures
c. Cases with severe anatomical and procedural difficulties
d. When the patient is physically unable to return for completion
Ans. c

14. **Patients scheduled for retreatment:**
a. May expect to have less interappointment pain
b. Should expect successful resolution
c. Should expect surgical intervention
d. May complain of thermal response on an adjacent tooth
Ans. d

15. **Surgical retreatment is indicated:**
a. For a persistent area of rarefaction at the apex of a retreated tooth
b. For the development of severe periodontal pocket formation
c. For juvenile diabetes patients
d. Before routine endodontic retreatment
Ans. a

PREPARATION FOR TREATMENT

1. **It has been established that:**
   a. Exposure to HIV is more likely than exposure to hepatitis B virus
   b. Transmission of tuberculosis is primarily blood-borne
   c. HIV is less fragile than the hepatitis B virus
   d. Each patient should be considered potentially infections
   Ans. d

2. **Endodontic files:**
   a. A are disposed of after one use
   b. Are considered reusable sharps
   c. May be picked up by hand before decontamination
   d. May be disposed of in "generic refuse"
   Ans. b

3. **To prevent cross-contamination after exposure of the X-ray film:**
   a. Gloves are superfolous
   b. Overgloves are placed over contaminated gloves
   c. Dispose of film packet in generic refuse
   d. Disinfect with sodium hypochlorite
   Ans. b

4. **Informed consent information for endodontic therapy excludes:**
   a. Alternatives to recommended treatment
   b. Procedure and prognosis
   c. A description of OSHA regulations
   d. Foreseeable and material risks
   Ans. c

5. **Radiographic exposure for purposes of endodontic therapy:**
   a. Has no place for fast, sensitive speed film
   b. Is minimized with Radio Visio Graphy
   c. Is unnecessary
   d. Does not require informed consent
   Ans. b

6. **X-ray units should be:**
   a. Optimally capable of utilizing 70 kVp
   b. Pointed in shape
   c. Collimated to reduce exposure level, not to exceed 7cm at the skin surface
   d. Collimated to reduce exposure level, not to exceed 9 cm at the skin surface
   Ans. c

7. **The American Heart Association recommends for prophylactic antibiotic coverage:**
   a. Penicillin V rather than amoxicillin
   b. Amoxicillin rather than penicillin V
   c. Keflex rather than penicillin
   d. Cephalosproins rather than erythromycin
   Ans. b

8. **Radiographic contrast can be directly affected by altering:**
   a. Milliamperage
   b. Exposure time
   c. Kilovoltage
   d. Angulation
   Ans. c

9. **An osterolytic lesion visualized on a radiograph could be mistaken for:**
   a. Granuloma
   b. Cyst
   c. Cementoma
   d. All of the above
   Ans. d

10. **The buccal object rule states:**
   a. That the object further from the buccal surface appears to move in the direction opposite the movement of the tube head
   b. That the object closest to the buccal surface appears to move in the same direction as the tube head
   c. That the object closest to the buccal surface appears to move in the direction opposite that of the tube head
   d. That objects closest to the lingual surface appear on the film to move in the direction opposite the movement of the cone
   Ans. c

11. **With the cone moved to the distal and facing towards the mesial, the mesiobuccal root of the first molar:**
   a. Will be projected mesially on the film
   b. Will be projected distallyon the film
   c. Will not move
   d. Appears to move lingually
   Ans. a

12. **To enhance tooth isolation to prevent contamination:**
   a. Isolation with cotton rolls is used
   b. Anticholinergic and systemic antibiotic drugs are used
   c. Isolation with rubber dam is used
   d. Direct access will achieve the goal
   Ans. c

13. **To enhance crown preparation and retention, crown lengthening is completed by:**
   a. Electrosurgery in the presence of infrabony defects
   b. Conventional gingivectomy in the presence of infrabony defects
   c. Laser surgery in the presence of infrabony defects
   d. Apically positioned flap, reverse bevel in the presence of infrabony defects
   Ans. d

ARMAMENTARIUM AND STERILIZATION

1. **Infection control procedures:**
   a. That protect against monilial infection protect against HBV
   b. That protect against HBV should protect against HIV
   c. That protect against HIV should protect against HBV
   d. Are controlled with the use of the rubber dam
   Ans. b

2. **Color change in a process indicator strip indicates:**
   a. Verification of sterilization
   b. Verification of completed sterilization cycle
   c. A change in pH
   d. A need to reprocess
   Ans. b

3. **The organism least resistant to thermal inactivation is:**
   a. Bacterial spores
   b. Virus

c. Streptococcus mutans
d. Spirochete
Ans. a

4. **Rapid-speed autoclaves:**
a. Require at least 30 minutes for sterilization
b. Require no antirust pretreatment
c. Destroy cloth products
d. Produce verifiable sterilization
Ans. d

5. **Chemiclave:**
a. A corrodes instruments
b. Solution can be recirculated
c. Sterilization is verifiable
d. Does not affect heat-sensitive materials
Ans. c

6. **Dry heat:**
a. Provides corrosion protection for dry instruments
b. Requires only 30 minutes
c. Has no mercury vapor effect
d. Does not destroy heat-sensitive materials
Ans. a

7. **Chairside dry heat glass bead or salt sterilization:**
a. Is verifiable
b. Serves as an emergency backup
c. Requires a brief time to warm up
d. Can sterilize a large number of instruments
Ans. b

8. **Glutaraldehyde:**
a. Requires a short period of sterilization
b. Is relatively noncorrosive
c. Results in verifiable sterilization
d. Is nonirritating and nontoxic
Ans. b

9. **The sterilizer:**
a. Is effective if the process indicator changes color
b. Should be checked weekly with a biologic indicator
c. Should be checked daily with a biologic indicator
d. Should be checked for sterilization of bacteria rather than spores
Ans. c

10. **Gutta-percha is best sterilized in:**
a. An autoclave
b. Dry heat
c. 5.5% sodium hypochlorite for 1 minute
d. Paraformaldehyde for I minute
Ans. c

TOOTH MORPHOLOGY AND ACCESS OPENING

1. **Kasahara and colleagues reported that:**
   a. Accessory canals are capable of being cleaned mechanically at least 60% of the time
   b. Over 60% of teeth examined showed accessory canals that were impossible to clean mechanically
   c. Apical foramina were located at the apex 80% of the time
   d. Canals terminate in the shape of a delta 45% of the time
   Ans. b

2. **Once the pulp chamber has been opened, canal orifices are located with:**
   a. A periodontal curette
   b. A spoon excavator
   c. An inverted cone bur
   d. An endodontic pathfinder
   Ans. d

3. **Access cavity preparation of anterior teeth:**
   a. Is completed using a K-type file
   b. Often can result in lateral cervical or root surface perforations
   c. Often can result in labial cervical or root surface perforations
   d. Arc initiated using a no.6 or 8 round bur
   Ans. c

4. **Fourth canals are usually found in:**
   a. Maxillary first premolars
   b. Maxillary second premolars
   c. Maxillary first molars
   d. Mandibular premobars
   Ans. c

5. **The fourth canal is often found in:**
   a. The mesiobuccal root of the maxillary first molar
   b. The mesial root of the maxillary first premolar
   c. The palatal root of the maxillary first molar
   d. The distobuccal root of the maxillary first molar
   Ans. a

6. **Entry into a maxillary central incisor is made:**
   a. Below (apical to) the cingulum in the direction of the long axis of the tooth
   b. Just coronal to the cingulum in the direction of the long axis of the tooth
   c. To include the marginal ridges
   d. With a slow-speed bur
   Ans. b

7. **Maxillary canines:**
   a. Are usually less than 25 mm long
   b. Are 35 mm or longer
   c. Possess extremely curved canals
   d. Have an anatomic apex distant from the apical foramen
   Ans. b

8. **Vertucci and colleagues describe that:**
   a. 50% of the maxillary second premolars have one canal at the apex
   b. Maxillary second premolars that have two canals have two distinct apical foramina
   c. 75% of maxillary second premolars have one canal at the apex
   d. Accessory canals are more prevalent in maxillary second premolars than in incisors
   Ans. c

9. **The maxillary first molar:**
   a. Has a palatal root that curves lingually
   b. Has a distobuccal root with two canals ending in a common orifice
   c. Should be approached for endodontic treatment with the assumption that two canals exist in the mesiobuccal root
   d. Should be approached for endodontic treatment with the assumption that one canal exists in the mesiobuccal root

   Ans. c

10. **Mandibular incisors:**
    a. Often have two separate apical foramina
    b. Two of five can have two separate canals
    c. Average 19 mm in length
    d. Are less likely to be perforated labially than lingually during access preparation

    Ans. b

11. **Mandibular premolars:**
    a. Can have more than one canal 12 to 23% of the time
    b. Are less prone to acute exacerbations
    c. Rarely present complex mechanical problems
    d. Are on average 19 mm long

    Ans. a

12. **Multiple accessory foramina:**
    a. Are more often present at the apex of the mandibular incisor
    b. Are more often present in the furcation of the maxillary premolar
    c. Are more often present in the furcation of the madibular first molar
    d. Are accessible for mechanical instrumentation

    Ans. c

13. **The mandibular first molar:**
    a. Has a fourth canal two-thirds of the time
    b. Has a fourth canal half the time
    c. Is the most difficult to treat
    d. Has a fourth canal one-third of the time

    Ans. d

14. **When a calcified root canal cannot be located or instrumented:**
    a. Extraction is the treatment of choice
    b. Retrograde and replantation procedures should be considered
    c. The dentist must proceed with the understanding that an unexplored or unfilled canal is worse than a perforation
    d. It is no longer accessible to bacterial infection

    Ans. b

CLEANING AND SHAPING OF THE ROOT CANAL SYSTEM

1. **Root canal morphology should be:**
   a. Conical
   b. Cylindrical
   c. Three dimensional
   d. Predictable

   Ans. c

2. **To achieve the objectives of vertical condensation, it is necessary to produce:**
   a. A cylindrical canal
   b. A conical canal
   c. A tapering conical canal
   d. A straight canal
   Ans. c

3. **To contain gutta-percha within the canal, instrumentation should result in:**
   a. Cleaning beyond the anatomic apex
   b. Cleaning beyond the radiographic apex
   c. A cylindrical canal shape
   d. The narrowest cross-sectional diameter at the terminus
   Ans. d

4. **To avoid external transportation of the root canal:**
   a. Precurve instruments
   b. Use large instruments
   c. Avoid the use of sodium hypochlorite
   d. Use vigorous instrumentation
   Ans. a

5. **According to the precepts of vertical condensation technology, the apical foramen should be:**
   a. As large as practicable
   b. As small as practicable
   c. Oval
   d. Circular
   Ans. b

6. **The projected success of creating patency relies principally on:**
   a. The choice of file type
   b. Irrigation
   c. The first instrument to reach the apical terminus
   d. The second instrument to reach the apical terminus
   Ans. c

7. **Reentry and/or reuse of previously utilized instruments is:**
   a. Capitulation
   b. Recapitulation
   c. Cleaning and shaping
   d. Reworking
   Ans. b

8. **Irrigation of the root canal achieves:**
   a. Debridement
   b. Dissolution of tissues
   c. Elimination of microbes
   d. All of the above
   Ans. c

9. **Each time the canal is flushed an appropriate volume of irrigant is:**
   a. 3 ml
   b. 1 ml
   c. 1 to 2 ml
   d. 4 ml
   Ans. c

10. **Debridement is most effective:**
    a. In large quantities
    b. When used with recapitulation
    c. When it remains in the canal between appointments
    d. Just prior to filling
    Ans. b

11. **Removal of the smear layer:**
    a. Is accomplished with irrigation
    b. Effectively reduces the microbial population
    c. is unnecessary for effective cementation during root canal filling
    d. is necessary for success
    Ans. b

12. **Biologic rationale dictates:**
    a. Overinstrumentation
    b. Undcrinstru mentation
    c. That the working length stop at the apical constriction
    d. Partial pulp removal
    Ans. c

13. **Blood at the tip of a paper point removed from the root canal indicates:**
    a. Possible hematoma
    b. Possible incomplete irrigation
    c. Possible incomplete instrumentation
    d. Possible root perforation
    Ans. d

14. **Filing with a Hedstrom file results in:**
    a. Effective cutting on insertion
    b. Effective cutting on withdrawal
    c. A lack of tactile sensation
    d. Narrower canal preparations
    Ans. b

15. **The crown-down preparation advocates beginning radicular access with:**
    a. Smaller instrument first
    b. Precurvaturc of a smaller instrument
    c. A larger instrument first
    d. Removal of the clinical crown
    Ans. c

16. **To improve accuracy, negotiate curved canals, and reduce force of instrumentation, the following tools are recommended:**
    a. Carbon steel files
    b. Nickel titanium instruments
    c. Reamers
    d. Hedstrom files
    Ans. b

17. **Radicular access can be achieved by:**
    a. First using a Gatcs-Glidden drill throughout half the canal length
    b. After instrumentation to no.10, employ the Gates-Glidden drill
    c. After instrumentation to no. 25, employ the Gates-Glidden drill
    d. Avoid Gates-Glidden drills when possible
    Ans. c

18. **Furcal perforation is often the result of:**
    a. Oversized radicular access preparations
    b. Use of Hedstrom files
    c. Natural occurrence
    d. Use of K-type files
    Ans. a

OBTURATION OF THE ROOT CANAL SYSTEM

1. **A well-lifted root canal:**
    a. Prevents microbial leakage
    b. Exhibits radiopacity
    c. Extends beyond the apical constriction
    d. Needs no root canal cement
    Ans. a

2. **Appropriate time for obturation is:**
    a. When the canal is free of hemorrhage
    b. When the canal has ceased to exude tissue fluids
    c. When the tooth is symptomatic
    d. Before post cementation
    Ans. c

3. **Rool-lilling materials must be:**
    a. Low cost
    b. Easily dissolved
    c. Rigid
    d. Biocompatible
    Ans. d

4. **Root canal cements should:**
    a. Be bactericidal
    b. Be bacteriostatic
    c. Be radiolucent
    Ans. b

5. **Tug-back is achieved and the canal is ready for filling:**
    a. When the gutta-percha has extended beyond the apex
    b. When the gutta-percha is easily removed from the root canal
    c. When the gutta-percha placed to apical constriction exhibits resistance on removal
    d. After cementation
    Ans. c

6. **Calcium hydroxide root canal sealers:**
    a. Are the most biocompatible
    b. Are irritating to the periapical tissue
    c. Should be used exclusively
    d. Preventpostobturation pain
    Ans. a

7. **The string-out test for root canal sealer is achieved when, using a spatula, the cement can be raised from the glass slab:**
    a. 0.5 inch
    b. 2 inches
    c. 1 inch
    d. 3 inches
    Ans. c

RECORDS AND LEGAL RESPONSIBILITIES

1. **Which of the following statements is true?**
   a. Alteration of records is forbidden
   b. Alteration of records is permitted if dated
   c. Additions to records are forbidden
   d. Additions to records are permitted if dated
   Ans. d

2. **Standard of care, as defined by courts:**
   a. Requires absolute perfection
   b. Describes what a reasonably careful and prudent clinician would do under similar circumstances
   c. Does not allow for individual variations of treatment
   d. Is equivalent to customary practice
   Ans. b

3. **The doctrine of informed consent does not:**
   a. Require that a patient be advised of reasonably foreseeable risks of treatment
   b. Require that the patient be advised of reasonable alternatives
   c. Require that the patient forfeit his right to do as he sees fit with his own body
   d. Require that the patient be advised of the consequences of non-treatment
   Ans. c

4. **To make sure a dentist to whom one refers a patient is not considered to be an agent of the referring dentist, the referring dentist should:**
   a. Verbally inform the patient of that fact
   b. Inform the patient in writing
   c. Enter a disclaimer in the patient's record
   d. Inform the patient that the referral is a suggestion only
   Ans. d

5. **A dentist may legally:**
   a. Refuse to treat a new patient despite severe pain and infection
   b. Be bound to see former patients on recall after treatment is completed
   c. Discharge a patient from his practice at any time
   d. Refuse to treat a patient who has an outstanding balance on his account
   Ans. b

6. **If a patient who is HIV seropositive requests that the dentist not inform the staff of his condition, the dentist should:**
   a. Refuse to treat the patient
   b. Tell the staff in private, then treat the patient using extra precautions
   c. Not teil the staff, but treat the patient with great caution
   d. Not tell the staff and require the patient to sign a private guarantee that the patient will be liable if someone contracts the virus
   Ans. a

7. **If a patient swallows a file and the dentist had not placed a rubber dam, the dentist should:**
   a. Offer to pay for any medical expenses incurred as a result
   b. Not offer to pay for medical expenses, which is an admission of guilt
   c. Nol mention who should pay medical expenses and try to infer that the patient is to blame (e.g., sudden movement, difficult case)
   d. Apologize for the mishap, and suggest that the patient have medical evaluation only if a problem develops as a result
   Ans. a

8. **An endodontist may be held liable who:**
   a. Informs the patient that her general practitioner is performing substandard care (the general practitioner may hold the endodontist liable)
   b. Fails to disclose to the patient and/or referring dentist evident pathosis other than the tooth they are treating
   c. Fails to locate a very small canal that is not evident radiographIcally
   d. Mistakenly initiates treatment on the wrong tooth in a difficult diagnosis situation
   Ans. b

9. **Of the following, the dentist's best approach to avoiding legal action by patients is to:**
   a. Tell all patients that he/she (the dentist) docs not carry malpractice insurance
   b. Attend Continuing Education courses frequently to remain informed of current techniques
   c. Refer all major patient complaints to peer review
   d. Demonstrate genuine interest in the welfare of each patient
   Ans. d

PULP DEVELOPMENT, STRUCTURE AND FUNCTION

1. **Blood vessels become established in the dental papilla:**
   a. Before the formation of the cervical loop
   b. During the bud stage of tooth formation
   c. During the bell stage of tooth formation
   d. During the cap stage of tooth formation
   Ans. c

2. **Root development begins:**
   a. Before enamel formation
   b. Concurrently with enamel formation
   c. After completion of enamel formation
   d. Before Hertwig's epithelial root sheath formation
   Ans. c

3. **The cell-rich zone:**
   a. Is more prominent in the radicular pulp than in the coronal pulp
   b. Exhibits increased mitotic activity following death of blasts
   c. Is the result of the central migration of cells from the periphery following completion of dentin formation
   d. Contains mainly macrophages and endothelial cells and few fibroblasts
   Ans. b

4. **Although similar in function, the odontoblast differs from the osteoblast and cemcntoblast in:**
   a. Morphologic characteristics
   b. Ultrastructurc
   c. Matrix production
   d. Being a protein-secreting cell
   Ans. a

5. **The extent to which the odontoblast process extends outward indentin:**
   a. Has been shown conclusively in recent years
   b. Varies with the age of the tooth
   c. Depends on continued mitotic activity of the odontoblast
   d. Is unrelated to the effects on the pulp of restorative procedures
   Ans. b

6. **Fibroblasts:**
   a. Are the least numerous cells of the pulp
   b. Are capable of giving rise to cells that may differentiate intomacrophages
   c. Increase in numbers as blood vessels and nerves decrease with age
   d. Undergo active differentiation in the pulp, as do fibroblasts of other connective tissues
   Ans. d

7. **The pathways of pulpal inflammation and infection arc strongly inilue need by:**
   a. The two structural proteins in the pulp: collagen and elastin
   b. Denial materials that depress pulpal metabolic activity
   c. The state of polymerization of the ground substance components in the pulp
   d. Osmotic pressures as regulated by proteoglycans
   Ans. c

8. **Water content of the pulp is approximately:**
   a. 30%
   b. 50%
   c. 70%
   d. 90%
   Ans. d

9. **Regardless of the nature of the sensory stimulus, all afferent impulses from the pulp result in the sensation of:**
   a. Proprioception
   b. Pain
   c. Heat
   d. Touch
   Ans. b

10. **The nerve fibers of the pulp are:**
    a. Mainly myelinated fibers at the time of tooth eruption
    b. Easily damaged by inflammation
    c. Only sensory
    d. Unevenly distributed throughout the pulp
    Ans. d

11. **Fluid movement in dentinal tubules is known as the:**
    a. Hydrodynamic theory
    b. Osmotic pressure
    c. Mechanical deformation theory
    d. Hydraulic theory
    Ans. a

12. **Painful pulpitis associated with an inflamed or degenerating pulp:**
    a. Is caused by a decrease in intrapulpal pressure
    b. Results from a reduction of nerve cell permeability
    c. Is associated with stimulation of A fibers
    d. Is most likely due to nociceptive C-fiber activity
    Ans. d

13. **Volume of blood flow in the pulp:**
    a. Is least in the regions of the pulp horns
    b. Is greater in the root portion than in the crown portion
    c. Is greater than the blood flow in most visceral organs
    d. Is largely under the control of the adrenergic sympathetic system
    Ans. d

14. A healthy dental pulp responds to an injury by:
   a. Developing an effective collateral circulation to transport inflammatory elements to the area
   b. Decreasing in blood flow throughout the pulp
   c. Initiating an inflammatory response, usually followed by patial or complete necrosis
   d. Forming reparative dentin at the pulpal surface corresponding to areas of irritation
   Ans. d

15. Pulpal calcifications:
   a. May compromise the pulpal blood supply
   b. Arc of no significance in root canal therapy
   c. Have an organic matrix of collagen in all sizes
   d. Occur only after eruption
   Ans. c

16. Calcific metamorphosis:
   a. Is caused by increased activity of odontoblasts
   b. May lead to complete obliteration of the pulp space
   c. Usually occurs in association with a constricted apical foramen
   d. Histologically resembles acellular cementum
   Ans. a

17. Growth factors arc likely to be involved in tooth formation. What is at least one probable function of these factors?
   a. Signaling epithelial-mescnchymal interactions
   b. One of the eruptive forces located in the apical region
   c. Disruption of Hcrtwig's epithelial root sheath
   d. Collagen maturation in the dental papilla
   Ans. a

18. The cell type to which the dendritic cell is most similar is:
   a. Fibroblast
   b. T-lymphocyte
   c. Mesenchymal cell
   d. Macrophage
   Ans. d

19. Lymphatics in the dental pulp:
   a. Have not been demonstrated
   b. Would not be necessary because of the extensive vascular network
   c. Cannot be demonstrated morphologically because they are identical to venules
   d. Participate in the removal of tissue fluids
   Ans. d

20. What would be the closest estimate of the number of tubules exposed with a full crown preparation of average depth that wail have a surface area of 100 mm^2?
   a. 5000
   b. 50,000
   c. 500.000
   d. 5,000,000
   Ans. d

21. When the pulp is injured it responds with inflammation. Why does it not have good capability for recovery if badly damaged?
   1. It has no collateral blood supply
   2. It lacks lymph drainage
   3. Pulp CT cells are incapable of mitosis
   4. It is encased in a noncompliant environment

a. 1 and 2 b. 1 and 3
c. 1 and 4 d. 2 and 3

Ans. c

PERIAPICAL PATHOLOGY

1. **In acute inflammation, the first cells to pass through the blood vessel walls into the tissue are:**
   a. Eosinophils
   b. Lymphocytes
   c. Monocytes
   d. Polymorphonuclear neutrophils (PMNs)
   Ans. d
2. **Following monocyte white cell migration from the vessel to the tissue, the monocyte becomes a :**
   a. Neutrophil
   b. Basophil
   c. Macrophage
   d. Histiocyte
   Ans. c
3. **In the inflammatory process, which of the following cell types function as phagocytes?**
   a. Macrophages and lymphocytes
   b. Lymphocytes and neutrophils
   c. Plasma cells and basophils
   d. Neutrophils and macrophages
   Ans. d
4. **Which of the following results may be expected following surgery when both the buccal and lingual cortical plates have been lost?**
   a. Ankylosis
   b. Scar tissue formation
   c. Osteosclerosis
   d. Normal bone regeneration
   Ans. b
5. **A foreign body reaction is characterized by the presence of:**
   a. Neutrophils
   b. Plasma cells
   c. Giant cells
   d. Fibroblasts
   Ans. c
6. **Acute osteomyelitis is typically characterized by:**
   a. A draining sinus tract
   b. A large diffuse radiolucency
   c. Necrotic bone
   d. Cellulitis
   Ans. c
7. **T-lymphocytes arise as immature cells in the:**
   a. Bone marrow
   b. Thymus
   c. Lymph nodes
   d. Inflammatory lesion
   Ans. a

8. Which of the following would predominate in the zone of irritation?
   a. Bacteria
   b. Chronic inflammatory cells
   c. Capillary buds
   d. Necrotic elements
   Ans. b

9. The periapical lesion that would most likely contain bacteria within the lesion is:
   a. Apical abscess
   b. Apical cyst
   c. Periapical granuloma
   d. Condensing osteitis
   Ans. a

10. Leukocytes move through the endothelium and into tissue by a process known as:
   a. Diapedesis
   b. Emigration
   c. Transudation
   d. Margination
   Ans. a

11. Opsonization facilitates:
   a. Mitosis of fibroblasts
   b. Chemotaxis of neutrophils
   c. Vasodilatation
   d. Phagocytosis
   Ans. d

12. A chemical mediator of inflammation that is responsible fereafy vascular response to injury is:
   a. C, a
   b. C_5a
   c. Histamine
   d. Bradykinin
   Ans. c

13. The factor that is responsible for stimulating nerve endings to cause the pain associated with acute apical periodontitis is:
   a. Fluid pressure
   b. Histamine
   c. Complement
   d. Neutrophilic enzymes
   Ans. a

14. A sinus tract associated with a suppurative apical periodontitis usually:
   a. Is lined with epithelium
   b. Should be cauterized or removed surgically
   c. Will not heal unless the microorganisms arc curetted from the apical area
   d. Requires no special treatment other than root canal treatment of the offending tooth
   Ans. d

15. What is the usual histologic picture of the pulp in a tooth with a chronic apical periodontitis (dental granuloma)?
   a. Pulpal abscess in the coronal pulp with chronic inflammatm in the radicular pulp
   b. Necrotic pulp
   c. The majority of the pulp exhibits chronic inflammation
   d. Chronic inflammation in the coronal pulp and the radicular pulp appears normal
   Ans. b

16. Chronic apical periodontitis (granuloma) presents a histologic picture that is most consistent with:
a. Infection
b. Early cyst formation
c. Healing
d. Immune response
Ans. d

MICROBIOLOGY AND IMMUNOLOGY

1. Most root canal infections involve:
a. A single obligate anaerobic species
b. Multiple anaerobic species only
c. Mixed aerobic and anaerobic microorganisms
d. Multiple aerobic species only
Ans. c

2. Studies have demonstrated a correlation between clinical and radiographic signs and symptoms of periapicalpathosis and the presence of:
a. Streptococcus mutatis
b. Prevotellamelaninogenicus
c. Staphylococcus aureus
d. No specific microorganism(s)
Ans. b

3. Which mediators of inflammation are considered also to be the main mediators of pain in inflammatory responses?
a. Vasoactive amines
b. Kinins
c. Complement
d. Arachidonic acid
Ans. b

4. The presence of which component of complement in the inflamed periapex suggests that the complement system participates in the pathogenesis?
a. CI
b. C3
c. C7
d. C9
Ans. b

5. Degranulation and release of histamine is usually stimulated by bridging which of the following on the mast cells?
a. IgA
b. IgE
c. IgG
d. IgM
Ans. b

6. Identification of lymphocytes in human periapical lesions has shown:
a. An absence of B lymphocytes
b. An absence of T lymphocytes
c. That T cells outnumber B cells
d. That B cells outnumber T cells
Ans. c

7. **In periapical lesions, suppressor T-cells are associated with:**
   a. Acute (developing) lesions
   b. Chronic lesions
   c. Healing lesions
   d. Foreign-body lesions
   Ans. b

8. **Routine culturing of the root canal system is generally not practiced in today's treatment regimens because:**
   a. It is time consuming
   b. Important anaerobes cannot be recovered
   c. Standard RCT techniques effectively eliminate the majority of microorganisms
   d. Microorganisms play a minor role in endodontic pathosis
   Ans. c

9. **When antibiotic therapy is indicated before, during, or after root canal treatment the drug of choice, is:**
   a. Clindamycin
   b. Erythromycin
   c. Penicillin
   d. Metronidazole
   Ans. c

10. **Long-term administration of clindamycin is contraindicaled because of the risk of developing:**
   a. Severe gastrointestinal conditions
   b. Urticaria
   c. Photosensitivity
   d. Hypersensitivity
   Ans. a

11. **Which one of the following is least likely to initiate an immuneresponse?**
   a. Necrotic tissue
   b. Endotoxins
   c. Autologous collagen
   d. Viable bacteria
   Ans. c

12. **What immunoglobulin predominates in a secondary humoral response?**
   a. IgA
   b. IgG
   c. IgM
   d. IgE
   Ans. b

13. **Elevated levels of IgE have been identified in a periapicalganuloma after canal instrumentation. This may represent which type of hypersensitivity reaction?**
   a. Type 1 (immediate hypersensitivity)
   b. Type II (immediate cytotoxic hypersensitivity)
   c. Type III (immune complex hypersensitivity)
   d. Type IV (delayed hypersensitivity)
   Ans. a

14. **The cytokine, interleukin-1 (IL-1), has been identified in the inflamed pulp and inflamed periapical lesion. One important faction is to:**
   a. Result in bone resorption
   b. Neutralize bacterial endotoxins
   c. Inhibit inflammation
   d. Promote phagocytosis by macrophages
   Ans. a

15. **The intracanal medication that has the best potential for effectiveness as an antimicrobial agent sealed in the canal is:**
    a. Formocresol
    b. 5.25% sodium hypochlorite
    c. Steroids
    d. Calcium hydroxide
    Ans. d

16. **Coronal exposure of gutta-percha/sealer obturation to bactaia has shown that, throughout the canal, the bacteria:**
    a. Penetrate very quickly (1 to 3 days) throughout obturation defects
    b. Penetrate very slowly (requires several months)
    c. Do not penetrate
    d. Penetrate fairly quickly (1 week to 1 month)
    Ans. d

17. **Regarding the presence of bacteria, most studies show that the majority of periapical granulomas are:**
    a. Supportive of numbers of anaerobes primarily
    b. Supportive of numbers of anaerobes only, primarily
    c. Supportive of numbers of variable, mixed flora,
    d. Bacteria free
    Ans. d

INSTRUMENTS, MATERIALS AND DEVICES

1. **The endodontic broach is used to:**
   a. Locate the orifices of the root canals
   b. Remove pulp tissue from the pulp spaces
   c. Smooth the walls of root canals
   d. Enlarge the root canal spaces
   Ans. b

2. **The basic difference between K-type files and reamers is:**
   a. The number of spirals or flutes per unit length
   b. The geometric cross section
   c. The depth of the flutes
   d. The direction of the spirals
   Ans. a

3. **The major determining factor that influences the efficacy of cd canal debridement is the:**
   a. Type of hand instrument used
   b. Irrigating solution
   c. Internal pulp space anatomy
   d. Instrumentation technique
   Ans. c

4. **The working portion of an endodontic condenser (plugger) is:**
   a. Smooth, tapered, and pointed
   b. Smooth, tapered, and flat-ended
   c. Smooth, of uniform width, and pointed
   d. Smooth, of uniform width, and flat-ended
   Ans. b

5. **Modification of the cross-sectional design of K-type files from square to rhomboid has resulted in significantly greater:**
   a. Torsional strength
   b. Tensile strength
   c. Stainless
   d. Flexibility
   Ans. d

6. **Significant deviations from circular canal preparations will occur when using a:**
   a. K-type reamer with a reaming action
   b. K-fype reamer with a filing action
   c. Krtype file with a reaming action
   d. K-type file with a filing action
   Ans. d

7. **The Hedstrom file is most commonly used to:**
   a. Flare the canal
   b. Establish a circular preparation
   c. Prepare post space
   d. Locate canal orifices
   Ans. a

8. **The temperature of the gutta-percha extruded from the "low-lemperalure," thermoplastic injection system is:**
   a. 160 °C
   b. 100 °C
   c. 70 °C
   d 40 °C
   Ans. a

9. **Some studies have reported that the most important aspect of irrigation is the:**
   a. Quantity of irrigant
   b. Chelating action of the solution
   c. Size of the needle
   d. Type of irrigant
   Ans. a

10. **Hardening of zinc oxide-eugenol is due to the:**
    a. Formation of zinc eugenolate
    b. Presence of water
    c. Evaporation of eugenol
    d. Heat generated during the chemical reaction
    Ans. a

11. **With time and with exposure to light and air, gutta-percha:**
    a. Does not change its physical properties significantly
    b. Will decompose and lose mass
    c. Becomes more brittle
    d. Alters, but can be restored by freezing
    Ans. c

12. **Temporary canal medications are of various types. Which of the following seems to satisfy more criteria as to desirable properties?**
    a. Formocresol
    b. Chlorhcxidinc
    c. Potassium iodide
    d. Calcium hydroxide
    Ans. d

13. **A disadvantage of Cavit as compared to IRM as a temporary restoration is that Cavit:**
    a. Does not have as much compressive strength
    b. Does not seal as well with time
    c. Is more susceptible to thermal changes
    d. Shrinks while setting
    Ans. a

14. **An inherent disadvantage of the gutta-percha/carrier systems is:**
    a. The carrier corrosion or disintegration products are toxic
    b. Difficulty in insertion
    c. Potential problems in retreatment
    d. No means arc available to prepare the post space
    Ans. c

15. **The Canal Master intracanal instrument has some disadvantages over conventional instruments in that the Canal Master:**
    a. Will enlarge the canal unevenly
    b. Will result in more transportation if not precurved
    c. Is more susceptible to breakage
    d. Cannot be utilized in all canal shapes
    Ans. c

16. **Thinking in terms of design, which of the following size-50 endodontic instruments made from the same steel would be most susceptible to fracture (separation)?**
    a. Triangular shaft file
    b. Square shaft reamer
    c. Rhomboid file
    d. Hedstrom file
    Ans. d

PULPAL REACTION TO CARIES AND DENTAL PROCEDURES

1. **The most common dentin response in the zone deep to caries is:**
    a. Increased permeability
    b. Alteration of collagen
    c. Dissolution of peritubular dentin
    d. Dentin sclerosis
    Ans. d

2. **Although each carious lesion is individual and influenced by multiple factors, the caries process is generally:**
    a. Continuous
    b. Rapid
    c. Intermittent
    d. Slow
    Ans. c

3. **Relatively few bacteria are found in a pulp abscess because of the:**
    a. Immune response of pulp tissue
    b. High tissue pH in the adjacent inflammation
    c. Mechanical blockage of sclerotic dentin
    d. Antibacterial products of neutrophils
    Ans. d

4. **Hyperplastic pulpitis:**
   a. Occurs only in permanent molars
   b. Occurs when there is.no damage
   c. Is not invaded by bacteria
   d. Is predominantly acute inflammation
   Ans. c

5. **A periodontal ligament injection of 2% lidocaine with 1:100,000 epinephrine will cause the pulp circulation to:**
   a. Cease for about 30 minutes
   b. Remain the same
   c. Increase markedly
   d. Decrease slightly
   Ans. a

6. **Of the following, the highest incidence of pulp necrosis is associated with:**
   a. Class V preparations on root surface
   b. Inlay preparations
   c. Partial veneer restorations
   d. Full crown preparations
   Ans. d

7. **According to the hydrodynamic theory of dentin sensitivity, the movement of fluid through dentinal tubules:**
   a. Stimulates the sensory nerve fibers of the underlying- pulp
   b. Displaces odontoblasts into the pulp tissue
   c. Has minimal effect on the odontoblasts
   d. Results in the death of many odontoblasts
   Ans. c

8. **Acid etching of dentin before insertion of the restorative material:**
   a. Protects the pulp from bacterial invasion
   b. Enhances bacterial penetration of the dentin
   c. Destroys odontoblastic processes in the tubules
   d. Decreases the pulp response to the restorative material
   Ans. b

9. **Pulpal blood flow is most increased by:**
   a. Impression taking using modeling compound with copper banding
   b. Fabrication of acrylic temporary restoration
   c. Rubber base impression
   d. Hydrocolloid impression
   Ans. a

10. **Dental tubules should be sealed before placement of restorations to:**
    a. Allow a calcium bridge to form in the pulp
    b. Reduce the pathogenicity of the microorganisms
    c. Decrease the number of dentinal tubules
    d. Decrease the permeability of underlying dentin
    Ans. d

11. **The smear layer on dentin walls acts to prevent pulpal injury by:**
    a. Reducing diffusion of toxic substance through the tubules
    b. Resisting the effects of acid etching of the dentin
    c. Eliminating the need for a cavity liner or base
    d. Its bactericidal activity against oral microorganisms
    Ans. a

12. A common histologic change in the pulp in response to moderately deep dentin caries is:
a. Chronic inflammation
b. Acute inflammation
c. Vasoconstriction
d. Increased numbers of odontoblasts
Ans. a

13. Application of frictional heat to exposed dentin may result in:
a. Severe postoperative symptoms
b. Vascular stasis or intrapulpal hemorrhage
c. Proliferation of cells in the cell-rich zone
d. Invariably chronic Inflammation
Ans. b

14. Hypersensitivity is best relieved or controlled by:
a. Opening tubules to permit release of intrapulpal pressure
b. Root planing to remove surface layers that arc hypersensitive
c. Applying antiinflammatory agents to exposed dentin
d. Blocking exposed tubules on the dentin surface
Ans. d

15. Deeper cavity preparations have more potential for pulp damage because:
1. Tubule diameter and density increase; therefore, there is increasing permeability
2. There is more vibration to pulp cells.
3. Odontoblastic processes are more likely to be severed
   a. 1 only
   b. 3 only
   c. 1 and 3
   d. 2 and 3

Ans. c

16. The pulp generally begins to show histologic changes of inflammation as soon as caries has entered:
a. The dentin
b. The enamel
c. The pulp
d. The reparative (irregular secondary) dentin
Ans. a

17. Of the following, which is the best way to prevent pulp damage during cavity preparation?
a. Retain the smear layer
b. Use diamond burs with a brush stroke
c. Use adequate air coolant
d. Use adequate water coolant
Ans. d

18. Which is the major reason why class 11 restorations with omposite is damaging to the pulp?
a. Microleakage at the occlusal
b. Microleakage at the gingival margin
c. Toxic chemicals are released from the composite and diffuse into the pulp
d. Polymerization shrinkage distorts the material at the occlusal and opens gaps which results in recurrent caries
Ans. b

19. A pulp has been damaged and is inflamed because of deep caries and cavity preparation. What material placed on the floor of the cavity aids the pulp in resolving the inflammation?
a. $Ca(OH)_2$
b. ZnOE base
c. Steroid formulations
d. There is no medication or material that actively promotes pulpal healing
Ans. d

20. A cusp fractures and exposes dentin but not the pulp. Whet is the probable response in the pulp?
a. Severe damage with irreversible inflammation
b. Mild-to-moderate inflammation
c. Pain but no inflammation
d. No pulp response
Ans. b

TRAUMATIC INJURIES

1. If several teeth are out of alignment following trauma, the most reasonable explanation is:
a. Luxation
b. Subluxation
c. Alveolar fracture
d. Contusion
Ans. c

2. Initial vitality testing of traumatized teeth is most useful to:
a. Establish a baseline for comparison with future testing
b. Determine whether or not root canal treatment is indicated
c. Determine if the blood supply to the pulp is compromised
d. Predict the prognosis
Ans. a

3. Initial radiographic examination of dental injuries that include lip lacerations:
a. Reveals hairline root fractures
b. Reveals facial-lingual diagonal root fractures
c. May reveal foreign objects in the lips
d. Should include occlusal views
Ans. c

4. Rubber dam application for the placement of a restoration at the emergency appointment:
a. Usually is not advisable
b. Is absolutely essential
c. Usually is possible
d. Is dictated by the restorative material
Ans. c

5. Which of the following radiographic film exposures is best for diagnosing root fractures in the apical third?
a. Parallel
b. Bisecting angle
c. Occlusal
d. Panoramic
Ans. c

6. The initial priority in treatment of a horizontal root fracture with significant mobility is:
a. Preservation of the pulp
b. Reduction and immobilization
c. Root canal therapy
d. Calcium hydroxide pulp therapy
Ans. b

7. **To prevent the onset of inflammatory resorption, the mature intruded tooth must:**
   a. Be allowed to reerupt
   b. Have the pulp removed within 1 to 2 weeks
   c. Have the pulp removed after the tooth is in position
   d. Have an immediate root canal filling completed
   Ans. b

8. **Inflammatory resorption is the mechanism of:**
   a. Rejection of autogenous protein
   b. Eliminating infected calcified tissue
   c. Scar tissue formation
   d. Sequestration of bone
   Ans. b

9. **Comparing dental trauma in boys and girls:**
   a. The rate of trauma is increasing more rapidly in girls
   b. Girls have more injuries as the result of fisttights
   c. Boys have more injuries.: in the maxilla, girls in the mandible
   d. Injuries are common in boys, rare in girls
   Ans. a

10. **A direct facial padded blow to the incisors is more likely to cause:**
    a. Enamel fracture
    b. Enamel-dcntin fracture
    e. Dentin fracture-pulp exposure
    d Luxation
    Ans. d

11. **Apulpotomy (coronal pulp removal) is indicated when there is a crown fracture and pulp exposure and:**
    a. Root formation is incomplete and the crown is fractured in the cervical one-third
    b. The pulp has been exposed longer than I week
    c. The puip is hypersensitive to cold
    d. Any portion of the fracture extends to the root
    Ans. a

12. **Nonunion of a root fracture and inflammatory response from pulp necrosis is indicated radiographically by:**
    a. A periapical lesion
    b. Marked separation of the segments
    c. Root resorption adjacent to the fracture
    d. Widening of the fracture and resorption of adjacent bone
    Ans. d

13. **Displaced teeth that had pulp necrosis with root resorption and Ihen had the appropriate endodontic treatment:**
    a. Often had continued resorption
    b. Occasionally had ankylosis
    c. Had a high rate of success
    d. Usually developed apical pathosis
    Ans. c

14. **Which medium of storage for an avulsed tooth is best for prolonged periods?**
    a Milk
    b. Distilled water
    c. Hank's balanced salt solution
    d. Patient's saliva
    Ans. c

15. After replantation of an avulscd tooth that has air dried, comparing RCT with immediate gutta-percha obturation vs. treatment with intracanal calcium hydroxide, the research:
  a. Shows that both arc doomed to failure
  b. Shows that RCT/immediate GP has the best success
  c. Shows that calcium hydroxide treatment first has the best success
  d. As yet is inconclusive

  Ans. d

16. A primary tooth whose crown is displaced lingually and the root facially:
  a. Is likely to damage the permanent successor
  b. Should be extracted
  c. Oflen will ankylosc, with resulting displacement of the erupting successor
  d. Generally requires no treatment and causes no damage to the successor

  Ans. d

17. If a fully formed tooth has suffered an intrusive injury and the crown is partially exposed, what is the recommended treatment?
  a. Leave alone and allow to erupt spontaneously
  b. Splint for 7 to 10 days; watchful waiting
  c. Orthodontially reposition into correct alignment within 3 to 4 weeks
  d. Reposition with forceps

  Ans. c

18. If calcific metamorphosis (reduction in canal space) is observed radiographically following a displacement, the treatment is:
  a. Immediate root canal treatment
  b. Root canal treatment only if the tooth is unresponsive to pulp tests
  c. Root canal treatment only if the tooth discolors
  d. Nothing unless signs and symptoms of periapicalpathosis develop in the future

  Ans. d

19. Alvused replanted teeth with incomplete root formation:
  a. Require pulp removal if the extraoral period is more than 2 hours
  b. Are prone to internal resorption
  c. Are tested for revascularization with the electric pulp tester
  d. In most cases develop roots

  Ans. a

20. Which is most likciy to result in severe pulp damage (necrosis)?
  a. Intrusion displacement
  b. Lateral displacement
  c. Enamel-dentin fracture
  d. Cervical one-third root fracture

  Ans. a

21. In a tooth that has been injured, a dramatic or distinct color change to purple or dark gray after a few weeks is usually indicative of:
  a. Internal hemorrhage that is reversible
  b. Internal resorption that is irreversible
  c. Internal resorption that is reversible
  d. Pulp necrosis

  Ans. d

22. A nonmobile asymptomatic root fracture with evidence of hypercalcification of the pulpal space of the coronal generally requires:
  a. No further treatment
  b. Root canal therapy with gutta-percha
  c. Root canal therapy with calcium hydroxide initially
  d. Extraction because there is likely to be pathosis

  Ans. a

23. The best way to treat a mature root fractured in the middle one third with mobility and no response to pulp testing is:
a. To reposition segments, splint, and monitor
b. To splint, begin access, pack with $Ca(OH)^-$
c. To extract immediately, because restoration is impossible
d. To perform root canal therapy, anchor segments together with cast post, and restore
Ans. a

ROOT RESORPTION

1. Internal resorption:
a. Radiographically is often confused with external replacement resorption
b. Is associated with systemic disease
c. Is usually associated with trauma
d. Usually results only if odontoblasts and/or predentin layer is lost or altered
Ans. a

2. Studies of internal resorption have shown:
a. Histologic differences in the process in primary and permanent teeth
b. No difference in rate of progression of the process in primary and permanent teeth
c. Normal pulp is replaced by a periodontal-like connective tissue
d. Resorption of dentin and no deposition of mineralized tissue
Ans. a

3. External resorption may be found in which one of the following systemic diseases?
a. Hypoparathyroidism
b. Diabetes
c. Leukemia
d. Parkinson's disease
Ans. c

4. Apical external resorption, as related to periapical pathosis:
a. Requires surgical intervention (apicoeetomy)
b. Is usually associated with a necrotic pulp
c. Is initially treated with conventional root canal treatment, although this has a questionable outcome
d. Is usually irreversible, has a poor prognosis, and requires extraction
Ans. b

5. Resorption following bleaching:
a. Is a reason not to treat tctracycline-stained teeth with root canal therapy and internal bleaching
b. May be due to erosion of dentin exposed at the cervical line
c. Is related to the use of heat and 30 % hydrogen peroxide
d. Docs not occur unless there is a history of trauma
Ans. c

6. Orthodontic treatment resorption is most prevalent in:
a. Maxillary incisors
b. Mandibular incisors
c. Maxillary premolars
d. Mandibular premolars
Ans. a

7. Avulsed teeth replanted without pulpectomy usually exhibit:
a. Revascularization of pulp space
b. Surface resorption
c. Inflammatory resorption
d. Ankylosis
Ans. c

8. **Cementum is more resistant than bone to resorption. A theory asto why this is true is that:**
   a. Cementum is more mineralized than bone
   b. Cementum contains an antiresorptive factor
   c. Bone is vascular; cementum avascular
   d. Liber patterns in cementum are different than in bone and tend to be more resistant to ciast-typc cells
   Ans. b

9. **The two major local causes of root resorption are:**
   a. Inflammation and excessive pressure
   b. Inflammation and cementoclast-activating factor
   c. Excessive pressure and increased pH of ground substance
   d. Cementoclast-activating factor and increased pH of ground substance
   Ans. a

10. **As related to root resorption during orthodontic movement root canal-treated teeth are:**
    a. More resistant to resorption
    b. Less resistant to resorption
    c. No different than untreated teeth
    d. More prone to resorption if there is a history of apical root resorption as related to apical pathosis
    Ans. c

11. **Lateral inflammatory root resorption is usually:**
    a. Related to a tooth injury that damages the PDL
    b. Related to sterile pulp necrosis
    c. Irreversible
    d. Successfully treated only if calcium hydroxide is placed in the canal prior to obturation
    Ans. a

12. **Clinical features of early stages of lateral inflammation root resorption include that usually it is:**
    a. Associated with normal pulp testing, visible radiographically
    b. Asymptomatic, not visible radiographically
    c. Associated with no (or abnormal) response to pulp testing, symptomatic
    d. Symptomatic, not visible radiographically
    Ans. b

13. **Cervical root resorption is in many (or most) cases:**
    a. Of unknown etiology
    b. Related to a subluxation injury
    c. Associated with a necrotic, infected pulp
    d. Unrelated to inflammation in the cervical periodontium
    Ans. c

14. **Treatment of medium depth cervical root resorption usually requires:**
    a. Root canal treatment alone
    b. Root canal treatment followed by surgery
    c. Surgery alone
    d. Surgery, followed if necessary by root canal treatment
    Ans. c

15. **These clinical features of internal resorption usually include:**
    a. Positive response to pulp testing, visible in the pulp spaceisdiographically
    b. Visible in both the pulp space and as a defect in 1he adjaoert bone
    c. Symptomatic, visible radiographically in the pulp space
    d. Asymptomatic, visible radiographically in (he pulp space, variable response to pulp testing)
    Ans. d

16. In the treatment of nonpcrlorating internal resorption, calcium hvdroxide may be used in the canal primarily to:
a. Sterilize the canal space
b. Reminerali/.e the resolved areas
c. Aid in breaking down inaccessible areas containing tissue
d. Lwer pH in the tissue to counteract the dentinobiasts
Ans. c

17. A common histologic feature of replacement resorption is:
a. Areas of fusion of bone with cemenlum/dentin
b. Inflammation in the adjacent periodontium
c. Pulp necrosis with bacteria deep into the tubules
d. Areas of necrotic bone and necrotic cementum
Ans. a

18. A treatment approach that will generally arrest replacement IB-sorption is:
a. Pulpectomy and placement of $Ca(OH)_2$
b. Surgery to expose and curette the defect
c. Pulpectomy and immediate obturation
d. Nonexistent. There is no known effective treatment
Ans. d

ENDODONTIC-PERIODONTAL RELATIONS

1. The highest percentage of lateral canals occurs:
a. In the coronal third of the root
b. In the middle third of the root
c. In the apical third of the root
d. Anywhere along Ihc root, depending on the tooth in question
Ans. b

2. Treatment of pulpal diseases that cause periodontal diseases usually requires:
a. Endodontic treatment alone
b. Both endodontic and periodontal treatment
c. Periodontal surgery and curettage
d. Combined pcriradicular and periodontal surgery
Ans. a

3. Studies on the effects of periodontal disease on the pulp have shown:
a. Pathologic pulp changes
b. Degenerative pulp changes
c. No pulp changes
d. All of the above
Ans. d

4. Which of the following statements concerning a sinus tract of pulpal origin is false?
a. The tract is usually thinner than an infrabony periodontal pocket
b. Vitality tests may evoke an unaltered, normal response
c. Pain is not often present
d. It can be traced to the source of irritation
Ans. b

5. **Which of the following statements concerning a primary endodoatic lesion with secondary periodontal disease is false?**
   a. This condition occurs with long-standing pulpal disease and chronic periapical drainage
   b. Radiographs may show- generalized periodontal disease with angular defects at the initial site of endodontic involvement
   c. Resolution of the lesion requires both endodontic and periodantal therapy
   d. If appropriate endodontic therapy is performed all bone loss will heal
   Ans. d

6. **In a primary periodontic lesion with secondary endodontic involvement:**
   a. There is a history of extensive periodontal disease
   b. The pulp always responds to vitality tests
   c. Pain is usually absent
   d. Periodontal therapy should precede endodontic therapy
   Ans. a

7. **The concomitant pulpal-pcriodontal lesion:**
   a. Is another name for the combined endodontic-periodontic lesion
   b. Requires either periodontal or endodontic treatment
   c. Radiographically may simulate a vertical fracture
   d. Depends for its prognosis on the success of periodontal treatment
   Ans. d

8. **The most common cause of root resection failures is:**
   a. Progressive periodontal disease
   b. Recurrent endodontic pathosis
   c. Root fracture
   d. Poor oral hygiene
   Ans. c

SURGICAL ENDODONTICS

1. **Unless the benefit-risk ratio is high, surgery should be avoided by:**
   a. Brittle diabetics
   b. Dialysis patients
   c. Immunocompromised patients
   d. All of the above
   Ans. c

2. **Which of the following statements regarding the presurgical workup is false?**
   a. It is performed by the surgical assistant
   b. The patient is informed of the nature of the procedure
   c. The patient's medical history is reviewed and blood pressure is checked
   d. None of the above
   Ans. a

3. **Maximum hemostasis is obtained by depositing anesthetic:**
   a. Into the attached gingiva
   b. Into the papillae
   c. Into the alveolar mucosa
   d. Into all of the above
   Ans. c

4. **2% Lidocaine with 1:50,001) Epinephrine:**
   a. Iscontraindicated in the medically compromised patient
   b. Is administered after anesthesia is obtained
   c. Provides anesthesia and analgesia
   d. Is deposited in multiple injections into the vestibular tissues apical to the root apices
   Ans. b

5. **The triangular/rectangular llap with suleular incision:**
   a. Provides the best access of all flaps
   b. Has no disadvantages
   c. Compromises the blood supply to the hap
   d. Elevation begins at the junction of the horizontal and vertical incision
   Ans. a

6. **Which of the following statements concerning the triangular/rectangular flap with mucogingival incision is false?**
   a. This flap is contraindicated with short roots
   b. Survival of marginal gingiva depends on secondary blood supply
   c. Because tissue reapproximation is simplified, scar formation is minimal
   d. It is popular because marginal gingiva is undisturbed
   Ans. c

7. **The most common cause of lip injury is:**
   a. Insufficient extension of releasing incisions
   b. Excessive tension by sutures
   c. Using undermining elevation
   d. Improper retractor positioning
   Ans. a

8. **Which of the following statements concerning apical curettage is true?**
   a. Apical curettage is definitive treatment
   b. Not all curetted soft tissue needs to be submitted for biopsy
   c. Bony access should be enlarged to remove the lesion in toto
   d Ml of the above
   Ans. c

9. **The angle of the beveled resected root:**
   a. Should be sufficient to provide access to perform the retropreparation
   b. Is rarely greater than it appears to be
   c. Should be at 45 degrees to the facial surface
   d. All of the above
   Ans. a

10. **Ferric subsulfatc:**
    a. Is used to identify the complete outline of the root
    b. Is painted on the wall of the bony crypt to provide hemostasis
    c. Acts by causing intravascular coagulation
    d. All of the above
    Ans. c

11. **All beveled root canal fillings:**
    a. Can be easily evaluated
    b. Leak
    c. Can be hermetically sealed by retrofilling without a magnification system
    d. Should be rctrofilled only if there is an apparent incompletely sealed root canal system
    Ans. b

12. **Which of the following is not a requirement for retropreparations:**
    a. All isthmus tissue must be removed
    b. In roots with one canal the shape is usually round
    c. It must be parallel to the anatomic outline of the pulpal space
    d. It must be at least 3 mm deep
    Ans. b

13. **Ultrasonic root end preparations:**
    a. Eliminate the bevel
    b. Facilitate idea! preparation
    c. Conserve root structure
    d. All of the above
    Ans. d

14. **Characteristics of an idea! retrofilling material include all of the following except:**
    a. Long-term sealing ability
    b. Unaffected by moisture
    c. Slight expansion on setting
    d. Nonresorbable
    Ans. c

15. **The retrofilling material that offers the most advantages to date is:**
    a. Amalgam and cavity varnish
    b. Composite resin
    c. IRM or EBA
    d. Polycarboxylate cement
    Ans. c

16. **Sutures:**
    a. Do not impede wound healing
    b. Ideally should be removed after 48 hours
    c. Are placed by proceeding from the attached tissue to the unattached tissue
    d. All of the above
    Ans. b

17. **Postoperative care does not include:**
    a. Continuous application of an ice pack
    b. Chlorhexidene mouth rinses
    c. Written postoperative instructions
    d. None of the above
    Ans. a

18. **The operating microscope can:**
    a. Enhance the ability of the surgeon to inspect, prepare, and seal the apex
    b. Be useful in patient education
    c. Provide a permanent record for insurance purposes
    d. All of the above
    Ans. d

THE MANAGEMENT OF PAIN AND ANXIETY

1. **The duration of action of a local anesthetic can be increased by:**
    a. Increasing its lipid solubility
    b. Increasing its protein-binding potential
    c. Decreasing its extra-neural tissue diffusibility
    d. Increasing its vasodilator activity
    Ans. b

2. **Inadequate anesthesia in some cases of inflamed or infected pulps is due to:**
    a. A decrease in the tissue pH around the involved tooth
    b. Availability of more cations for binding at the receptor site
    c. A larger proportion of the free base
    d. A smaller proportion of the cation
    Ans. a

3. **Supraperiostcal anesthesia is:**
   a. Most effective in areas of infection
   b. Generally used for pulpal anesthesia of maxillary teeth
   c. Not effective for primary teeth in the mandibular arch
   d. Effective in areas of dense cortical bone
   Ans. b

4. **The infraorbital nerve block does not anesthetize:**
   a. The maxillary premolar
   b. The maxillary incisors
   c. The palatal mucosa
   d. The maxillary cuspid
   Ans. c

5. **Partial anesthesia to the mesial of the mandibular first molar can be alleviated by:**
   a. Anesthetizing the motor fibers of the mylohyoid nerve
   b. Depositing anesthetic on the buccal side at the level of the mesial apex
   c. Depositing anesthetic on the lingual side at the level of the apex of the second molar
   d. All of the above
   Ans. c

6. **Electronic dental anesthesia (EDA):**
   a. Has not been approved by the FDA for intraoral pain control
   b. Can be used without local anesthesia for pulp extirpation
   c. Has been successful as a technique for post-endodontic surgery patient management
   d. Has not been successful as an adjunct in treating hot man dibular molars
   Ans. c

7. **Conscious sedation is a technique designed to:**
   a. Control pain
   b. Control anxiety
   c. Control pain and anxiety
   d. Affect the patient's protective reflexes
   Ans. b

8. **Oral sedation:**
   a. Is the most frequently employed technique of pharmacosedation
   b. Is quick acting
   c. Is short acting
   d. Is least accepted by patients compared with other routes of drug administration
   Ans. a

9. **Disadvantages of intramuscular sedation include:**
   a. Inability to titrate to the ideal level of sedation
   b. Inability to deepen the level of sedation
   c. Inability to lighten the level of sedation
   d. All of the above
   Ans. d

10. **When sedation is required the most advantageous route of administration is:**
   a. Oral
   b. Inhalation
   c. Intramuscular
   d. Intravenous
   Ans. b

11. **Compared to diazepam (Valium), midazolam (Versed):**
    a. Provides an amnesic effect
    b. Is not as potent
    c. Requires no local anesthetic for pain control
    d. Provides a greater degree of sedation
    Ans. a

12. **Which route of administration of conscious sedation requires no one to escort the patient from the office?**
    a. Oral
    b. Intravenous
    c. Inhalation
    d. None of the above
    Ans. c

BLEACHING OF VITAL AND PULPLESS TEETH

1. **Which of the following is not helpful in determining if a patient is appropriate for bleaching?**
    a. Recent periapical radiographs
    b. Vitality tests
    c. Transillumination
    d. An intraoral camera
    Ans. d

2. **The most difficult stains from dental treatment to bleach successfully are from:**
    a. Amalgam restoration
    b. Root canal sealers
    c. Composite restorations
    d. Gold restorations
    Ans. b

3. **Teeth are most susceptible to tetracycline staining from:**
    a. Four months in utero to eight years of age
    b. Birth to seven years of age
    c. Seven months in utero until the third molars are formed
    d. Anytime during life
    Ans. a

4. **As described by Jordan and Boksman, third degree tetracycline staining is:**
    a. Dark gray or blue in color, with banding
    b. Dark yellow or gray in color
    c. Too dark to bleach
    d. Light yellow or gray in color
    Ans. a

5. **Minocycline, in contrast to other tetracyclines:**
    a. Causes staining of enamel
    b. Causes discoloration in teeth after calcification
    c. Chelates with calcium to form tooth pigmentation
    d. All of the above
    Ans. b

6. **Fluorosis:**
    a. Affects ameloblasts resulting in defective enamel development
    b. Most commonly affects premolars
    c. Is caused by drinking water containing fluoride concentrations in excess of one part per million
    d. All of the above
    Ans. d

7. **Which of the following is not a contraindication to bleaching?**
   a. Dentin hypersensitivity
   b. Teeth with white spots
   c. Patients over 70 years of age
   d. Patients who are perfectionists
   Ans. c

8. **Which of the following statements concerning microabrasion is false?**
   a. It is effective in treating white spots
   b. The active ingredient is hydrochloric acid
   c. It permanently removes surface stains
   d. It can successfully treat some tetracycline stains
   Ans. d

9. **Etching the enamel prior to bleaching:**
   a. Enhances the penetrability of the bleaching solutions
   b. Shortens the appointment time
   c. Retains the fluoride-rich surface layer of enamel
   d. All of the above
   Ans. a

10. **The usual range of temperatures for bleaching vital teeth with a heat or light source is:**
    a. 100 to 115 degrees
    b. 115 to 140 degrees
    c. 140 to 160 degrees
    d. 160 to as high as the patient can tolerate
    Ans. b

11. **With vital bleaching:**
    a. Both arches should be treated simultaneously
    b. Treatment should proceed from the less discolored teeth to the most discolored
    c. Incisal halves of teeth respond quicker than cervical halves
    d. Yellow-brown and gray stains are equally difficult to remove
    Ans. c

12. **Which of the following is not necessary for vital bleaching?**
    a. Patient wears safety glasses
    b. Local anesthesia
    c. Pumice prophylaxis
    d. Polish teeth after last treatment
    Ans. b

13. **The barrier material for bleaching pulpless teeth should be:**
    a. IRM
    a. Dental sealant
    c. Glass ionomer cement
    d. Zinc oxyphosphate
    Ans. c

14. **Cervical resorption in bleached pulpless teeth may result from:**
    a. Bleach placed apical to the CEJ
    b. Tooth becoming pulpless before patient reaches age 25
    c. A defect in the CEJ
    d. All of the above
    Ans. d

15. The most common treatment for cervical resorption following intracoronal bleaching is:
a. Surgical repair
b. Orthodontic extrusion
c. Extraction
d. Calcium hydroxide therapy
Ans. a

16. Which of the following is not part of the bleaching procedure for endodontieally treated teeth?
a. Rubber dam isolation
b. Acid etching
c. Superoxolor sodium perborate
d. A heat source
Ans. b

17. With nightguard vital bleaching:
a. The reported success rate is 75%
b. Fluorosed teeth are the least responsive
c. The bleaching agent is 10% carbamide peroxide
d. Patients with removable partial dentures can wear the night-guard only at night
Ans. c

18. Unknowns about nightguard bleaching include all of the following except:
a. Longevity
b. Effects on restorations
c. Efficacy
d. None of the above
Ans. b

19. Patient instructions during nightguard bleaching include:
a. Replace bleaching solution every 3 to 4 hours
b. Wear nightguard as long as possible
c. Discontinue treatment and contact the dentist if teeth become hypersensitive
d. All of the above
Ans. c

20. Following the second appointment, the nightguard bleaching patient should return to the office when:
a. The desired shade is achieved
b. Six weeks have passed
c. If side effects need attention
d. All of the above, whichever comes first
Ans. d

RESTORATION OF THE ENDODONTICALLY TREATED TEETH

1. Pulpal degeneration increases:
a. With the complexity of the restoration
b. With the degree of periodontal disease
c. With time, following insertion of the restoration
d. All of the above
Ans. d

2. Endodontic access through existing crowns:
a. Usually has no effect on porcelain strength
b. Does not cause separation of the porcelain veneer from the metal substructure
c. Often leads to excessive removal of coronal tooth structure
d. Should not be performed
Ans. c

3. **During the restorative examination prior to endodontic therapy:**
   a. The strategic value of the tooth is of minor significance
   b. A critical amount of solid coronal dentin is required
   c. The ferrule has no effect on the incidence of root fracture
   d. If insufficient tooth structure remains to withstand functional forces, the tooth should always be extracted
   Ans. b

4. **Inendodontically treated teeth:**
   a. Decreased strength is due to the loss of coronal tooth structure
   b. Decreased strength is a direct result of the endodontic treatment
   c. Mandibular teeth are stronger than maxillary teeth
   d. All of the above
   Ans. a

5. **The dowel functions primarily:**
   a. To retain the core material
   b. To strengthen the tooth
   c. To distribute forces along the length of the root
   d. To decrease the risk of root fracture
   Ans. a

6. **Guidelines for dowel length in a tooth with normal periodontal support include:**
   a. Two thirds of the length of the canal
   b. The coronal length of the tooth
   c. One half the bone-supported length of the tooth
   d. All of the above
   Ans. d

7. **Dowel features that contribute the greatest retention are:**
   a. Increased length, parallel sides, and moderate diameter
   b. Increased length, taper, and serrated surface
   c. Increased length, parallel sides, and serrated surface
   d. Increased length, taper, and smooth surface
   Ans. c

8. **Compared to nickel-chrome dowels, titanium dowels are:**
   a. Stronger
   b. Less radiopaque
   c. More allergenic
   d. More economical
   Ans. b

9. **The microleakage phenomenon is greatest with:**
   a. Composite resin core
   b. Amalgam core
   c. Glass ionomer core
   d. Cast post and core
   Ans. a

10. **Which material should be avoided in teeth with high esthetic value?**
   a. Composite resin
   b. Glass ionomers
   c. Amalgam
   d. Cast post and core
   Ans. c

11. **Composite cores:**
    a. Are anticariogenic
    b. Should be used only in teeth with significant remaining structure
    c. Are dimensionally stable
    d. All of the above
    Ans. b

12. **Which endodontically treated teeth always require a dowel, a core, and crown?**
    a. Fixed partial denture abutments
    b. Removable partial denture abutments
    c. Individual teeth
    d. None of the above
    Ans. b

13. **The ferrule:**
    a. Significantly reduces the incidence of fracture
    b. Must not terminate on restorative material
    c. Is a metal band encircling the external dimension of the residual tooth
    d. All of the above
    Ans. d

14. **For dowel space preparation:**
    a. Gutta-percha is removed using heat, rotary instruments, or solvents
    b. Gutta-percha removal should be done 48 hours or more after root canal filling
    c. Intimate contact of the dowel and dentin is not necessary for passive dowel systems
    d. To refine the dowel space dowel drills must be used in a dental handpiece
    Ans. c

15. **Regarding cementation of the dowel:**
    a. Zinc phosphate and glass ionomer cements increase resistance to fracture
    b. Zinc phosphate and resin cements inhibit marginal leakage
    c. Retention is greatest when both the dowel and canal are coaled with cement
    d. the dowel is seated with finger or biting pressure
    Ans. c

16. **The major cause of failure of endodontically treated posterior teeth that are periodontally compromised is:**
    a. Recurrent periodontal disease
    b. Root fracture
    c. Endodontic failure
    d. Caries
    Ans. b

PEDIATRIC ENDODONTIC TREATMENT

1. **The basic morphologic difference between primary and permanent teeth is that:**
    a. The thickness of dentin between the pulp and enamel is greater in primary teeth
    b. The enamel is thicker on primary teeth
    c. The pulp chamber is comparatively smaller in primary teeth than in permanent teeth
    d. The pulp horns arc higher in primary molars than in permanent molars
    Ans. d

2. **Radiographically, in primary teeth:**
    a. Pathologic changes in the periradicular tissues are most often apparent at the apices rather than the furcation in molars
    b. The presence of calcified masses within the pulp is indicative of acute pulpal disease
    c. The treatment of choice for internal resorption is extraction
    d. Pathologic bone and root resorption is always indicative ofnonvital pulp
    Ans. c

3. **Which of the following diagnostic tests are usually reliable fir determining pulpal status in primary teeth?**
   a. Thermal pulp tests
   b. Electric pulp tests
   c. Percussion testing
   d. None of the above
   Ans. d

4. **Indirect pulp therapy:**
   a. Is indicated only in the treatment of teeth with deep carious lesions in which there is no clinical evidence of pulpal degeneration or periapical pathology
   b. Removes all the bacteria but not all the caries
   c. Includes placing calcium hydroxide or ZOE over the remaining caries and permanently restoring the tooth with amalgam
   d. All of the above
   Ans. a

5. **Direct pulp capping is recommended for primary teeth with:**
   a. Carious exposures
   b. Mechanical exposures
   c. Calcification in the pulp chamber
   d. All of the above
   Ans. b

6. **Calcium hydroxide:**
   a. Is the material of choice for direct pulp capping
   b. May cause calcification of the remaining pulp tissue
   c. Does not enter into the formation of the dentin bridge
   d. All of the above
   Ans. d

7. **Formocresol pulpotomy on a primary tooth is indicated when:**
   a. There is a history of spontaneous toothache
   b. The inflammation or infection is confined to the coronal pulp
   c. The pulp docs not hemorrhage
   d. Hemorrhage following coronal pulp amputation is uncontrollable
   Ans. b

8. **Which of the following usually is not an indication of failure for a formocresol pulpotomy:**
   a. Pain
   b. Internal resorption of the root adjacent to the area where the formocresol was applied
   c. Development of a periradicular radiolucency
   d. Loosening of the tooth
   Ans. a

9. **Formocresol pulpotomy as compared to glutaral dehyde pulpotomy:**
   a. Is more successful
   b. Has more undesirable effects
   c. Is the technique taught at most dental schools
   d. All of the above
   Ans. c

10. **Which of the following statements concerning primary root canal anatomy is false?**
   a. Root/crown ratio is smaller than that of permanent teeth
   b. Roots are narrower than those of permanent teeth
   c. Molar roots are more divergent than those of permanent molars
   d. Roots are shorter than those of permanent teeth
   Ans. a

11. Considerations for endodontic treatment on primary teeth include:
a. Profound anesthesia at the fill appointment
b. Prevention of overinstrumentation and overfilling
c. Three-dimensional obturation with gutta-percha
d. All of the above
Ans. b

12. Which of the following is not a contraindication for root canal therapy of primary teeth?
a. Radiographic evidence of internal resorption in the roots
b. Apical restoration involving the roots
c. Presence of a dentigerous or follicular cyst
d. Mechanical or carious perforation of the floor of the pulp chamber
Ans. b

13. Access openings on primary incisors:
a. Are from the facial surface
b. Are from the lingual surface
c. Are from the incisal surface
d. Differ in location for maxillary and mandibular incisors
Ans. c

14. Apexification is the treatment of choice for a permanent tooth with a wide-open apex when:
a. The pulp is necrotic
b. There is a history of spontaneous pain with a carious exposure
c. There is a large mechanical exposure with profuse pulpal bleeding
d. All of the above
Ans. a

GERIATRIC ENDODONTICS

1. Periapical radiographs should be reviewed:
a. Before discussion of the chief complaint
b. After discussing the chief complaint with the patient
c. Just before the clinical examination
d. After completing the clinical examination
Ans. d

2. With aging:
a. Lateral canals become more clinically significant
b. Gingival recession exposes cementum and dentin, which is less resistant to decay
c. The cementodentinal junction moves closer to the radiographic apex with continuous apical remodeling
d. All of the above
Ans. b

3. Which pulp tests have limited diagnostic value in geriatric patients?
a. Electric pulp tests
b. Test cavity
c. Selective anesthesia
d. All of the above
Ans. d

4. Cracked teeth:
a. Are rare in geriatric patients
b. Will not have pulpal or periodontal disease unless the cause of pulpal irritation is evident
c. With periapical disease and normal pocket depths have an excellent prognosis following root canal therapy
d. When associated with periodontal pockets have a poor prognosis
Ans. d

5. **In geriatric patients:**
   a. There is a direct correlation between the degree of response to electric pulp testing and the degree of inflammation
   b. There is a reduced volume and increased neural component of the pulp
   c. Tooth discoloration usually is not indicative of pulpal death
   d. Diffuse pain of vague origin is common
   Ans. c

6. **In the geriatric patient, with increasing age, radiographically:**
   a. The incidence of condensing osteitis increases
   b. The incidence of odontogenic and nonodontogenic cysts increases
   c. The apical constriction is closer to the radiographic apex
   d. All of the above
   Ans. b

7. **Regarding endodontic treatment in aged patients:**
   a. One appointment procedures are advantageous
   b. Frequent appointments of short duration are preferable
   c. Root canal treatment is more traumatic than extraction
   d. Intraligamentary injection is the recommended technique for obtaining anesthesia
   Ans. a

8. **The frequency and intensity of discomfort following instrumentation is *not* related to:**
   a. The amount of preparation
   b. Pulp or periapical status
   c. Whether or not the root canal is tilled at the same appointment
   d. All of the above
   Ans. d

9. **In evaluating success and failure of endodontic therapy in aged patients, one must consider that:**
   a. The bone of the aged patient is more mineralized than that of a younger patient
   b. Overlooked canals are seldom a problem because they are usually calcified
   c. As long as 2 years may be necessary to produce healing that would occur at 6 months in an adolescent
   d. Cold sensitivity is the only symptom that may indicate a missed canal
   Ans. c

10. **Endodontic surgery in geriatric patients:**
    a. Requires more anesthetic and vasoconstrictor than in younger patients
    b. Is usually indicated to establish drainage or for relief of pain
    c. Produces postoperative eechymosis more commonly than in younger patients
    d. Seldom requires the placement of a retrograde filling
    Ans. c

ENDODONTIC FAILURES AND RETREATMENT

1. **Which of the following is not significant in evaluating treatment results:**
   a. The extension of filling material
   b. The location of the treated tooth
   c. The obturation quality
   d. The presence of periapicalpathosis before treatment
   Ans. b

2. **In evaluating treatment results, the consensus on the minimum period of observation was:**
   a. At least 6 months
   b. 6 months to a year
   c. At least 1 year
   d. At least 2 years
   Ans. c

3. **Pitfalls associated with radiographic interpretation of success or failure include:**
   a. Change in angulation
   b. Lack of radiographic changes
   c. Personal bias
   d. All of the above
   Ans. d

4. **Which of the following statements concerning radiographs is true?**
   a. Swelling and pain, necessitating incision and drainage, may occur without any radiographic indication
   b. At least 30% of the bone must be decalcified for a lesion to. be evident radiographicaily
   c. The size of the lesion on the radiograph is indicative of the actual amount of bone destruction
   d. Complete denudation of bone over the root apex is always evident radiographicaily
   Ans. a

5. **Undcrextending the access cavity preparation may lead to:**
   a. A missed canal
   b. Breakage of endodontic instruments
   c. Discoloration of the crown
   d. All of the above
   Ans. d

6. **Bony lesions that may be associated with vertical root fracture include:**
   a. A widened periodontal ligament space on one or both sides of the root
   b. A halo-like lesion around the root apex extending to midroot
   c. An angular periodontal defect extending apically from the crcstal bone
   d. All of the above
   Ans. d

7. **Endodontic retreatment:**
   a. Is as technically challenging as original treatment
   b. Has a poorer prognosis than original treatment
   c. Is performed only on endodontic failures
   d. Has different objectives than primary treatment
   Ans. b

8. **Clinically successful cases with radiographicaily unsatisfactory obturation:**
   a. Should always be retreated
   b. Should be retreated only if a new prosthetic restoration is planned
   c. Should be considered for retreatment or follow-up if a newprosthetic restoration is planned
   d. Should only be considered for follow-up if no new restorationis planned
   Ans. c

9. **Which of the following aspects of the root canal filling is not a factor in determining whether anendodontic failure should be retreated or surgically treated?**
   a. Time since obturation
   b. Apical extension of filling material
   c. Density of filling material
   d Type of filling material
   Ans. a

10. **Removal of existing prosthetic restorations before retreatment:**
   a. Is always indicated
   b. Permits more radiographic information to be obtained
   c. Will not aid in revealing a vertical fracture
   d All of the above
   Ans. b

11. **To remove soft-settina pastes, they should initially be penetrated by:**
    a. Sonic instruments
    b. Ultrasonic instruments
    c. Routine endodontic instruments
    d. Solvents
    Ans. c

12. **Overextended gutta-percha should be removed:**
    a. By pulling it out in one piece
    b. Surgically
    c. With rotary instruments
    d. With solvents
    Ans. a

13. **During retreatment the coronal portion of gutta-percha should be:**
    a. Dissolved with solvents
    b. Drilled out
    c. Removed by heat
    d. Removed using ultrasonics
    Ans. b

14. **Chloroform:**
    a. Is the most effective gutta-percha solvent
    b. Is prohibited for use in dentistry in most countries
    c. Has no adverse effects on clinicians
    d. All of the above
    Ans. a

15. **Which solvent, when heated, is as effective as chloroform?**
    a. Xylene
    b. Methyl chloroform
    c. Halothane
    d. Eucalyptol
    Ans. d

16. **The technique of choice for removing poorly condensed guttapercha is:**
    a. Automated instrumentation
    b. Hand instrumentation
    c. Ultrasonic instrumentation
    d. Rotary instrumentation
    Ans. b

17. **The Masserann kit technique for removing solid objects:**
    a. Is not time consuming
    b. Is more successful in posterior teeth than in anterior ones
    c. Requires frequent radiograph monitoring
    d. Is better than the ultrasonic technique
    Ans. c

High-yield Facts

1. Enameloid conglomerates seen in H/P of **Regional Odontodysplasia**
2. Nasoalveolar cyst is also called **Klestadt cyst**
3. Functionally generated path technique in complete occlusal rehabilitation by **Pankey and Mann**
4. **Sky furcation** is done in maxillary molars
5. **PKT** Instruments:

   No. 1: Creating mesial distal and buccal ridges

   No. 2: Adding wax

   No. 3: Smoothening grooves

   No. 4: Smoothing lingual ridges

   No. 5: Refining triangular ridges
6. Dancing eye syndrome seen in **neuroblastoma**
7. Salmon patch is also called as **Stork Bites**
8. **Double pot method** is used to disinfect wells
9. Mixing waste with cement is called **Inertisation**
10. **THETA:** Booklet of a Dental Education Programme
11. **RED CROSS** formed by Henry Durant
12. Father of Dental Hygiene—**Alfred Fones**
13. **Choking Off** Seen with NaF
14. Flouride in human enamel found by **Morichini**
15. Post with antirotational lock—**Parkell Post System**
16. Chrome Cobalt wire as a post with a gold core cast—**Wiptam Technique**
17. Small straight elevator is also called **SHOEHORN FORCEPS**
18. **McGregor's Patch** refers to Zygomatic ligament
19. Incisal guidance and Condylar guidance are prefixed and mathematically derived in **HOBO'S TECHNIQUE**
20. **Broyle's ligament**: Seen in inner surface of thyroid cartilage
21. **ANNEXIN V** dye recognises apoptosis
22. Subcondylar osteotomy to correct prognathism by **Robinson and Hinds**
23. C factor was developed by **Feilzer**
24. PRR for recently erupted teeth was described by **Henderson and Setcos**
25. Bioresorbable plated excretes as **WATER + CO_2**

26. Castable apatite ceramic is called **CERAPEARL**
27. **Blue Daper syndrome** is Tryptophan malabsorption
28. **KOZAK CONSENSUS SEQUENCE** is presence of purine at positions -3 and + 4 relative to the AUG
29. The protein that acts by modulating the expression of Hepcidin is **HEMOJUVELIN**
30. Most Common site of Ivory Osteoma—**Frontal Sinus**
31. **Rosenthal Syndrome** due to deficiency of clotting factor XI
32. Sleep apnoea lasts for atleast **10 seconds**
33. Reversal of shunt is not possible in **Tetralogy of Fallot**
34. Commonest site of Hematogenous Osteomyelitis—**Metaphysis**
35. Ribs associated with triangle of auscultation—**6th and 7th**
36. Non progressive contractions of oesophagus are—**Tertiary**
37. Tongue worms an arthropod causes a disease called **Porocephalosis**
38. Night Terrors: **NREM** and Night mares: **REM**
39. Ion used in PCR: **Magnesium**
40. Hb Yakima seen in **Polycythemia**
41. Hb Kansas seen in **Pseudoanemia**
42. Hb Iwata seen in **Methemoglobinemia**
43. **Holdaway analysis** measures upper lip strain
44. Appropriate method to evaluate intraoperator Cephalometric errors is by **Dahlberg's formula**
45. Technique used to demonstrate Negri bodies—**Seller's technique**
46. Scorpion venom belongs to **Class B** of local anaesthetics
47. C shaped canal configuration was first reported by **Cooke and Cox**
48. Adverse effect of Efavirenz is **Crystalluria**
49. **MIC 2** and **CD 99** are markers for Ewing's Sarcoma
50. **UV Bleaching** was developed by Rosenthal
51. Root Canal Anatomy Laws are developed by **Krasner and Rankow**
52. Pin holes are prepared using **KODEX DRILL**
53. The only teeth showing all the eight root canal configurations is **Maxillary second premolar**
54. Clove Oil is used as sedative by **Lazare Rivere**
55. **Rule of Mixtures** is associated with dental composites
56. Mesenteric Line was described by **Pickrell**
57. Pan T lymphocyte marker is **CD 3**
58. Candle flame and Blade of grass appearance seen in the radiographic appearance of **Paget's Disease**
59. .Onlay graft described as thick free gingival graft by **Siebert**
60. **Port wine colored urine** seen in electrical burns

61. **Protostylid** is seen in buccal surface of mesiobuccal cusp of mandibular molars
62. **12 Peck Rule** is related with Light Speed RCT Instruments
63. **Sector classification** for canine impaction was given by Ercison and Kurol and modified by Lindauer
64. **Bergland index** to evaluate success of bone graft based on height of interdental septum

    Type I Normal

    Type II 75 % of normal bone height

    Type III Less than 75 %

    Type IV No bony ridge
65. **Insta Nance** for Molar Distalisation was developed by Hilgers
66. Mushroom shaped arch wire was by **Fujita**
67. Merrifield profile line is also called **Z angle**

    Normal Value is 80+/- 9 degrees
68. **GULL IN FLIGHT CONTOUR** seen in base of nose
69. **V8** area associated with color vision
70. **SDA (Shortened Dental Arch)** Concept was by Arnd Kayser
71. Chondroma is mostly seen in **Anterior Maxilla**
72. **PAX-6** associated with Aniridia
73. **Clay Shoveler's fracture** associated with cervical vertebrae-C 6 and C 7
74. **Second window of infectivity** of Caries at age 6–12 Years and was described by Klock and Kroske
75. **Dutcher bodies** are seen in Multiple Myeloma
76. BRCA-1, BRCA-2 hMSH2, etc. affects genomic stability and is called **CARETAKER GENES**
77. Rb, NF-1, APC, VHL, etc. directly regulates the growth of tumour and is called **GATEKEEPER GENES**
78. **Klatskin tumours** are seen at confluence of left and right hepatic ducts
79. Tufting of terminal phalanges seen in **Hyperparathyroidism**
80. **Vanishing Bile Duct Syndrome** is associated with Chlorpromazine
81. Welder's flash is due to **Gamma Rays**
82. ADA number for water based dental cements is **96**
83. Reichenbach and Taatz used **Shoe and Foot Analogy** for Maxilla and Mandible
84. **Stacked brick pattern** of adherence to epithelial cells seen in EAEC
85. **3** Antiepileptics used for the prophylaxis of Migraine-**Topiramate**

    Valproate and Gabapentin
86. PTERION is called **GOD'S LITTLE JOKE**
87. **JW-17** used to identify calcifying canals
88. **Imaginary Audience Concept** was by David Elkind
89. First event of puberty occurs in **brain**

90. Best anesthesia for **TTXR channels**—Bupivacaine
91. **Exotic metal** is NiTi
92. **SAF** belongs to **Group 4** of endodontic instruments
93. **Multiaxis grinding** seen in H type instruments
94. **Tetraclean** contains Polypropylene glycol detergent
95. **Terminal Hinge Axis Theory** was by McCollum
96. A test based on counting the direction of each within pair difference- **Y sign test**
97. Removable Distal Shoe appliance by **Starkey**
98. **Blue Teeth** seen in Parkinson Disease patients
99. **Molar Triangle** is seen in Maxillary first molar
100. **M2 NiTi** instrument has Italian S cross section.
101. **Party wall** appearance seen in canalicular adenoma
102. **Tower Skull** seen in Apert's Syndrome
103. **Pyronine bodies** seen in Periapical granuloma
104. **Kuttner's tumour** is chronic sclerosing sialadenitis
105. Father of Public Health is **Cholera**
106. Multiple teeth can be isolated using **Silker-Glickman clamp**
107. Bur used for placement of chamfer—**Tinker bur**
108. Too low a current in an electrosurgical electrode can be detected by **Tissue Drag**
109. Predictive index for sports related injury was given by **Peter.J.Fos**
110. The model describing remineralisation demineralisation process is **MORENO MODEL**
111. The model describing GCF production is **PASHLEY'S MODEL**
112. Visible particles more than 50 mm are called **SPATTERS**
113. Droplets more than 50 mm are called **MISTS**
114. Alpha, beta and Gamma types of thumb sucking classification was given by **COOK**
115. **Ballista spring** used for treatment of impacted teeth
116. **PINT CLASP** used for retention under a molar tube
117. **DELTA CLASP** used in Twin Block Appliance
118. **RESTA CLASP** is a modified version of Adam's Clasp with squash loop
119. Enamel Flourosis was described by **BERZELIUS**
120. **Sheath of Neuman** seperates peritubular dentin from inter tubular dentin
121. Step child of Permanent Dentition—**Third molar**
122. **Crystal Growth Technique** was developed by Smith and Cartz
123. **Premolar Classification** of Malocclusion by **Katz**
124. **Law of Minimum** by Justin Von Liebig

125. **Theory of Canalisation of Growth** by Waddlington
126. **DENTAL CRUTCH** refers to Hawley's appliance
127. **Finite Element Analysis** is done to carry out stress distribution in a material
128. **Occlusogram** was developed by Marcotte and Burstone
129. **Double Flare Technique** was by Fava
130. **Anticurvature filing** was by AbouRass
131. **Balanced Force Technique** by Roane and Sabala
132. The **subgluteal vacuum concept** was by Sicher
133. **Ingle's Syndrome** is related to protrusive bruxism
134. **Spoon Denture** is used in Maxillary Kennedy Class IV in children
135. **Third day fever** is due to infection caused by an IV catheter
136. Contact Inhibition is shown by **GORE TEX**
137. Mid Crestal Split of Anterior Ileum Harvest is called **Clamshell Technique**
138. Medial or Lateral Pedicled Cortical Osteotomy is called **Trapdoor approach**
139. Crestal Pedicled Osteotomy is called **Tschopp approach**
140. Medial and Lateral Oblique Crestal Osteotomy is called **Tessier Approach**
141. **Pseudomonas aeroginosa** is the main pathogen in Septic Arthritis from malignant otitis externa in poorly controlled diabetes patients
142. **Mushroom shaped mass** seen in CT in TMJ Ankylosis
143. **Holmium-Y AG** laser used in fibrous ankylosis cases
144. **Steiger Burr** used to perform gap arthroplasty and condylectomy
145. **Blade Implants** developed by Linkow
146. **Zero in Kernahan Stark Classification** refers to Incisive Foramen
147. **Cayler's syndrome** affects Depressor AnguliOris
148. **Stapedial Artery Hematoma Theory** By Poswillo
149. **Treacle gene** – 5q32-33.1
150. Premaxilla also called as **Median Septal System**
151. **Miss Piggy Nose** seen after LeFort 1 osteotomy
152. **Second Messenger Concept in Orthodontics** by Sutherland and Roll
153. Material which doesn't flow until a critical shear stress is reached is **BINGHAM**
154. Suggested viral etiology for Paget's Disease- **MYXOVIRUS**
155. **Indian File Cells** are seen in Low Grade Polymorphic Adenocarcinoma
156. **Pseudoshave biopsy** is done in Melanoma
157. Cranial graft best taken from **Parietal** and is avoided from **Temporal**
158. Suggested organism for Parry Romberg Syndrome is **Borrelia**

159. **Cupping Effect** is seen in Verucca Vulgaris
160. **Tyndall effect** is seen in blue nevus
161. **Erlenmeyer flask deformity** seen in Gaucher disease
162. **Spitz nevus** also called as Juvenile Melanoma
163. Three rooted mandibular first premolars—**TOME'S ROOT**
164. Actinomycoses species shows **FRUSTRATED PHAGOCYTOSIS**
165. Term Zip coined by **Weine**
166. Three rooted maxillary first premolars is called **minimolars**
167. **Ratio measurement method** used in third generation apex locators
168. Gutta-percha is also called **MAZERWOOD**
169. **ENDODONTIC PANACEA** refers to Ca $(OH)_2$
170. Medial confluence of stress lines on the ramus that represents the arcial growth of the surface of the mandible is called **EVA'S POINT**
171. The best current source of hematopoetic stem cells is **umbilical cord blood**
172. **Confabulation** is associated with lesion in the ventromedial portions of the Frontal Lobe
173. Metabolic Pump Actvity is shown by **Retrodiskal Pad**
174. **POWER DRIVE** electronic Instrument is used with CARISOLV
175. **SLEEPERS** are implants inserted only to maintain crestal bone height
176. Acetyl Choline Theory by **DETT BARN**
177. Calcium Displacement Theory by **GOLDMAN**
178. Surface Charge Repulsion Theory by **WEI**
179. Membrane Expansion Theory by **LEE**
180. Specific Receptor Theory by **Strichartz**
181. CARIOGRAM developed by **Brathall**
     Dark Blue-Diet
     Light Blue-Susceptibility
     Yellow-Circumstances
     Green-Chance of avoiding caries
     Red-Bacteria
182. **Functional Measure Index** = Filled + Sound Teeth/28
183. **Haberman Feeder** and **Hazelbake finger feeder** used for Cleft patients
184. **Shoulder Hand Syndrome** is Adverse effect of INH
185. Fourth Dimension of habit along with Duration, Intensity, Frequency- Direction introduced by **Pinkham**
186. **Cheating muscle** is Superior Oblique
187. **RHINO ROCKET** is guaze pack for Epistaxis
188. Concept of Extreme Magnification In Dentistry by **Apotheker**

189. Heavy artillery of pediatric conscious sedation is **NARCOTICS**
190. **MCEWOY** preparation is used for esthetic resin placement in primary incisors
191. Almond Eyes seen in **PRADER WILLI SYNDROME**
192. **Pitchfork Analysis** was by LYSLE JOHNSTON
193. **TRIBOCHEMICAL COATING:** Fusing a microscopic layer of ceramic to the metal with special silica particle material called ROCATEC PLUS
194. **WATER TREES** refers to porosities in the Polymerised adhesive layer
195. **Ionic Seesaw Concept** was by LEVINE
196. Incremental Dental Care concept By **George Cunningham**
197. **YURKSTAS METHOD** is the use of U shaped metal occlusal template that is slightly convex on the lower surface
198. **HEX-LOCK** type implants are used in Cleft patients
199. A weaker fourth buttress in the midface: **ETHMOID VOMERIAN PILLAR**
200. **COMMA** shaped incision used to remove impacted teeth
201. Stereolithography in trauma uses **ARGON LASER**
202. **Christensen prosthesis** and **Kent-Vitek Prosthesis** used in TMJ Reconstruction
203. **ACUVOL** measures composite shrinkage
204. **WILHELMY METHOD** is the use of tensiometers to record forces of immersed impression specimens
205. **SUGGAMADEX** has a doughnut structure
206. **CHANDY MANEUVER** is used in Intubating LMA
207. ICU patients are monitored for **FAST HUG** protocol by Vincent

    F-Feeding

    A-Analgesia

    S-Sedation

    T-Thrombocytopenia

    H-Head of bed

    U-Ulcer prophylaxis

    G-Glycemic Control

208. Index used in Cleft Patients: **Great Ormond Street London Index** (GOSLON)
209. Artificial line that runs from medial canthus to the angle of mandible separating maxillary sinus into inferior and superior parts- **OHNGREN'S LINE**
210. **FACIT** collagens are **Type IX, XII and XIV**
211. Anchoring fibril collagen—**Type VII**
212. Endostatin forming collagens—**Type XV and XVIII**
213. **Loricin** in keratohyaline granules contain Sulphur
214. **ZISMAN PLOT** is used for determining critical surface energy of a solid

215. **Canine Model** was suggested for pathogenesis of Vibrio Cholera
216. The percentage of incisor show on posed smile with respect to clinical crown height is **MORLEY'S RATIO**
217. Envelope of Discrepancy coined by **EPKER**
218. **Key Ridge** term was by Atkinson
219. **BJORK SUM** = NSAr + SArGo + ArGoMe = 396 +/- 6 degrees
220. **Moire Diffraction** is used to determine facial asymmetry
221. **DENTAL HEMOGRAM** was developed by GUTHRIE
222. Maxillary lateral incisors are most commonly involved teeth in **apical scar formation**
223. **WHITE LINE TEST** is used to recognise extra canals
224. **RED LINE TEST** is used to know the underlying anatomy
225. **STUNNED PULP** refers to non responsive pulp for a period of 6–8 weeks
226. Ashleaf spots and Shagreen patch seen in **TUBEROUS SCLEROSIS**
227. **Full Mouth Disinfection** was by Quirynen et al.
228. Pitch of Hyrax Screw is **1 mm**
229. **Lines of Luder** seen in AMALGAM as well as acrylic in dental decompression syndrome
230. Oral site of lymphogranuloma venerum is **tongue**
231. **Galen's Nerve** is branch of SLN to Recurrent LN
232. **Zellballen or nests** are seen in Carotid body tumour
233. Fomepizole is a classical example of **ORPHAN DRUG**
234. **Trochlear** is also called PATHETIC NERVE
235. Abducent nerve passes through **DORELLO'S CANAL**
236. Four Zones of 4 handed dentistry

     MNEMONIC : OATS

     *__O__perating Zone

     *__A__ssistant Zone

     *__T__ransfer Zone

     *__S__tatic Zone
237. Tobramycin is C/I in **Myasthenia gravis**
238. **Phosphotungstic acid** stains mitochondria blue
239. **Exner's nerve:** Nerve from pharyngeal plexus to cricothyroid membrane
240. **Off label use** refers to the use of therapeutic use of fluoride varnish in U.S
241. **Apical Barrier Technique** as an alternative to Apexification was developed by HARBERT
242. First observation of dental mottling by **KUHNS**
243. Father of Forensic Odontology is **Dr OSCAR AMEDO**
244. 5 Step Panoramic Radiographic Analysis was by **CHOMENKO**

245. Top bottom Outside in approach in Panfacial fractures is by **GRUSS**
246. A combination of natural and synthetic molecule used to stimulate bone growth in injuries **GELRIN**
247. **SUNNY 16 RULE** is used in Cameras
248. Button Wiring technique by **LEONARD**
249. **Litchenstein Theory** was suggested as cause for OSTEOCHONDROMA
250. **Kubelka Munk Equation** is used to describe the OPTICAL properties of restorative materials
251. Hobo classified **DISOCCLUSION** into 4 types
252. Lithium disilicate crystals are seen in **IPS IMPRESS 2**
253. Plasma Prekallikrein is called CLOTTING FACTOR 15 **FLETCHER FACTOR**
254. High Molecular Weight (HMW) Kininogen is called CLOTTING FACTOR 14 **FITZGERALD FACTOR**
255. **Eppendorf tube** is used to store unused MTA
256. Kennedy Applegate Classification modified by **FISET** to Class VII to X

    Class VII In which all remaining natural teeth are located on one side of arch or of median line

    Class VIII All remaining natural teeth are at one anterior corner of the arch

    Class IX The functional and cosmetic requirements require the use of telescoped prosthesis

    Class X The arch must be restored with an overdenture
257. **TWIST**: Positive regulator of osteoblast differentiation
258. **Bird's Eye View** taken at 45 degrees
259. Pre eruptive caries was described by **Muhler**
260. **Intersystem crossing** is seen in Phosphoresecence
261. Teeth with smaller dowels exhibit greater resistance to fracture **CONSERVATIONIST**
262. Atleast 1 mm of sound dentin should be maintained circumferentially to resist the fracture- **PRESERVATIONIST**
263. Post width should not exceed 1/3rd of root width at its narrowest dimensions to resist fractures- **PROPORTIONIST**
264. **Magnetic Telescopic Device** also called Ritto Appliance
265. SABG was by **Boyne and Sands**
266. **AHI** (Apnoea Hypopnea Index) for grading Obstructive Sleep Apnea (OSA)

    ***10–20** Mild

    ***20–40** Moderate

    ***40 and above** Severe
267. Self ligating brackets by **Stolzenberg**
268. **Hamman's crunch** seen in Cervicofacial Emphysema
269. **Grapefruit juice** is an enzyme inhibitor
270. MTAD contains **Tween 80** Detergent

271. **Briault Probe** is used to identify pulp horns
272. **Tooth Slooth** is used to identify levels of tooth fracture
273. Hidden receptors in acquired pellicles for bacterial adhesion is referred to as **CRYPTITOPES**
274. Inventor of Dental Floss is **LEVI SPEAR PARMLY**
275. Term **Blow out Fracture** by Smith and Regan
276. Potential nociceptor during pulpal inflammation **LTB4**
277. Bonded Injectable Autopolymerising Composites used in **CANAL PROJECTION TECHNIQUE**
278. **SEMAPHORIN 3A** controls dental trigeminal axon fasciculation
279. Champagne Bubble test is for **NaOCl**
280. Overfilling of canals result in **SPHAGETTI PHENOMENON**
281. Matrix vesicles concentrate **Calcium and Lanthanum**
282. **Kasabach Meritt syndrome** associated with Hemangioma
283. String of Pearls seen in **Lichenoid Reaction**
284. **Chrysiasis** refers to pigmentations of GOLD
285. **Javelle's water** is NaOCl
286. Only appliance still made from gold is **CROZAT**
287. Opus Loop was by **SIATKOWSKI**
288. Height is measured by using **STADIOMETER**
289. **Musical Instruments** cause Class II malocclusion
290. Adrenarche is due to formation of **DHEA**
291. Neural crest cells are called as **FOURTH GERM LAYER**
292. **HYPERPLASIA** is the prominent feature of all forms of growth
293. Z line to plasma membrane connected by **DESMIN**
294. Actin to Z line by **ACTININ**
295. Z line to M line by **TITIN**
296. Silver Cones was introduced by **JASPER**
297. **THUMB SUCKING BOOK** was developed by Dragan Antolos
298. Term Timely Extraction was coined by **STEMM**
299. Anatomic similarity between ipsilateral anterior ileum and hemimandible is explained **by MANCHESTER PRINCIPLE**
300. RVG was developed by **Dr Francis Mouyen**
301. Mickey Mouse Ears are seen in Paracoccidiomycosis

Numerical Corner

- Size of sand particles in slow sand filter: 0.4–0.7 mm
- Size of sand particles in rapid sand filter: 0.2–0.3 mm
- Depth of supernatant water above sandbed: 1–1.5 metre
- Uneconomical to run filter when loss of head exceeds: 1.3 metre
- Air Prevention and Control of pollution Act 1981
- Normal conversation: 60–65 decibels
- World Ozone Day: September 16
- First Census of India: 1881
- Number of medical officers required for community health centres: 4
- ICDS Scheme 1975
- Quarantine act 1825
- India joined WHO in 1948
- Official birth of WHO: 7th April 1948
- Red Cross started in 1920
- Training of Dental Nurses at Wellington, NZ – 1921
- Shoe Leather Survey 1934
- World's first artificial fluoridation 1945
- Reduction percentage by community water fluoridation: 50–65%
- Concentration of NaF in duraphat: 2.26%
- Knutson technique at ages: 3, 7, 11, 13
- SnF2 used at concentration of 8%
- APF used at concentration of 1.23%
- Certainly lethal dose (CLD) for Fluoride: 32–64 mg/kg body weight
- Safely tolerated dose (STD): 8–16 mg/kg body weight
- Fluor protector: 0.7% Fluoride
- NaF daily used in concentration of 0.05%
- NaF weekly used in concentration of 0.2%
- Recommended school water fluoridation when community water supply is not fluoridated: 4.5 pppm
- Antiplatelet dose of aspirin: 0.5–1.5 mg/kg/day
- Analgesic dose of aspirin: 5–10 mg/day

- Antiinflammatory: 30 mg/kg/day
- Risk of dry socket for women having oral contraceptives: 20%
- Maximum dose of lignocaine without adrenaline: 4.4 mg/kg body weight
- Maximum dose of lignocaine with adrenaline: 7 mg/kg body weight
- Amount of vasoconstrictor in 1 ml of 2% lignocaine solution with 1: 2,00,000 adrenaline: 0.005 mg
- Safe dose of adrenaline in cardiac patient: 0.04 mg
- ECG changes can be pobserved when level of lignocaine more than: 5–6 μg/ml
- Amount of dye that can be injected into the ductal system of parotid gland during sialography: 1–1.5 ml
- Gap between the base of the skull and ramus of the mandible during arthroplasty to prevent reankylosis should be at least: 1–1.5 cm
- The outermost holes of an eccentric dynamic compression plate are angled at 75 degree
- Wire used for figure of eight wiring for stabilisation of subluxated teeth in alveolar injuries: 0.35 mm stainless steel wire
- Blow out fracture needed for surgical intervention when enophthalmos exceeds 3 mm
- Thickness of split skin graft used in OMFS: 0.3–0.5 mm
- Chlorhexidine percent used in full mouth disinfection: 1% for 1 minute
- Spectrum of health has dimensions 7
- Average value of palatal height index 42%
- Scrub time with CHX soap: 3–5 minutes
- Morely's ratio is usually 75–100%
- Maximum plaque accumulation takes place in 30 days
- Energy range required to fracture mandible is in the range of 44.6–74.4 kg/m
- Temperature of recovery room: 19–22 degree Celsius
- Period of Na excretion shutdown can last up to 48 hours
- Ideal temperature of cooling water for burns: 15 degree Celsius
- Guage of needle used in the Trifecta system of obturation: 22 guage
- The inherent filtration of X-ray machines range from .... thickness of Aluminium: 0.5–2 mm
- The overall accuracy of sensitivity of bitewing to detect caries is estimated to be 40–65%
- The detection limit for mercury in water is 0.02 microgram/ml
- The minimum output of QTH should be never less than 300 Mw/cm^2
- The incidence of secondary caries in composite after 10 years is 3%
- Tests for safety of biomaterials are described as parts of ISO 7405:1997
- Minimum interpin distance for Minikin and Minim are 3 mm and 5 mm
- One grain is equal to 65 mg
- Freedom of centric is 0.5–1.5 mm

- The amount of epinephrine lost (and presumed absorbed) from 2.5 cm of typical retraction cord during 5–15 minutes in the gingival sulcus is 71 micrograms
- A minimum urinary output required to excrete the end products of protein metabolism is 400 ml
- Normal anion gap is 8–16 Mm/l
- Peak of dental caries is at ....% of sugar concentration: 15
- Pantograph tracing utilises ...... styli: 6
- The intercondylar distance in Whipmix articulator is 88–112 mm
- Sleep apnoea lasts for at least 10 seconds
- Fracture of base of skull may cause injury to all cranial nerves except: II and XII
- Forsus available in length of: 25 mm, 29 mm, 32 mm, 35 mm and 38 mm
- T loop 0.017 × 0.025 TMA wire
- Mushroom loop by Nanda 0.017 × 0.025 CNA wire
- Active stabilisation can overcome forces up to 5–10 gm/cm^2
- Merrifield line or Z angle normal value is 80 +/- 9 degrees
- The total height of both casts in occlusion is 7–7.5 cm
- ADA 57 sealers
- ADA 32 orthodontic wires
- ADA 119 manual toothbrushes
- Colour vision area: V8
- Anticipated degree of error which is bound to occur while orienting a cast on a surveyor after tripoding: 0.2 mm
- Clay shoveler's fracture affects cervical vertebra: C6 and C7
- Rickett's spring for canine retraction: 0.016 × 0.016 blue Elgiloy wire
- Gjessing spring: 0.16 × 0.22 SS/TMA wire
- Marker for hypertophic chondrocytes: Type IX collagen
- Adam's clasp in canine made of 24 mil
- Fetal alcohol syndrome Day 17
- Total eruption path of first permanent molar: 2.5 cm
- For conversion from flush terminal to class I .... Movement of lower molar is needed: 3.5 mm
- Adrenarche age 6
- When nose blocked there is 5 degrees change in craniovertebral angle
- The change from nasal to oral breathing crossover varies, but usually reaches a resistance of about 3.5–4 cm H_2O/L/min
- Latex elastics are 4–6 times better
- Drag loop made using 14 mil SS wire

- Potato chip wire used for levelling uses 16 mil NiTi wire
- Opus loop of Siatkowski made from 16 × 22 SS, 18 × 25 SS, 17 × 25 TMA
- Play same for 17 × 25 (18 slot) and 21 × 25 (22 slot) brackets

Tipping	35–60 gms
Translation	70–120 gms
Root uprighting	50–100 gms
Rotation	35–60 gms
Extrusion	35–60 gms
Intrusion	10–20 gms

- Cold test maximum 15 seconds
- Heat test maximum 150 degree Celsius
- LDF HeNe 632.8 mm
- Pulse oximetry 640 mm
- ISO 3630-1 K type files
- SAF 20 K file available in 3 lengths: 21 mm, 25 mm and 31 mm
- Apexum: 330 micrometres and uses 30 file
- Residual antimicrobial activity of CHX in root canal: 12 weeks
- Tetraclean contains: 50 mg/5 ml doxycycline and polypropylene glycol
- Endovac: Size 55 with 2% taper
- Intralight UV disinfection: 254 nm
- Tolerance of endodontic file: +0.05 mm
- ADA 41: Protocols for biologic evaluation of dental materials
- Cavit placed at thickness of at least 4–5 mm
- PMMA transmit light into UV range of wavelength: 0.25 micrometres
- Half life of MMA in blood at 37 degree Celsius: 20–40 minutes
- Classical alloy mercury ratio: 5 parts alloy to 8 parts mercury
- Complete wax elimination occurs at: 480 degree Celsius for 45 minutes
- Endosequence: 600 rpm
- Flexmaster: 0.15-0.7 mm diameter
- Hot Shot instrument available in 3 guages: 20, 23 and 25
- Odontoblasts consume Oxygen at the rate of 3.2+/- 0.2 ml/min/100 gm of pulp tissue
- Interstitial fluid volume in pulp is 0.6+/- 0.03 ml/g wet weight
- Resting pulpal blood flow is 0.15–0.60 ml/min/gm of tissue
- Stabident and X tip intraosseous anaesthesia uses 27 guage wire
- X-rays collimated not to exceed 7 cms at skin surface

- Actisite has tetracycline 12.7 mg/9 inches
- Restorative materials may change in dimension by up to ..... times more than enamel for every degree of temperature change 4.4
- ISO TC 106 SC1: Filling and restorative materials
- SC2: Prosthodontic materials
- SC3: Terminology
- SC4: Dental instruments
- SC 6: Dental equipment
- SC 7: Oral hygiene products
- SC 8: Dental implants
- For testing the ductility of dental materials the standard guage length is usually 51 mm
- ISO 10993: For testing biocompatibility of dental materials
- While doing a casting the pressure should be maintained for at least 4 seconds
- The minimum thickness of the dentin bonding agent to avoid oxygen inhibition should be 50 micrometres
- The degree of conversion for restorative resin is 50–60%
- Maximum permissible thickness of cements for restorative purpose is 40 micrometres
- The acid content of the liquid of zinc phosphate cement is about 33+/-5%
- Gamma phase: Ag3Sn
- Gamma 1: Ag2Hg3
- Gamma 2: Sn8Hg
- Eta: Cu6Sn5
- Epsilon: Cu3Sn
- Homogenising of amalgam is done for 24 hours
- Critical mercury content for both high and low copper amalgams above which there is a marked reduction in strength is 54%
- Vapour pressure of mercury at room temperature is 20 mg/m^3
- Minimal thickness of metal coping required in the occlusal surface of a PFM crown is 0.3 mm
- Inclination of lower incisors by 1 degree labially increases arch length by 0.8 mm
- Voltage at which welding machine operates: 2–10 Volt
- Maximum retraction of incisors achieved by orthodontic treatment is 7 mm
- Depth of cure achieved with visible light cure unit for orthodontic bonding material polymerisation is close to 2.5 mm
- Sliding teeth along an arch wire would require a clearance of at least 0.05 inches
- Bracket slot for Begg bracket is 0.020 × 0.045 inch
- Approximate daily secretion of cortisol by adrenal cortex is 15 mg

AIIMS Anesthesia Question Bank

1. **Which of the following is correct regarding color coding of anesthetic gases?**
   a. Oxygen – Black with grey shoulders
   b. Nitric oxide – Blue
   c. Cyclopropane – Red
   d. Helium – Orange

   Ans. b
   - **Oxygen – Black with white shoulders**
   - **Nitric oxide – Blue**
   - Cyclopropane – Orange
   - Carbon Dioxide – Grey
   - Nitrogen – Black
   - Helium – Brown
   - Air – Grey body with white & black quartered shoulder

2. **Anesthetic agent contraindicated in hypertensives is:**
   a. Propofol
   b. Thiopentone sodium
   c. Diazepam
   d. Ketamine

   Ans. d
   - **Ketamine** increases heart rate, cardiac output and blood pressure
   - These effects are due to stimulation of the sympathetic nervous system and decrease in reuptake of noradrenaline
   - Hence it is contraindicated in:
     - Hypertensives
     - Ischemic heart disease
     - Congestive cardiac failure
     - Arterial aneurysms
   - It is also contraindicated in patients with increased intracranial tension
   - It produces dissociative anesthesia

3. **Contraindications to vasoconstrictors in local anesthesia:**
   a. Spinal anesthesia
   b. Epidural anesthesia
   c. Digital nerve block
   d. Regional anesthesia

   Ans. c
   - Vasoconstrictors like adrenaline are used with local anesthetics for decreasing the systemicabsorption and to increase the local anesthetic concentration and duration of nerve block
   - But adrenaline should not be used with lignocaine when infiltrating areas of **end arterial supply**
   - These sites include:
     - Fingers
     - Toes
     - Pinna
     - Penis
     - Nose
   - The use of adrenaline is these areas can compromise the blood flow and result in ischemic injury

4. **Which anesthetic agent is preferred in a patient taken for surgery with bilirubin of 8.6 mg/dl and serum creatinine of 2.1 mg/dl?**
   a. Atracurium
   b. Vecuronium
   c. Pancuronium
   d. Rocuronium
   Ans. a
   - Atracurium is the preferred muscle relaxant in a patient with liver dysfunction/renal failure
   - It undergoes non specific ester hydrolysis and non enzymatic degradation (Hoffman degradation)
   - It does not depend on the liver/kidney for its deactivation
   - Other muscle relaxants that can be given in liver/renal disease are Cisatracurium and Mivacurium
5. **A Lower Segment Caesarean section (LSCS) can be carried out under all the following techniques of anesthesia except:**
   a. General anesthesia
   b. Spinal anesthesia
   c. Caudal anesthesia
   d. Combined Spinal Epidural anesthesia
   Ans. c
   - Caudal anesthesia is used only for perineal surgery.
6. **The following modes of ventilation may be used for weaning off patients from mechanical ventilation except:**
   a. Controlled Mechanical ventilation (CMV)
   b. Synchronized intermittent mandatory ventilation (SIMV)
   c. Pressure support ventilation (PSV)
   d. Assist-control ventilation (ACV)
   Ans. a
7. **In CMV, the ventillator delivers the tidal volume. The patient effort is the most appropriate circuit for ventilating spontaneously breathing infant during anesthesia:**
   a. Jackson Rees modification of Ayre T piece
   b. Mapleson A or Mgill's circuit
   c. Mapleson C or Waters' to and fro canister
   d. Bains circuit
   Ans. a
8. **The following are used for treatment of postoperative nausea and vomiting following squint surgery in children except:**
   a. Ketamine
   b. Ondansetron
   c. Propofol
   d. Dexamethasone
   Ans. a
   - Ketamine can cause nausea and vomiting following administration.
9. **Which one of the following anesthetic agents causes a rise in the Intracranial pressure:**
   a. Sevoflurane
   b. Thiopentone sodium
   c. Lignocaine
   d. Propofol
   Ans. a
   Some anesthetic agents which increase Intracranial pressure
   - Sevoflurane
   - Isoflurane
   - Halothane

- Nitrous oxide
- Ketamine

10. Which one of the following is the fastest acting inhalational agent?

a. Halothane
b. Isoflurane
c. Ether
d. Sevoflurane

Ans. d Sevoflurane

Sevoflurane is the fastest acting among the options given. Desflurane is THE fastest acting inhalational agent.

11. Which of the following agents is used for the treatment of postoperative shivering?

a. Thiopentone
b. Suxamethonium
c. Atropine
d. Pethidine

Ans. d

- Drug of choice – Tramadol
- Alternate drugs – pethidine, pentazocine

Supportive treatment – oxygen inhalation (there is increased oxygen consumption during shivering)

12. Which of the following intravenous induction agents is the most suitable for day care surgery?

a. Morphine
b. Ketamine
c. Propofol
d. Diazepam

Ans. c

Propofol is the induction agent of choice in day care surgery

- Early induction
- Smooth recovery
- Decreased incidence of post operative nausea and vomiting

13. Which of the following anesthetic agents does not trigger malignant hyperthermia?

a. Halothane
b. Isoflurane
c. Suxamethonium
d. Thiopentone

Ans. d

Anesthetic agents implicated in malignant hyperthermia:

- Succinyl choline
- Halothane
- Isoflurane

14. Which of the following statements is not true about etomidate?

a. It is an intravenous anesthetic
b. It precipitates coronary insufficiency
c. It inhibits cortisol synthesis
d. It causes pain at site of injection

Ans. b

Disadvantages of etomidate:

- Decrease cortisol synthesis
- Painful injection
- Nausea and vomiting during recovery period
- Produce restlessness and rigidity

15. Which one of the following agents sensitizes the myocardium to catecholamines?

a. Isoflurane
b. Ether
c. Halothane
d. Propofol

Ans. c

- Halothane sensitizes the myocardium to the action of catecholamines and can produce severe ventricular arrhythmia.

16. Which of the following inhalational agents is the induction agent of choice in children?

a. Methoxyflurane
b. Sevoflurane
c. Desflurane
d. Isoflurane

Ans. b

- Sevoflurane has a fast, smooth and pleasant induction. Hence it is preferred in children. Sevoflurane reacts with soda lime to produce toxic products. Hence it cannot be used in a closed circuit

17. Which one of the following local anesthetics belongs to the ester group?

a. Procaine
b. Bupivacaine
c. Lignocaine
d. Mepivacaine

Ans. a

Other ester linked local anesthetics:

- Cocaine
- Tetracaine
- Benzocaine
- Chlorprocaine

18. Which one of the following antibacterials should not be used with d-tubocurarine?

a. Norfloxacin
b. Streptomycin
c. Doxycycline
d. Cefotaxime

Ans. b Streptomycin

- Streptomycin can potentiate the action of d-tubocurarine and cause prolonged apnoea.

d-tubocurarine is a muscle relaxant. All aminoglycosides including streptomycin reduce ACh release from motor nerve endings. This is usually not manifested clinically. But the effect is more pronounced when given along with curare like muscle relaxants

19. Which of the following is the muscle relaxant of choice in renal failure?

a. Rapacurium
b. Pancuronium
c. Atracurium
d. Rocuronium

Ans. c

Atracurium undergoes Hoffman degradation. So elimination does not depend upon liver or kidney function.

20. Which one of the following muscle relaxant has the maximum duration of action?

a. Atracurium
b. Vecuronium
c. Rocuronium
d. Doxacurium

Ans. d

21. Which of the following is not an indication for endotracheal intubation?

a. Maintenance of a patent airway
b. To provide positive pressure ventilation
c. Pulmonary toilet
d. Pneumothorax

Ans. d

Pneumothorax should be treated with intercostal drainage/needle thoracocentesis.

22. Which one of the following is the description used for the term allodynia during pain management?

a. Absence of pain perception
b. Complete lack of pain sensation
c. Unpleasant sensation with or without a stimulus
d. Perception of an ordinarily non noxious sitmulus as severe pain.

Ans. d

Perception of an ordinarily non noxious sitmulus as severe pain Allodynia is the perception of an ordinarily non noxious sitmulus as severe pain

23. Which side effect is commonly seen with fentanyl?

a. Chest wall rigidity
b. Tachycardia
c. Pain in abdomen
d. Hypertension

Ans. a

- Chest wall rigidity is an important side effect of opioids like fentanyl. It may even impair ventilation.

24. Which of the following drugs is contraindicated in a patient with raised intracranial pressure?

a. Thiopentone
b. Propofol
c. Midazolarn
d. Ketamine

Ans. d

- Ketamine increases cerebral blood flow and intracranial pressure. Hence it is contraindicated in patients with increased intracranial pressure.

25. The following anesthetic drug causes pain on intravenous adminstration:

a. Midazolam
b. Propofol
c. Ketamine
d. Thiopentone sodium

Ans. d

- Inadvertent intra arterial injection of thiopentone sodium produces pain, not intravenous injection. Propofol causes pain with intravenous injection.

26. Which of the following fluorinated anesthetics corrodes metal in vaporizers and breathing systems?

a. Sevoflurane
b. Enflurane
c. lsoflurane
d. Halothane

Ans. d

27. Which of the following inhalational agents has the minimum blood gas solubility coefficient?

a. Isoflurane
b. Sevoflurane
c. Desflurane
d. Nitrous oxide

Ans. c

28. **Which of the following is the neuromuscular blocking agent with the shortest onset of action?**
    a. Mivacurium
    b. Vecuronium
    c. Rapacuronium
    d. Succinylcholine
    Ans. d
29. **In general, the last muscle to be rendered akinetic with a retrobulbaranesthetic block is:**
    a. Superior rectus
    b. Superior oblique
    c. Inferior oblique
    d. Levator palpebral superioris
    Ans. b
30. **A 20-year-old patient presented with early pregnancy was admitted for Medical Termination of Pregnancy (MTP) in day care facility. What will be the anesthetic induction agent of choice?**
    a. Thiopentone
    b. Ketamine
    c. Propofol
    d. Diazepam
    Ans. c
31. **Which of the following produces dissociative anesthesia?**
    a. Ketamine
    b. Propofol
    c. Thiopentone
    d. Enflurane
    Ans. a
32. **Which of the following in anesthesia will produce decreased EEG activities?**
    a. Hypothermia
    b. Early hypoxia
    c. Ketamine
    d. N2O
    Ans. a
33. **Which of the following is not true about Xenon anesthesia?**
    a. Non explosive
    b. Minimal cardiovascular side effects
    c. Slow induction and slow recovery
    d. Low blood gas solubility
    Ans. c
    - Xenon is very close to being an ideal anesthetic agent with multiple advantages like:
        - Inert
        - Non toxic
        - Minimal cardiovascular effects
        - Low blood solubility
        - Fast induction and recovery
        - Non explosive
        - Does not cause malignant hyperthermia
34. **Merits of nasotracheal intubation is:**
    a. Good oral hygiene
    b. Less infection
    c. Less mucosal damage and bleeding
    d. More movement or displacement of endotracheal tube
    Ans. a

35. Most common nerve used for monitoring during anesthesia:
   a. Ulnar nerve
   b. Facial nerve
   c. Radial nerve
   d. Median nerve

   Ans. a

36. All are seen in Malignant hyperthermia except:
   a. Bradycardia
   b. Hyperkalemia
   c. Metabolic acidosis
   d. Hypertension

   Ans. a

37. Side effects of oxygen therapy are all except:
   a. Absorption atelactasis
   b. Increased pulmonary compliance
   c. Decreased vital capacity
   d. Endothelial damage

   Ans. b

38. Muscle relaxant of choice in hepatic and renal failure:
   a. Cisatracurium
   b. Rocuronium
   c. Vecuronium
   d. Rapacuronium

   Ans. a

39. A young boy undergoes eye surgery under day care anesthesia with succinyl choline and propofol and after 8 hours he starts walking and develops muscle pain. What is the likely cause?
   a. Early mobilisation
   b. Due to the effects of eye surgery
   c. Succinyl choline
   d. Propofol

   Ans. a

   Muscle pain is a common adverse effect

40. Which of the following is not an amide linked local anesthetic?
   a. Lignocaine
   b. Procaine
   c. Bupivacaine
   d. Dibucaine

   Ans. b

   It is an ester linked anesthetic

AIIMS Physiology SR Papers

GENERAL FUNCTIONAL ORGANIZATION OF THE NERVOUS SYSTEM

1. **The central nervous system includes all the following components, except:**
   a. Spinal cords
   b. Medulla oblongata
   c. Autonomic ganglia
   d. Diencephalon
   Ans. c
2. **The central nervous system is connected with the peripheral nervoussystem by all the following types of nerve fibers, except:**
   a. Postganglionic autonomic fibers
   b. Preganglionic autonomic fibers
   c. Somatic motor fibers
   d. Autonomic sensory fibers
   Ans. a
3. **The sensory system is involved in all the following, except:**
   a. Initiation of reflex movements
   b. Initiation of voluntary movements
   c. Learning processes
   d. Initiation of emotional responses
   Ans. b

SENSORY SYSTEM AND SENSORY RECEPTORS

1. **The two-element sensory receptors differ from other types of receptors in being:**
   a. More numerous
   b. More widely spread in the body
   c. More sensitive
   d. Composed of specialized cells at the sensory nerve terminals
   Ans. d
2. **Sensory receptors are classified functionally according to the following criteria, except:**
   a. Their location in the body
   b. The nature of tissues in which they are found
   c. The nature of stimuli acting on them
   d. Their connection with cerebral coretx
   Ans. a
3. **Most sensory receptors:**
   a. Are stimulated by different types of stimuli
   b. Are stimulated only by specific stimuli
   c. Posses a high threshold for their specific stimuli
   d. Pnly 'b' and 'c' are correct
   Ans. b
4. **A specific stimulus produces a receptor potential by:**
   a. Inhibiting Na^+ influx into receptor
   b. Inhibiting K^+ efflux from receptor
   c. Enhancing Na^+ influx into receptor
   d. Enhancing K^+ efflux from receptor
   Ans. c

5. **Receptor potential initiated by an adequate stimulus:**
   a. Develops always at it full magnitudes
   b. Undergoes temporal summation only
   c. Undergoes spatial summation only
   d. Could initiate an action potential
   Ans. d
6. **Once initiated, the receptor potential:**
   a. Spreads to a long distance along the sensory nerve fiber
   b. Amplitude is not related to the strength of the stimulus
   c. Always generates an action potential from the receptor
   d. Stays for a variable period depending on the type of the receptor
   Ans. d
7. **Receptor potential generates:**
   a. An electrotonic current which is transmitted along sensory fibers to the CNS
   b. A nerve impulse at the receptive region of the receptor
   c. A state of hyperpolarization of the receptor membrane
   d. A nerve impulse at the spike initiating region of the receptor
   Ans. d
8. **When stimulated by effective steady stimuli, sensory receptors?**
   a. Continuously discharge impulses
   b. Stop discharging after a short time
   c. Produce an initial high rate of impulse discharge followed by decline of this rate
   d. Differ in their response; some types discharge continuously, while other types do not respond at all
   Ans. c
9. **Slowly adapting receptors include all the following types, except:**
   a. Golgi tendon organs
   b. Warmth receptors
   c. Free nerve endings
   d. Meissner corpuscles
   Ans. d
10. **Slowly adapting receptors differ from rapidly adapting receptors in:**
   a. Stopping to discharge after a relatively longer period of constant stimulation
   b. Detecting the dynamic properties of stimuli
   c. Detecting velocity of stimuli
   d. Generating receptor potentials with different properties
   Ans. d
11. **Rapidly adapting receptors are involved in:**
   a. Initiation of rapid reflex responses
   b. Detection of joint movements
   c. Regulation of heart rate
   d. Pnly 'a' and 'b' are correct
   Ans. b
12. **Receptors detect stimulus intensity by:**
   a. Lowering the threshold for receptor stimulation
   b. By generating receptor potentials having higher magnitudes
   c. By generating nerve impulses that are transmitted along sensory fibers at higher velocities
   d. By enhancing the central effects of sensory impulses
   Ans. b

SENSATION AND CODING OF SENSORY INFORMATION

1. **General sensations:**
   a. Originate from all sensory receptors of the body
   b. Are mediated by somatic sensory fibers only
   c. Include the sense of movement
   d. Include the sense of equilibrium
   Ans. c
2. **Detection of the stimulus modality depends upon:**
   a. The location of the receptors in the body
   b. The magnitude of the stimulus
   c. The anatomical connections between the receptors and specific sensory areas in the cerebral cortex
   d. The magnitude of the receptor potential
   Ans. c
3. **Receptors detect stimulus intensity by:**
   a. Lowering the threshold for stimulating receptors
   b. Raising the threshold for stimulating receptors
   c. Decreasing the magnitude of receptor potential
   d. Raising the magnitude of receptor potential
   Ans. d
4. **The ability to localize the site of stimuli depends upon:**
   a. The type of the stimulated receptor
   b. Connections between the receptor and the sensory cortex
   c. The rate of adaptation of the stimulated receptors
   d. The nature of the stimulus
   Ans. b

MECHANORECEPTIVE SENSATIONS

1. **Touch receptors:**
   a. Are found only in the skin
   b. Are all encapsulated receptors
   c. Include two-element receptors
   d. Are stimulated by vibration
   Ans. d
2. **Tactile receptors include all the following receptors, except:**
   a. Free nerve endings
   b. Hair follicle receptors
   c. Hair cell receptors
   d. Ruffini nerve endings
   Ans. c
3. **Rapidly adapting tactile receptors include all the following types, except:**
   a. Merkel discs
   b. Meissner corpuscles
   c. Pacinian corpuscles
   d. Hair end organs
   Ans. a
4. **Fine touch:**
   a. Is detected by slowly adapting touch receptors
   b. Is transmitted by the spinothalamic tract
   c. Is characterized by it emotional affect
   d. Is not involved in feeling the texture of touched objects
   Ans. a

5. **Crude touch is more effective than fine touch in evoking an emotional response because:**
   a. Its provoking stimuli are stronger
   b. Its central pathway connects with the limbic system
   c. It is stimulated during emotional excitement
   d. The provoking stimuli have an emotional nature
   Ans. b
6. **A more developed two-point tactile discrimination:**
   a. Indicates a greater threshold distance for feeling of two points of touch applied simultaneously
   b. Is seen in the proximal regions of the body compared with the distal regions
   c. Is inversely related to the size of the receptive fields of the stimulated sensory units
   d. Depends upon the type of the involved touch
   Ans. c
7. **Proprioceptive sensations include all the following, except:**
   a. Position sense
   b. Equilibrium sense
   c. Movement sense
   d. Kinesthetic sense
   Ans. b
8. **Proprioceptors include all the following types of receptors, except:**
   a. Muscle spindles
   b. Pressure receptors
   c. Vestibular receptors
   d. Joint receptors
   Ans. c
9. **Proprioceptive sensations are transmitted by all the following pathways, except:**
   a. Spinothalamic tracts
   b. Spinocerebellar tract
   c. Gracile tract
   d. Cuneocerebellar tract
   Ans. a
10. **Astereognosis:**
   a. Indicates inability to localize the site of touch on the body surface
   b. Results from lesions of the secondary somatic sensory area
   c. Associates parietal lobe neglect
   d. Results from loss of crude touch sensation
   Ans. c
11. **Parietal lobe neglect:**
   a. Is characterized by inability to use skeletal muscles on the opposite side of the body
   b. Is characterized by inability to use skeletal muscles on the same side of the body
   c. Causes loss of sensations on the opposite side of the body
   d. Causes loss of sensations on the same side of the body
   Ans. a

PAIN SENSATION

1. **Pain sensation:**
   a. Is evoked by strong stimulation of specific receptors
   b. Produces reactions that block transmission of pain impulses
   c. Arises from small encapsulated receptors
   d. Pccurs when the stimulus causes damage of the sensory receptors
   Ans. a

2. **Reaction to pain includes all the following, except:**
   a. Increased heart rate
   b. Depression
   c. Withdrawal reflexes
   d. Depressed transmission of pain impulses along sensory pain fibers
   Ans. d
3. **Pain receptors:**
   a. Become more sensitive with prolonged stimulation
   b. Are stimulated by prostaglandins
   c. Are more numerous in viscera than other tissues
   d. Include different morphological types
   Ans. a
4. **Pain threshold:**
   a. Is the highest intensity of stimulus that causes pain
   b. Is the lowest intensity of stimulus that causes pain
   c. Differs markedly among different individuals
   d. Is elevated by substance P
   Ans. b
5. **Fast pain differs from slow pain in:**
   a. Being transmitted in the dorsal column pathway
   b. Evoking a depressor autonomic reaction
   c. Having a sharp quality
   d. Arising from encapsulated pain receptors
   Ans. c
6. **Double pain sensation that is occasionally felt following painful stimulation of the skin is due to:**
   a. Repetition of the painful stimulus
   b. Presence of dual pain pathways
   c. Perception of pain at two different higher centers
   d. Application of two painful stimuli simultaneously at two different sites
   Ans. b
7. **Cutaneous pain:**
   a. Is always sharp in character
   b. Is transmitted by A sensory fibers
   c. Is always followed by hyperalgesia
   d. Evokes spasm of nearby muscles
   Ans. b
8. **Primary cutaneous hyperalgesia:**
   a. Develops in the normal skin region around the area of flare
   b. Is an abnormal condition in the skin in which painful stimuli become more severe
   c. Is due to changes in threshold of pain receptors
   d. Is associated with throbbing type of pain
   Ans. c
9. **Deep pain shows the following characteristics, except:**
   a. Dull aching
   b. Throbbing
   c. Evokes flexor reflexes
   d. Diffuse
   Ans. c

10. **Intermittent Claudications evoke:**
    a. Visceral pain
    b. Deep pain
    c. Cutaneous hyperalgesia
    d. Colicky pain
    Ans. b
11. **Pain produced by muscle spasm results from:**
    a. Mechanical stimulation of pain receptor by muscle spasm
    b. Decreased release of lactic acid from the spastic muscle fibers
    c. Release of compounds from the spastic muscle which increase the threshold for stimulation of pain receptors
    d. Decreased oxygen supply to the muscle
    Ans. d
12. **Visceral pain:**
    a. Is more common than the other types of pain
    b. Arises only from wall of the visceral organs
    c. Is often well localized
    d. Evokes depressor autonomic reactions
    Ans. d
13. **Stimuli which evoke true visceral pain include all the following, except:**
    a. Sharp cutting
    b. Stretching
    c. Spasm
    d. Chemical irritation
    Ans. a
14. **Visceral pain is usually felt:**
    a. Deeply in the diseased viscera
    b. In deep tissues close to the diseased viscera
    c. In skin areas that just overlie the diseased viscera
    d. In skin areas remote from the diseased viscera
    Ans. d
15. **Intracranial headache could result from painful stimuli applied on:**
    a. The dura lining the inner surface of the bones of cranial vault
    b. The brain tissue
    c. Wall of big intracranial veins
    d. Arachnoid mater
    Ans. c
16. **Intracranial headache may result from all the following clinical causes, except:**
    a. Decreased CSF pressure
    b. Spasm of scalp muscles
    c. Distension of big venous sinuses
    d. Pressure upon tentorium cerebelli
    Ans. b
17. **Transmitters in pain control system include all the following, except:**
    a. Serotonin
    b. Acetylcholine
    c. Enkephalin
    d. Norepinephrine
    Ans. b

18. **Enkephalin binds best with:**
    a. Delta 'δ' opiate receptors
    b. Muta 'μ' opiate receptors
    c. Kappa 'κ' opiate receptors
    d. All opiate receptors with equal affinity
    Ans. a
19. **Pain control system:**
    a. Is activated whenever a painful stimulus is applied to body tissues
    b. Is never activated naturally
    c. Is activated only by administration of opiate drugs
    d. Is activated naturally under conditions associated with strong emotional excitement
    Ans. d
20. **Enkephalin blocks pain transmission by:**
    a. Blocking the response of pain receptors to painful stimuli
    b. Slowing down transmission of pain impulses through synapses in the pain pathway
    c. Inhibiting the response of the cerebral cortical somatic sensory area to pain signals
    d. Blocking Ca^{++} channels in the central terminals of pain sensory fibers
    Ans. d
21. **The spinal pain gate is:**
    a. Ligand controlled
    b. Voltage controlled
    c. Ppened by enkephalin
    d. Closed by substance P
    Ans. a

THERMAL SENSATIONS

1. **Thermal sensations:**
    a. Are evoked by all changes in environmental temperatures
    b. Are evoked by stimulation of thermo-sensitive pain receptors
    c. Are involved in regulation of metabolic activity
    d. Are transmitted by Aβ sensory fibers
    Ans. c
2. **Thermal receptors are:**
    a. Slowly adapting receptors
    b. Rapidly adapting receptors
    c. Biphasic receptors
    d. All encapsulated receptors
    Ans. a

SYNAPSES OF THE CENTRAL NERVOUS SYSTEM

1. **Connexons of gap junctions in electric synapses:**
    a. Are Ligand gated
    b. Are voltage-gated
    c. Allow transmission of potential changes in both directions between the pre and post-synaptic neurons
    d. Close whenever the presynaptic neuron becomes hyperpolarized
    Ans. c
2. **Chemical synapses in the nervous system:**
    a. Allow diffusion of chemical substances form the presynaptic neuron into the postsynaptic neuron
    b. Allow transmission of potential changes in one direction only; from the presynaptic to the postsynaptic neurons
    c. Have potential-gated ionic channels
    d. Are more numerous in the peripheral nervous system than the central nervous system
    Ans. b

3. **Synaptic cleft:**
   a. Is the space between two synapses on the surface of neurons
   b. Allow diffusion of transmitters between neurons
   c. Is filled with intracellular fluid
   d. Ranges between 20–30 μm in width
   Ans. b
4. **Synaptic knobs:**
   a. Synthesize different types of neurotransmitters
   b. Release neurotransmitters by diffusion across their membranes
   c. Have ligand gated Ca^{++}
   d. Are located at the terminal end of dendrites
   Ans. a
5. **Synaptic transmission depends upon:**
   a. Direct transmission of impulses from the presynaptic neuron to the postsynaptic neuron
   b. Diffusion of neurotransmitters from synaptic knobs into the soma and dendrites of postsynaptic neurons
   c. Presence of voltage-gated Ca^{++} channels in membrane of synaptic knobs
   d. Presence of voltage-gated Ca^{++} channels in the subsynaptic membrane
   Ans. c
6. **Postsynaptic receptors include all the following types, except:**
   a. G-protein coupled receptors
   b. Ligand gated cation channels
   c. G-protein regulated K^+ channels
   d. Voltage-gated Cl- channels
   Ans. d
7. **When opened, the ligand gated cation channels do not allow diffusion of Cl^- because:**
   a. The size of Cl- is bigger than the bore of the channels
   b. Intracellular negativity causes complete inhibition of Cl^- influx
   c. The channels are specific for diffusion of Na^+ only
   d. The inner surface of the channels is negatively charged
   Ans. d
8. **Opening of ligand gated Cl- channels causes:**
   a. Inhibition of the postsynaptic neuron
   b. Depolarization of the postsynaptic neuron
   c. Initiation of an action potential
   d. Block of ligand gated cation channels
   Ans. a
9. **IPSP differs from EPSP in:**
   a. Being of shorter duration
   b. Being unable o summate spatially
   c. Moving the membrane potential away from threshold
   d. Depending upon opening of voltage K^+ channels
   Ans. c
10. **When EPSP and IPSP occur simultaneously the postsynaptic membrane:**
   a. Becomes depolarized
   b. Becomes hyperpolarized
   c. Initiates an action potential
   d. Shows potential changes that depend upon the summation of their effects
   Ans. d

11. **When a postsynaptic neuron is adequately stimulated, action potentials develop at the initial segment of the axon because:**
    a. It contains many voltage-gated Na^+ channels
    b. It contains the highest concentration of ligand gated cation channels
    c. It contains many voltage-gated Ca^{++} channels
    d. It is more sensitive to the direct stimulant effect of neurotransmitters
    Ans. a
12. **IPSP could result from:**
    a. Opening of K^+ channels
    b. Ppening of ligand gated cation channels
    c. Closure of Cl- channels
    d. Closure of potential-gated Ca^{++} channels
    Ans. a
13. **Synaptic transmission s terminated by:**
    a. Block of postsynaptic receptors
    b. Elevation of Ca^{++} concentration in synaptic cleft
    c. Reuptake of neurotransmitters by postsynaptic neurons
    d. Degradation of neurotransmitters by specific enzymes
    Ans. d
14. **Presynaptic inhibition is characterized by all the following, except:**
    a. Increased Cl- influx into presynaptic terminals
    b. Increased Ca^{++} influx into presynaptic terminals
    c. Decreased response of postsynaptic receptors
    d. Hyperpolarization of presynaptic terminals
    Ans. b
15. **Presynaptic inhibition depends upon:**
    a. Augmented release of chemical transmitter from presynaptic terminals
    b. Continued depolarization of presynaptic terminals
    c. GABA receptors in presynaptic terminals
    d. Ppening of voltage-gated Ca^{++} channels in presynaptic terminals
    Ans. c
16. **In chemical synapses, transmission occurs in a forward direction because:**
    a. Neurotransmitter receptors are found only in the postsynaptic membrane
    b. The subsynaptic membrane does not contain neurotransmitter vesicles
    c. The subsynaptic membrane is more sensitive than the membrane of synaptic knob to the effect of neurotransmitters
    d. The subsynaptic membrane contains both ligand gated and voltage-gated ionic channels
    Ans. b
17. **Synaptic delay:**
    a. Is the time needed for release of neurotransmitter from synaptic vesicles
    b. The minimal delay time in the central nervous system is about 0.5 millisecond
    c. Is determined by the type of the neurotransmitter
    d. Is determined by the number of postsynaptic receptors
    Ans. b
18. **Synaptic fatigue is due to:**
    a. Decreased synthesis of neurotransmitters
    b. Inability to release neurotransmitters by exocytosis
    c. Failure of action potentials to open voltage-gated Ca^{++} channels in presynaptic terminal
    d. Imbalance in between rates of synthesis and release of neurotransmitters
    Ans. d

19. **Synaptic transmission is inhibited by all the following, except:**
    a. Oxygen lack
    b. Alkalosis
    c. Acidosis
    d. Prolonged activity of synapse
    Ans. b
20. **Post-tetanic Potentiation in synapses:**
    a. Is due to increased Ca^{++} concentration in postsynaptic neurons
    b. Is due to increased Ca^{++} influx into presynaptic neurons
    c. Results from slow prolonged stimulation of synapse
    d. Causes fatigue of the synapse
    Ans. b
21. **Long-term potentiation of synaptic transmission:**
    a. Is involved in pain control system
    b. Results from fast prolonged stimulation of synapses
    c. Results from fast repetitive stimulation of synapse
    d. Is associated with decreased Ca^{++} concentration in postsynaptic neurons
    Ans. c
22. **Drugs which open Cl- channels in synapses:**
    a. Cause depolarization of postsynaptic membrane
    b. Cause hyperpolarization of postsynaptic membrane
    c. Enhance release of neurotransmitters from synaptic knobs
    d. Enhance response of postsynaptic neurons
    Ans. b
23. **Small-molecule neurotransmitters include all the following types, except:**
    a. Substance P
    b. Gamma amino butyric acid
    c. Acetylcholine
    d. Norepinephrine
    Ans. a
24. **Neuropeptides:**
    a. Are synthesized in the synaptic knobs
    b. Consist of small molecules
    c. Interact with ligand receptors
    d. Could produce prolonged changes in the structure of postsynaptic neurons
    Ans. d
25. **All the following transmitters are neuropeptides, except:**
    a. Neuropeptide Y
    b. Somatostatin
    c. Dopamine
    d. Encephalin
    Ans. c
26. **Actions of neuropeptides include all the following, except:**
    a. Inhibition of gene transcription
    b. Decreased cyclic AMP synthesis
    c. Changing intracellular Ca^{++} level
    d. Activation of ligand gated receptors
    Ans. d

MOTOR FUNCTIONS OF THE SPINAL CORD: SPINAL REFLEXES

1. **Higher motor commands originate in all the following centers, except:**
   a. Cerebral cortex
   b. Thalamus
   c. Caudate nucleus
   d. Cerebellum
   Ans. b
2. **A reflex action:**
   a. Is a fast brief response to a sensory stimulus
   b. Is involved in regulation of voluntary movements
   c. Includes at least three sequential sets of neurons in its pathway
   d. Is always initiated whenever its specific receptors are effectively stimulated by a specific stimulus
   Ans. d
3. **Reflex actions could be classified according to:**
   a. The type of sensory receptors initiating them
   b. The type of afferent nerves mediating them
   c. The type of efferent nerves mediating them
   d. The type of neurotransmitters mediating them
   Ans. c
4. **Events of reflex actions include all the following, except:**
   a. Stimulation of sensory receptors
   b. Stimulation of central synapses
   c. Inhibition of sensory receptors d.Inhibition of central synapses
   Ans. c
5. **A reflex arc includes:**
   a. At least two sets of sequential neurons
   b. At least two sequential sets of central synapses
   c. At least two types of sensory receptors
   d. At least two types of efferent neurons
   Ans. a
6. **The central terminals of afferent neurons mediating spinal reflexes are distributed within the spinal cord, so that:**
   a. All of them terminate in the same spinal segment of their entry to the cord
   b. All of them terminate on interneurons
   c. All of them subserve spinal reflexes
   d. They provide pathways for divergence of the incoming sensory impulses
   Ans. d
7. **Interneurons:**
   a. Provide communication between the central ends of afferent neurons
   b. Provide communication between dendrites of the efferent neurons
   c. Influence the rate of discharge from the alpha motor neurons
   d. Participate in ascending sensory pathways
   Ans. c
8. **The divergence function of interneurons is involved in:**
   a. Temporal summation
   b. Spatial summation
   c. Reverberation
   d. Irradiation
   Ans. d

9. **Interneuron after-discharge circuits prolong the duration of:**
   a. Sensory input to the spinal motor centers
   b. Synaptic delay in central synapses
   c. Discharge of efferent neurons
   d. Conscious perception of the evoked sensation
   Ans. c
10. **A flexor withdrawal reflex shows all the following properties, except:**
   a. Recruitment
   b. Prepotent
   c. Non-fatigable
   d. Irradiation
   Ans. c
11. **Flexor reflexes do not involve:**
   a. Flexor muscles
   b. Extensor muscles
   c. Reciprocal inhibition
   d. Reflex spasm of the involved muscles
   Ans. d
12. **The ability of stronger stimuli to produce wider range of reflex responses depends upon:**
   a. Presence of reverberating circuits in reflex pathway
   b. Presence of parallel-chain circuits in reflex pathway
   c. Convergence of interneurons
   d. Divergence of interneurons
   Ans. d
13. **Recruitment of a reflex response is due to:**
   a. Difference in the amount of presynaptic inputs to the various efferent neurons initiating the reflex
   b. Difference in the conduction velocity of the various afferent neurons mediating the reflex
   c. Delay at the neuromuscular junction
   d. Presence of inhibitory interneurons in the reflex pathway
   Ans. a
14. **After-discharge of reflex responses:**
   a. Increase the magnitude of the reflex responses
   b. Delays the onset of fatigue of reflex responses
   c. Involves interneuron circuits
   d. Depends upon spatial summation
   Ans. c
15. **Central delay of reflex actions:**
   a. Is due to presence of inhibitory interneurons in the reflex pathway
   b. Is the time between stimulation of receptors and response of the effector muscle
   c. Is longer in the flexor reflex than in the stretch reflex
   d. Is determined by the velocity of conduction of impulses along the afferent and efferent neurons in the reflex pathway
   Ans. c
16. **Fatigue of reflexes:**
   a. Develops gradually and recovers rapidly
   b. Develops rapidly and recovers slowly
   c. Develops gradually and recovers slowly
   d. Develops rapidly and recovers rapidly
   Ans. c

17. In flexor withdrawal reflexes contraction of flexor muscles is associated with reciprocal inhibition of:

a. Synergistic flexor muscles
b. Contralateral extensor muscles
c. Ipsilateral extensor muscles
d. Both 'a' and 'b' are correct

Ans. c

18. Reciprocal inhibition between reflexes depends upon all the following, except:

a. Presence of inhibitory interneurons in the reflex pathways
b. Presence of excitatory interneurons in the reflex pathways
c. Presence of anion channels in membranes of the involved neurons
d. Release of inhibitory transmitters which block cation channels in the reflex pathways

Ans. d

19. When a reflex action inhibits another reflex, it:

a. Releases an inhibitory transmitter at the synapses of the pathway of the inhibited reflex
b. Blocks the effect of excitatory transmitters at synapses of the inhibited reflex
c. Depletes the excitatory transmitters in synapses of the inhibited reflex
d. All the above are correct

Ans. a

20. Stretch of an innervated muscle evokes:

a. Contraction of its spindles
b. Contraction of its extrafusal fibers
c. Contraction of antagonistic muscles
d. Relaxation of synergistic muscles

Ans. b

21. Muscle spindles:

a. Are found in all skeletal muscles
b. Are found only in large skeletal muscles
c. Consist of small numbers of extrafusal muscle fibers
d. Consist of a large number of extrafusal muscle fibers

Ans. a

22. The nuclear-bag fibers of muscle spindles are innervated by:

a. Aγ nerve fibers
b. Aβ nerve fibers
c. Aδ nerve fibers
d. Ia nerve fibers

Ans. d

23. The nuclear-chain fibers of spindles are innervated by:

a. Aα and Aδ nerve fibers
b. Aδ and C nerve fibers
c. Ia and II nerve fibers
d. Only type II nerve fibers

Ans. c

24. The central ends of afferents from muscle spindles synapse with all the following types of neurons, except:

a. α-motor neurons of the same muscle
b. γ-motor neurons of the same muscle
c. Local interneurons
d. 2nd order neurons of ascending sensory pathways

Ans. b

25. γ-motor innervation of muscle spindles produces:
   a. Contraction of the central region of the spindle fibers
   b. Increased sensory discharge from the central region of the spindle fibers
   c. Decreased sensory discharge from the central region of the spindle fibers
   d. Relaxation of the peripheral regions of the spindle fibers
   Ans. b

26. Discharge from muscle spindles could be increased by all the following, except:
   a. Increased α-motor neuron discharge
   b. Increased γ-motor neuron discharge
   c. Stretch of the intrafusal muscle fibers
   d. Stretch of the extrafusal muscle fibers
   Ans. a

27. Increased γ-motor neuron discharge stimulates muscle spindles, because:
   a. It produces stretch of the extrafusal muscle fibers
   b. It causes stretch of the peripheral regions of the intrafusal fibers
   c. It causes stretch of the central region of the intrafusal fibers
   d. It stimulates directly the sensory fibers innervating muscle spindles
   Ans. c

28. γ-motor neuron discharge to a muscle is inhibited by impulses reaching the γ-motor neurons from all the following source, except:
   a. Golgi tendon organs of the same muscle
   b. Spindles of antagonistic muscles
   c. Medullary reticular formation
   d. Pontine reticular formation
   Ans. d

29. When the γ-motor neuron discharge to a muscle decreases, it causes:
   a. Increased muscle spindle discharge
   b. Shortening of the spindle fibers
   c. Stronger contraction of the extrafusal muscle fibers
   d. Decreased spindle sensitivity to stretch
   Ans. d

30. The role of muscle spindles in the maintenance of the upright posture depends upon all the following, except:
   a. Contraction of the spindle fibers
   b. Increased sensory discharge from spindles of postural muscles
   c. Increased supraspinal facilitation to the γ-motor neurons of postural muscles
   d. Presence of greater numbers of spindles in postural muscles
   Ans. d

31. The role of γ-motor neurons in regulation of equilibrium is achieved by:
   a. Initiating contraction of spindle fibers which directly antagonize postural deviation
   b. Increasing spindle sensitivity to stretch
   c. Directly stimulating extrafusal muscle fibers to antagonize postural deviation
   d. Directly adjusting the discharge of γ-motor neurons innervating the extrafusal muscle fibers to antagonize postural deviation
   Ans. b

32. Interruption of γ-motor neuron discharge to a skeletal muscle produces:
   a. Contraction of the muscle
   b. Contraction of the spindle fibers
   c. Relaxation of the spindle fibers
   d. Increased sensory discharge from the spindle fibers
   Ans. c

33. Co-activation of α and γ-motor neurons:

a. Increases γ-motor neuron discharge whenever the activity of α-motor neurons rises to a high level
b. Is mediated by interneurons that link the α and γ-motor neurons
c. Maintains the proprioceptive information to higher centers during muscle contraction
d. Increases the α-motor neuron discharge whenever the activity of γ-motor neurons rises to a high level

Ans. c

34. Increased sensory discharge from muscle spindles:

a. Decreases muscle tone
b. Increases muscle tone
c. Could either increase or decrease muscle tone
d. Has no effect on muscle tone

Ans. c

35. Interruption of spindle discharge from a muscle causes contraction of the muscle to become jerky and irregular due to:

a. Increased activity of reverberating circuits causing fluctuation of the motor discharge to the muscle
b. Increased activity of inhibitory interneurons causing oscillating inhibition of the α-motor neurons of the muscle
c. Irregular response of the α-motor neurons of the muscle to excitatory inputs
d. Post-tetanic potentiation of the α-motor neurons of the muscle

Ans. c

36. Whenever the position of a joint is stabilized at a certain attitude, the nervous system produces this by:

a. Increasing the α-motor neuron discharge to all muscles attached to the joint
b. Increasing the γ-motor neuron discharge to all muscles attached to the joint
c. Increasing γ-motor neuron discharge to postural muscles
d. Co-activation of α and γ-motor neurons innervating the involved muscles

Ans. d

37. The highly localized nature of stretch reflex is due to:

a. The limited number of interneurons in the reflex pathway
b. All the central ends of afferents from spindles of the stretched muscle terminate on the α-motor neurons of the muscle
c. The α-motor neurons of the stretched muscle receive most of the central terminals of afferents coming from spindles of the muscle
d. Activation of inhibitory interneurons which inhibit the motor neurons of the surrounding muscles

Ans. c

38. The shortest reflex time is recorded with:

a. A flexor withdrawal reflex
b. An inverse stretch reflex
c. A stretch reflex
d. A scratch reflex

Ans. c

39. When a skeletal muscle is suddenly stretched:

a. It relaxes suddenly
b. It develops a static stretch reflex
c. It develops a dynamic stretch reflex
d. It develops clonic contractions

Ans. c

40. Sensory impulses from spindles of a stretched muscle could inhibit antagonistic muscles by:

a. Directly inhibiting γ-motor neurons of the antagonistic muscles
b. Directly inhibiting the α -motor neurons of the antagonistic muscles

c. Inhibiting the transmitter release from the central terminals of afferents from the spindles of the antagonistic muscles
d. Activation of inhibitory interneurons
Ans. d

41. Antigarvity muscles maintain stretch reflex for prolonged periods without fatigue, because:
a. They are heavily innervated by α-motor neurons
b. They obtain their energy needs mainly from anaerobic metabolic processes
c. They contain exceptionally high levels of creatine phosphate
d. They are rich in mitochondria
Ans. d

42. The discharge from Golgi tendon organs initiated by excessive stretch of a skeletal muscle produces:
a. Inhibition of α-motor neurons of antagonistic muscles
b. Inhibition of γ-motor neurons of antagonistic muscles
c. Inhibition of α -motor neurons of the same muscle
d. Stimulation of γ-motor neurons of the same muscle
Ans. c

43. Inverse stretch reflex:
a. Increases the possibility of avulsion of the excessively stretched muscle from its bony attachments
b. Has no reciprocal innervation circuits
c. Is clinically manifested by lengthening reaction
d. Is clinically tested by examining the tendon jerks
Ans. c

44. Skeletal muscle tone:
a. Is a dynamic stretch reflex
b. Has a dynamic state
c. Is increased during rest
d. Is decreased during standing upright
Ans. b

45. γ-motor neurons control muscle tone by:
a. Adjusting the supraspinal facilitatory discharge
b. Adjusting the α-motor neuron discharge
c. Adjusting the muscle spindle discharge
d. Adjusting the activity of interneurons in the reflex arc of muscle tone
Ans. c

46. Adequate level of muscle tone is essential for the accurate performance of voluntary movements, because:
a. It adjusts the α-motor neuron discharge initiating voluntary movements
b. It adjusts posture of proximal joints of the acting limbs
c. It adjusts the upright posture of the whole body during voluntary movements
d. It adjusts sensitivity of the spindles of the involved muscles
Ans. b

47. A tendon jerk:
a. Is a dynamic stretch reflex
b. Is a static stretch reflex
c. Is evoked by gradually stretching the muscle
d. Is evoked by stimulation of tendon receptors
Ans. a

48. The tendon jerk which has its center in the 5th and 6th cervical segments of the spinal cord is:
a. The jaw jerk
b. The deltoid jerk
c. The biceps jerk
d. The triceps jerk
Ans. c

49. **Tendon jerks are clinically examined to assess:**
    a. Integrity of muscle spindles
    b. Integrity of reflex pathway
    c. The total reflex time of the jerk
    d. Central delay time of the jerk
    Ans. b
50. **Absence of a tendon jerk could result from any of the following conditions, except:**
    a. Lesions of supraspinal facilitatory centers
    b. Lesions of the efferent neurons
    c. Lesions of the afferent neurons
    d. Lesions of the spinal nerve centers
    Ans. a
51. **Exaggeration of tendon jerks could result from any of the following conditions, except:**
    a. Lesions of supraspinal facilitatory centers
    b. Lesions of supraspinal inhibitory centers
    c. Increased γ-motor neuron discharge
    d. Anxiety
    Ans. a
52. **Clonus:**
    a. Is a sign of decreased supraspinal facilitation
    b. Initiated by briefly stretching the tendon of the muscle
    c. Is manifested as oscillating mechanical vibrations following tendon jerks
    d. Associates exaggeration of tendon jerks
    Ans. d

THE DESCENDING MOTOR SYSTEMS

1. **All of the following are descending motor tracts, except:**
    a. Rubrospinal tract
    b. Spinotectal tract
    c. Reticulospinal tract
    d. Corticobulbar tract
    Ans. b
2. **Corticospinal tract originates from all the following areas, except:**
    a. Premotor area in the frontal lobe
    b. Prefrontal area in the frontal lobe
    c. Supplemental motor area in the frontal lobe
    d. Somatic sensory area in the parietal lobe
    Ans. b
3. **The cranial motor nuclei which receive innervation only from the contralateral corticobulbar tract are:**
    a. Nuclei of the trigeminal and vagus nerves
    b. Nuclei of the vagus and glossopharyngeal nerves
    c. Nuclei of the facial and hypoglossal nerves
    d. Nuclei of the facial and glossopharyngeal nerves
    Ans. c
4. **Axons of the lateral corticospinal tract synapse mainly with:**
    a. Lateral motor neurons
    b. Medial motor neurons
    c. Intermediolateral neurons
    d. Interneurons
    Ans. a

5. **The lateral motor system includes:**
   a. The lateral Reticulospinal tract
   b. The lateral corticospinal tract
   c. The lateral vestibulospinal tract
   d. All the above tracts
   Ans. b
6. **The corticobulbospinal tract is involved in all the following, except:**
   a. Voluntary movements
   b. Postural adjustment
   c. Automatic movements
   d. Tendon jerks
   Ans. d
7. **The Rubrospinal tract:**
   a. Originates from the pontine reticular formation
   b. Descends contralaterally
   c. Controls activity of axial muscles
   d. Is a component of the medial motor system
   Ans. b
8. **The reticulospinal tracts:**
   a. Are inhibitory to muscle tone
   b. Are excitatory to muscle tone
   c. Are either excitatory or inhibitory to muscle tone
   d. Have effect on muscle tone
   Ans. c
9. **Vestibulospinal tracts:**
   a. Adjust the discharge of vestibular receptors
   b. Adjust muscle tone
   c. Antagonize the effects of rubrospinal tract
   d. Terminate on the lateral motor neurons in the spinal cord
   Ans. b
10. **Tectospinal tract:**
   a. Originate mainly from the inferior colliculus
   b. Priginate mainly from the medial geniculate body
   c. Mediate responses initiated by sudden changes of head position
   d. Terminate in the cervical segments of the cord
   Ans. d
11. **Representation of the body in the primary motor area:**
   a. Is ipsilateral
   b. Is upright
   c. Is disproportionate to the actual anatomical size of the represented region
   d. All the above are correct
   Ans. c
12. **The primary motor area receives inputs arising from all the following centers, except:**
   a. Basal ganglia
   b. Cerebellum
   c. Hypothalamus
   d. Thalamus
   Ans. c

13. **The primary motor area projects efferent fibers to all the following centers, except:**
    a. 1ry somatic sensory area
    b. Premotor area
    c. Supplemental motor area
    d. Brainstem motor nuclei
    Ans. a
14. **The premotor area includes all the following, except:**
    a. Broca's area
    b. Head rotation area
    c. Supplemental motor area
    d. Hand skills area
    Ans. c
15. **Supplemental motor area is involved in all the following functions, except:**
    a. Adjusting posture
    b. Prienting responses
    c. Motor programming
    d. Coordinating bilateral movements
    Ans. b

LMN LESIONS, UMN LESIONS, AND SPINAL CORD LESIONS

1. **Lower motor neuron lesions cause all the following, except:**
    a. Decreased number of transmitter receptors in the denervated muscle
    b. Atrophy of the denervated muscle
    c. Flaccid paralysis of the denervated muscle
    d. Loss of flexion withdrawal reflex
    Ans. a
2. **Fasciculations of lower motor neuron lesions:**
    a. Are caused by injury currents initiated in the denervated muscle fibers
    b. Can be recorded by electromyogram
    c. Consist of asynchronous contraction of the muscle fibers composing a motor unit
    d. Develop later than fibrillations of the muscle fibers
    Ans. b
3. **Denervation super sensitivity of the muscle in LMN lesions is due to:**
    a. Increased release of neurotransmitter from the degenerating nerve terminals
    b. Decreased release of neurotransmitter from the degenerating nerve terminals
    c. Increased number of transmitter receptors in fibers of the denervated muscle
    d. Decreased number of transmitter receptors in fibers of the denervated muscle
    Ans. c
4. **When compared to normal muscle, the response of the denervated muscle to electrical stimulation shows:**
    a. Decreased chronaxie
    b. Greater response to faradic stimulation
    c. Slower response to galvanic stimulation
    d. CCC becomes greater than ACC
    Ans. c
5. **The most dramatic effects of an UMN lesion occurs with lesions at the level of:**
    a. The 1ry motor area
    b. Internal capsule
    c. Medullary pyramids
    d. Lateral column of spinal white mater
    Ans. b

6. **Motor defects that result from an internal capsular lesion include:**
   a. Paralysis of all skeletal muscles on the opposite side of the body
   b. Paralysis of all skeletal muscles on the same side of the body
   c. Paresis of axial muscles on the same side of the body
   d. Paralysis of the distal muscles on the opposite side of the body
   Ans. d
7. **Internal capsular lesions cause marked paralysis of the following muscles, except:**
   a. Tongue muscles
   b. Upper facial muscles
   c. Lower facial muscles
   d. Distal limb muscles
   Ans. b
8. **Hypertonia of UMN lesions is characterized by:**
   a. Increased inhibitory discharge from the premotor area
   b. Inhibition of pontine reticular formation
   c. Increased γ-motor neuron discharge
   d. Decreased muscle spindle discharge
   Ans. c
9. **In UMN lesions the response to plantar reflex:**
   a. Becomes exaggerated
   b. Becomes inhibited
   c. Becomes modified
   d. Is absent
   Ans. c
10. **In UMN lesions the response of the paralyzed muscles to electrical stimulation is:**
    a. Exaggerated
    b. Inhibited
    c. Not changed
    d. Is absent
    Ans. c
11. **Spasticity of the paralyzed muscles in UMN lesions is associated with:**
    a. Inhibition of tendon jerks
    b. Remarkable wasting of the muscle
    c. Clonus
    d. Non of the above
    Ans. c
12. **Spinal shock is due to:**
    a. Severe pain felt at the site of the lesion
    b. Severe hypotensive shock
    c. Interruption of the ascending sensory pathways
    d. Interruption of the descending facilitatory tracts
    Ans. d
13. **The stage of spinal shock is characterized by:**
    a. Loss of sensations from the body
    b. Paralysis of all skeletal muscles innervated by the spinal cord
    c. Exaggerated tendon jerks
    d. Failure of spinal reflexes
    Ans. d
14. **In humans the usual duration of the stage of spinal shock is:**
    a. From 2–6 hours
    b. From 2–6 days
    c. From 2–6 weeks
    d. From 2–6 months
    Ans. c
15. **Failure of spinal reflexes during the stage of spinal shock causes:**
    a. Automatic micturition
    b. Hypotension
    c. Babinski sign
    d. Spasticity of the paralyzed muscles
    Ans. b

16. **Complete transection of the spinal cord produces all of the following effects, except:**
    a. Permanent loss of all sensations mediated by the cord below level of lesion
    b. Permanent loss of voluntary movements by muscles innervated by the cord below level of lesion
    c. Permanent loss of reflexes mediated by the cord below level of lesion
    d. Temporary loss of micturition reflexes
    Ans. c
17. **Complete transection of the spinal cord did not affect arterial blood pressure when the lesion occurs at level of:**
    a. Mid cervical segments
    b. Upper thoracic segments
    c. Lower thoracic segments
    d. Mid lumbar segments
    Ans. d
18. **The earliest spinal reflex that recovers after the stage of spinal; shock is:**
    a. The micturition reflex
    b. The scratch reflex
    c. The stretch reflex
    d. The flexor reflex
    Ans. d
19. **With recovery of arterial blood pressure following spinal cord transection, the recovered blood pressure tends to:**
    a. Be higher than normal
    b. Be lower than normal
    c. Show abnormal oscillations
    d. Drop progressively
    Ans. c
20. **Recovery of micturition reflexes following the stage of shock:**
    a. Is due to recovery of supraspinal facilitation to the micturition center in the sacral segments
    b. Is due to recovery of activity of the micturition center
    c. Causes retention with overflow
    d. Causes normal micturition
    Ans. b
21. **Failure of the spinal reflexes is manifested by:**
    a. Automatic micturition
    b. Appearance of Babinski sign
    c. Loss of sensations from regions innervated by the cord below the level of the lesion
    d. Disappearance of the tendon jerks
    Ans. d
22. **Brown-Sequard syndrome is characterized by all the following, except:**
    a. Loss of vibration sense on the opposite side below level of the lesion
    b. Loss of voluntary movements on the same side below the level of the lesion
    c. Loss of reflex movements on the same side at the level of the lesion
    d. Loss of pain sensation on the opposite side below the level of the lesion
    Ans. a

Trauma MCQs Set A

1. **In acute traumatic head injury in the emergency department setting which of the following is true?**
   a. Paediatric subdural hemorrhage is always accidental
   b. Primary cellular death results mainly from an increase in cellular glutamate
   c. Diffuse axonal injury is most likely with delayed coma onset
   d. Hypocapnia should be avoided
   Ans. d
2. **Sternal fractures remain ununited in:**
   a. 50%
   b. 30%
   c. 2%
   d. 10%
   Ans. b
3. **With traumatic chest injury and 'flail segment' which of the following statements is incorrect:**
   a. Pulmonary contusion is the most common associated injury
   b. Ribs 4–9 are most commonly involved
   c. Pendulluft is the movement of air between injured and uninjured lung especially in setting of partial upper airway obstruction
   d. Mechanical ventilation does not mandate placement of an inter costal catheter in absence of pneumothorax
   Ans. d
   Flail segments are high risk for tension-pneumothorax with mechanical ventilation
4. **In regard to spinal X-rays:**
   a. In the upper thoracic spine the posterior height is usually 1.5 mm less than the anterior height
   b. In a true lateral cervical spine film taken at 1.8 m there may be up to 3 mm of anterior subluxation in a normal uninjured adult
   c. In a lateral cervical spine film the space between the anterior arch of C1 and the odontoid process of C2 (pre-dental space) should not exceed 3 mm in adults and 5 mm in children
   d. A Chance fracture through the lumbar spine is best seen on axial CT scans
   Ans. c
5. **The following are true about Traumatic Aortic Injury except:**
   a. The isthmus is the most common location
   b. Commonly associated with crush or deceleration injuries
   c. The aortic tear is most often transverse
   d. It is a non-survivable injury
   Ans. d
6. **Regarding blow our fractures of the orbit which is true?**
   a. Horizontal diplopia indicates inferior rectus muscle entrapment
   b. They are often associated with intracranial injuries
   c. Antibiotics are of proven benefit
   d. Enophthalmos will always require surgical management
   Ans. d
7. **Regarding LeFort III fractures which is correct?**
   a. They commonly involve the temporal bones
   b. Nasal packing is relatively contraindicated

c. They are usually an isolated injury
d. They are often associated with a CSF leak
Ans. b

8. **Which of the following is true in regard to Le Fort fractures?**
   a. A Le Fort 2 fracture separates the palate from the maxilla
   b. A Le Fort 2 fracture results in craniofacial dysfunction
   c. In Le Fort 2 fractures, the upper jaw and nose are mobile
   d. All facial fractures are easily classified into a Le Fort category
   Ans. c
9. **Which part of the mandible is fractured the most frequently in trauma?**
   a. Condyle
   b. Symphysis
   c. Body
   d. Ramus
   Ans. a
   Emedicine-mandibular fractures
10. **Which of the incomplete spinal cord syndrome patterns is correct?**
    a. Central cord syndrome-Bilateral impairment of dorsal columns (DS), Spinothalamic tracts (ST) and the motor tracts (MT), legs>arms
    b. Anterior spinal artery syndrome-Bilateral motor function loss and pain sensation loss with preservation of position sense
    c. Dorsal Column syndrome: Position sense preserved below the lesion and motor function and pain lost
    d. Brown Sequard syndrome: Loss of motor function and pain sense on the same side and contralateral position sense loss
    Ans. b

    Ref: Cameron Fig 2.3.1 Spinal cord and syndromes
11. **Which of the following is correct with regards to a normal X-ray appearance of the C spine?**
    a. The prevertebral soft tissue distance at C2 should be less than 22 mm
    b. You should be able to see down to C7
    c. Intervertebral lines can have steps in them
    d. In true pseudo subluxation there is preservation of the spinolaminar view in all lateral views
    Ans. d

    Ref: Cameron et al p91
12. **According to the Canadian CT Head rules, a CT head is indicated in all of the following situations except:**
    a. Retrograde amnesia of 15 minutes or less
    b. Suspected open skull fracture
    c. Vomiting 2 or more times
    d. CSF otorrhoea or rhinorrhoea
    Ans. a
    Canadian CT head rules.

    Ref: Dunn p811
13. **Which of the following is not a CXR sign of aortic injury?**
    a. Widened mediastinum (mediastinum to chest ratio > 0.25)
    b. Loss of the aortic knob
    c. Deviation of the trachea to the left
    d. Depression of the left main bronchus to below 40 degrees from the horizontal
    Ans. c
    Trachea deviates to the right.

    Ref: p95 Cameron et al

14. Regarding small bowel injury which of the following is true?
a. RBC/WCC ratio higher in lavage fluid then peripheral blood
b. Free intraperitoneal gas is present in the majority of cases
c. Serial erect CXR's don't increase sensitivity
d. Peritonism may be delayed
Ans. d

Ref: Dunn

15. X-ray findings in duodenal injuries may include all except:
a. Intraperitoneal gas
b. Retroperitoneal gas
c. Biliary tree gas
d. Obliteration of left psoas shadow
Ans. d

Ref: Dunn

16. In regard to traumatic chest injuries in children, which is FALSE?
a. Flail chest injuries are rare in children
b. Rib fracture under the age of three should raise the concern of child abuse
c. A CT scan is the best test to fully evaluate the rib cage for further injury when investigating possible child abuse
d. Children are more prone to hypoxia after injury than adults because of physiological differences
Ans. c

Ref: Cameron Textbook of Paed EM p72

17. With regards the need for cervical spine X-rays, which of the following is NOT part of the NEXUS criteria?
a. No midline tenderness
b. No distracting injury
c. Age < 65 yrs
d. Alert patient
Ans. c
C is part of Canadian c-spine rules NOT NEXUS

18. Which of the following is FALSE with regards paediatric trauma?
a. Trauma is not the most common cause of death in children < 1 year
b. Spleen is the most commonly injured abdominal organ
c. Duodenum injury is most commonly associated with LAP belt injuries
d. SCIWORA is more common than in adults
Ans. c
Jejunum is most commonly injured – Tintinalli

19. Features suggestive of decompensation of a previously stable patient with a penetrating neck injury DO NOT include:
a. Dyspnoea
b. Dysphonia
c. Distended Neck Veins
d. Bruit
Ans. c

Ref: Rosen 66/e p443

20 Principles of Trauma Management include all of the below except:
a. Organised team approach
b. Transfer to Trauma Centre
c. Assumption of most serious injury
d. Frequent reassessment
Ans. b

Ref: Rosen 6/e p304

21. **In regards to the Canadian Cervical Spine rule and published paper, which is TRUE?**
    a. It is less sensitive than CT in not missing fractures
    b. Those who did not have an X-ray ordered by the treating physician were excluded from the study analysis
    c. Can be utilized to guide the necessity for X-rays in all major trauma
    d. Is more specific than the Nexus criteria

    Ans. d

    D is incorrect, as Professor Stiel was a co author only

22. **When using the Canadian C-spine rules to make a decision regarding the need to perform imaging to exclude clinically important cervical spine injury following blunt trauma, the following statements are true, except:**
    a. The sensitivity is close to 100%
    b. The specificity is less than 50%
    c. All patients presenting after rear-end collisions of more than 10 kilometres per hour should undergo imaging because of the "whiplash" phenomenon
    d. A patient that develops new neck pain two days following an injury (after initially being alert and pain-free) unlikely has a clinically important neck injury

    Ans. c

    Ref: JAMA, Vol 286, No 15, p 1847

23. **The following is TRUE regarding head injuries:**
    a. Acute subdural hematoma most commonly develops due to a skull fracture overlying the middle meningeal artery
    b. Intracerebral hematomas in the occipital lobes are more common than in the other parts of the brain, because of the backwards motion of the brain during acceleration-deceleration injury
    c. In more than 80% of cases a unilateral fixed dilated pupil is the result of ipsilateral cerebral herniation
    d. The administration of prophylactic anti-epileptic drugs does not reduce the incidence of seizures in the long term, but it does reduce the incidence of early post-traumatic seizures

    Ans. d A,B,D,E

    Ref: Tintinalli p1568 C: Cameron, p 77

24. **Which of the following is NOT high risk according to the Canadian CT Head Rules?**
    a. Vomiting > = 2 episodes
    b. Any sign of basal skull #
    c. Age > = 60 years
    d. Suspected open or depressed skull #

    Ans. d

    Ref: Cameron, 3rd Ed, pg 118

25. **With regard to Odontoid #'s which statement is TRUE:**
    a. A Type I # is through the dens below the transverse ligament
    b. Type III #'s are most common
    c. Type II #'s with < 6 mm displacement have a 10% non-union rate
    d. They account for only 2–5% of all cervical spine #'s

    Ans. c

    Ref: Dunn, 4/e, p1019 A – above the transverse ligament B – type II are most common. D – account for 10-15% of all Cx spine #s

26. **With respect to myocardial contusion which is FALSE?**
    a. It is usually of no clinical significance
    b. VF does not occur as a delayed rhythm
    c. AF is the most common clinically significant rhythm in this situation
    d. Troponin level is a reliable test for myocardial injury

    Ans. d

    Ref: Dunn

27. With respect to diaphragm injury which is FALSE?
   a. Up to 10% are diagnosed after 48 hours
   b. Left side affected more than the right
   c. Usually an isolated finding
   d. Most CXRs in this context are not diagnostic
   Ans. c

Ref: Dunn

28. Which of the following statements is CORRECT regarding Intracranial Hematomas?
   a. Epidural hematomas are crescent shaped on CT
   b. Subarachnoid hematomas are commonly seen in the elderly and in alcoholics
   c. Intracerebral hematomas usually involve the anterior temporal or posterior frontal lobe
   d. Subdural hematomas are commonly caused by skull fracture and tearing of the middle meningeal artery
   Ans. c

Ref: Tintinalli 6/e p1568

29. Which of the following is NOT a 'hard' sign of penetrating neck trauma?
   a. Non expanding hematoma
   b. Shock not responsive to fluids
   c. Airway obstruction
   d. Cerebral ischemia
   Ans. a

Ref: Rosens 7/e p379

30. Which of the fallowing is FALSE in regards to trauma in Australia:
   a. The most significant reduction in trauma deaths has been due to improvements in hospital trauma patient management
   b. Trauma is the leading cause of death from 1–44 yrs
   c. Suicide causes more deaths than MVAs
   d. Age >55 is a high-risk factor for life threatening injury in trauma
   Ans. a
   A Prevention strategies have reduced trauma deaths.

Ref: Cameron – Ch 3.1

31. Regarding neck trauma:
   a. Horner's syndrome may indicate ipsilateral carotid artery injury
   b. Most vital structures lie in the posterior triangle of the neck
   c. Cervical spine injury is common in blunt neck trauma
   d. Clinical assessment is most reliable for injuries in Zone III
   Ans. a

Ref: Neck trauma handout

32. Radiographic features of an isolated orbital blow-out fracture include all of the following except:
   a. Widening of the zygomatico-frontal suture
   b. Teardrop sign in the maxillary antrum
   c. 'Black-eyebrow' sign
   d. Fluid level in the maxillary antrum
   Ans. a
   Maxillofacial Trauma: Challenges in ED diagnosis and Management
   Ref: Emergency Medicine Practice February 2008 Volume 10, Number 2 and Accident & Emergency Radiology 2nd edition

33. Regarding blunt cervical spine injury, which of the following statements is FALSE?
   a. Pseudosubluxation of C2–C3 is common in children and may persist up to age 14 years
   b. Nexus criteria are more specific than the Canadian cervical spine rule for a clinically important injury

c. C2 is the most commonly fractured vertebra in elderly patients (> 65 years)
d. Disruption of the posterior vertebral body line on CT is indicative of an unstable injury

Ans. b

Cervical Spine Injury: An Evidence-based evaluation of the patient with blunt cervical trauma.

Ref: Emergency Medicine Practice. April 2009 Vol 11, Number 4

34 Which of the following is FALSE in regard to nasal fractures?

a. Aseptalhematoma if missed is frequently complicated by septal necrosis
b. Naso-orbito-ethmoid complex fractures cause medial displacement of the medial palpebral fissure
c. Reduction should be performed at 5–10 days post injury
d. X-ray are of no use in uncomplicated nasal fractures

Ans. b

Ref: Dunn p1029

35. Regarding thoracolumbar injuries, which statement is TRUE?

a. The most common mechanism of injury is compression
b. Isolated pars fractures are usually unstable
c. A Chance fracture is caused by compression and extension
d. T12–L1 bony injuries have a proportionally high incidence of spinal cord injury

Ans. d

Ref: Dunn p1021-1024

36. Regarding facial trauma:

a. Up to 10% of head, neck and facial injuries sustained by women may be the result of domestic violence
b. Malocclusion is a poor indicator of mandibular fracture
c. Coexisting severe brain injury is the major cause of death in facial trauma
d. Traumatic facial hemorrhage is potentially life threatening in 5% of midfacial fractures

Ans. d

Ref: Cameron (2009) p94-95

37. Which of the following statements is FALSE?

a. There is little evidence for replacement of clotting factors where blood loss is less than 5L
b. Concussion is bruising of the brains substance associated with head trauma
c. Over 50% of trauma deaths are associated with head injury
d. On the AVPU scale, a response to painful stimuli correlates to a GCS of 6–8

Ans. b

This is the definitions of contusion.

Ref: Cameron (2009) p 72, 75

38. With respect to myocardial contusion which is FALSE?

a. It is usually of no clinical significance
b. VF does not occur as a delayed rhythm
c. AF is the most common clinically significant rhythm in this situation
d. Troponin level is a reliable test for myocardial injury

Ans. d

Ref: Dunn

39. With respect to diaphragm injury which is FALSE?

a. Up to 10% are diagnosed after 48 hours
b. Left side affected more than the right
c. Usually an isolated finding
d. Most CXRs in this context are not diagnostic

Ans. c

Ref: Dunn

40. Which of the following statements is CORRECT regarding Intracranial Hematomas?
   a. Epidural hematomas are crescent shaped on CT
   b. Subarachnoid hematomas are commonly seen in the elderly and in alcoholics
   c. Intracerebral hematomas usually involve the anterior temporal or posteriorfrontal lobe
   d. Subdural hematomas are commonly caused by skull fracture and tearing ofthe middle meningeal artery

Ans. c

Ref: Tintinalli 6th ed p1568

41. Which of the following is NOT a 'hard' sign of penetrating neck trauma?
   a. Non expanding hematoma
   b. Shock not responsive to fluids
   c. Airway obstruction
   d. Cerebral ischemia

Ans. a

Ref: Rosens 7/e p379

42. Which of the fallowing is FALSE in regards to trauma in Australia?
   a. The most significant reduction in trauma deaths has been due to improvements in hospital trauma patient management
   b. Trauma is the leading cause of death from 1-44 yrs
   c. Suicide causes more deaths than MVAs
   d. Age > 55 is a high-risk factor for life threatening injury in trauma

Ans. a

Prevention strategies have reduced trauma deaths.

Ref: Cameron – Ch 3.1

43. Regarding neck trauma:
   a. Horner's syndrome may indicate ipsilateral carotid artery injury
   b. Most vital structures lie in the posterior triangle of the neck
   c. Cervical spine injury is common in blunt neck trauma
   d. Clinical assessment is most reliable for injuries in Zone III

Ans. a

Ref: Neck trauma handout

44. Radiographic features of an isolated orbital blow-out fracture include all of the following except:
   a. Widening of the zygomatico-frontal suture
   b. Teardrop sign in the maxillary antrum
   c. 'Black-eyebrow' sign
   d. Fluid level in the maxillary antrum

Ans. a

Maxillofacial Trauma: Challenges in ED diagnosis and Management.

Ref: Emergency Medicine Practice. February 2008 Volume 10, Number 2 and Accident & Emergency Radiology 2nd edition

45. Regarding blunt cervical spine injury, which of the following statements is FALSE?
   a. Pseudosubluxation of C2–C3 is common in children and may persist up to age 14 years
   b. Nexus criteria are more specific than the Canadian cervical spine rule for a clinically important injury
   c. C2 is the most commonly fractured vertebra in elderly patients (> 65 years)
   d. Disruption of the posterior vertebral body line on CT is indicative of an unstable injury

Ans. b

Cervical Spine Injury: An Evidence-based evaluation of the patient with blunt cervical trauma.

Ref: Emergency Medicine Practice. April 2009 Vol 11, Number 4

46. Which of the following is FALSE in regard to nasal fractures?
   a. Aseptalhematoma if missed is frequently complicated by septal necrosis
   b. Naso-orbito-ethmoid complex fractures cause medial displacement of the medial palpebral fissure

c. Reduction should be performed at 5-10 days post injury
d. X-ray are of no use in uncomplicated nasal fractures
Ans. b

Ref: Dunn p1029

47. Regarding thoracolumbar injuries, which statement is TRUE?
a. The most common mechanism of injury is compression
b. Isolated pars fractures are usually unstable
c. A Chance fracture is caused by compression and extension
d. T12-L1 bony injuries have a proportionally high incidence of spinal cord injury
Ans. d

Ref: Dunn p1021–1024

48. Regardicng facial trauma:
a. Up to 10% of head, neck and facial injuries sustained by women may be the result of domestic violence
b. Malocclusion is a poor indicator of mandibular fracture
c. Coexisting severe brain injury is the major cause of death in facial trauma
d. Traumatic facial hemorrhage is potentially life threatening in 5% of midfacial fractures
Ans. d

Ref: Cameron (2009) p94-9549. B This is the definitions of contusion. Cameron (2009) p72, 75

49. Which of the following statements is FALSE:
a. There is little evidence for replacement of clotting factors where blood loss is less than 5L
b. Concussion is bruising of the brains substance associated with head trauma
c. Over 50% of trauma deaths are associated with head injury
d. On the AVPU scale, a response to painful stimuli correlates to a GCS of 6-8
Ans. d

Ref: Emergency Medicine Practice
Cervical Spine Injury: An evidence-based evaluation of the patient with blunt cervical trauma

50. Which of the following is NOT an unstable fracture of the vertebral column?
a. Flexion tear drop fracture
b. Bilateral facet joint dislocation
c. Unilateral facet joint dislocation
d. Odontoid fracture with lateral displacement
Ans. c

Ref: Emergency Medicine Practice. Cervical Spine Injury: An Evidence –Based Evaluation of the Patient With Blunt Cervical Trauma

51. Which statement regarding the Canadian C-spine rule is incorrect?
a. Previous C-spine surgery is an exclusion criteria
b. The specificity of the Canadian C-spine rule is lower than the NEXUS criteria
c. Age 65 years is a High-risk feature
d. It includes consideration of the mechanism of injury
Ans. b

Ref: Emergency Medicine Practice. Cervical Spine Injury: An evidence-based evaluation of the patient with blunt cervical trauma

52. When resuscitating the major trauma victim:
a. Platelets should be given if > 10 units of blood are used
b. Hypothermia < 32 degrees is recommended for cerebro protection
c. Clotting factors should be transfused if total blood loss > 3 litres
d. Micropore filters reduce complications of transfusion
Ans. a

Ref: Cameron 3/e p72-73, Mild hypothermia may be beneficial, but below 32 deg interferes with coagulation, decreases myocardial contractility and predisposes to arrhythmias Replace clotting factors if blood loss > 5 litres or after 5-6 units PRBCs given (4 units FFP for every 6 units PRBCs) Micropore filters slow transfusion and do not appear to reduce complications in MTV

53. A hyperextension injury of the neck associated with bilateral upper limb weakness is most consistent with:

a. Anterior cord syndrome
b. Brown-Sequard syndrome
c. Central cord syndrome
d. Dorsal column syndrome

Ans. c

Ref: Dunn 4/e p1160

54. A dental fracture that is exquisitely tender and is bleeding from a central pinkish area is most likely an:

a. Ellis I dental fracture
b. Ellis II dental fracture
c. Ellis III dental fracture
d. Ellis IV dental fracture

Ans. c

Ref: Dunn 4/ e p1179

55. Which of the following is TRUE of facial injuries?

a. Bilateral mandibular condyle fractures result in protrusion of the jaw
b. In mandibular fractures the symphysis is the most common site of fracture
c. Nasal fracture reduction should occur within 48 hours of injury
d. Le Forte II fracture results in mobile maxilla and zygoma

Ans. a

Ref: Dunn chapter 29

56. Which of the following is TRUE of head injury?

a. Extradural hematomas commonly occur without skull fracture
b. Papilloedema is an early sign of raised intracranial pressure
c. CSF leak occurs in 20% of base of skull fractures
d. Adults are more likely than children to develop cerebral oedema in head trauma

Ans. c

Ref: Dunn 3/e, p342

Trauma MCQs Set B

1. **All of the following are causes of compartment syndromes except:**
   a. Crush injuries
   b. Electrocution
   c. Vigorous exercise
   d. Decompression illness
   Ans. d
2. **Which is the least likely to be affected by compartment syndrome?**
   a. Peroneal compartment of the leg
   b. Extensor compartment of forearm
   c. Anterior compartment of thigh
   d. Intrinsic muscle compartments of the hand
   Ans. c
3. **The compartmental pressure at which muscle ischemia first occurs is?**
   a. 5–10 mm Hg
   b. 10–25 mm Hg
   c. 35–45 mm Hg
   d. 55–100 mm Hg
   Ans. c
4. **Penetrating Neck Injuries, all the following are true except:**
   a. The patient with Hemodynamic instability or obvious aero-digestive injury requires urgent Operating Theatre management
   b. Esophageal injuries are at risk of being missed clinically with subsequent delayed presentation and very high mortality
   c. Zone 3 injuries are best assessed using Angiography
   d. Exploration of penetrating neck injuries beyond the platysma does have arole in the ED
   Ans. d
5. **In the third trimester of pregnancy:**
   a. The resting HR has returned to baseline
   b. Tidal volume and residual volume are increased due to high levels of progesterone
   c. Plasma volume has increased by 25%
   d. T wave inversion is normal in V1, V2 and III
   Ans. d
6. **In the secondary survey of the pregnant trauma patient:**
   a. Abdominal examination is unreliable and may cause premature labour in the irritable uterus so should not be performed
   b. A vaginal examination is contraindicated if there is evidence of vaginal blood loss
   c. A stethoscope is inadequate for auscultation of the fetal HR. Doppler ultrasound should be performed
   d. The uterine fundus can reliably be palpated for contractions
   Ans. d
7. **Regarding pelvic fracture classification, all the following are true except:**
   a. Lateral compression type I has 4% rate of bladder rupture
   b. Mortality is roughly 25% for vertical shear injuries

c. Malgaigne fractures show symphyseal diastasis
d. Anteroposterior compression type III have 75% chance of severe hemorrhage
Ans. d

8. Signs of major pelvic fractures include all of the following except:
a. Destot's sign
b. Roux's sign
c. Earle's sign
d. Bucholz's sign
Ans. d

9. Which of the following is false with regards to cervical spine fractures:
a. Clay shoveller's fracture is a flexion injury
b. Bilateral facet joint dislocation is a rotation type-injury
c. Anterior tear drop fracture is mechanically unstable
d. A type II fracture is the most common type of odontoid fracture
Ans. b

10 With regard to SCIWORA (spinal cord injury without radiological abnormality):
a. If recovery of neurological deficit has occurred prior to arrival then no further spinal precautions are required
b. Can only be diagnosed if neurological deficits persist without change
c. Occurs in children with incompletely calcified vertebral columns
d. Has a good prognosis regardless of level of injury
Ans. c

11. In assessment of penetrating neck wounds:
a. Zone 1 refers to the region from the angle of the jaw to the lower mandible
b. Zone 3 injuries can be observed if there is no clinical evidence of major structure damage
c. All should have a full cervical spine XRay series and CXR
d. Combined oesophagoscopy and oesophagram for Zone 2 injuries has a > 90% sensitivity for detecting oesophageal injuries
Ans. d

12. Which statement is TRUE regarding Fractures of the Pelvis?
a. Associated Hemodynamic instability carries a 25% mortality
b. CT is not helpful to evaluate suspected injuries to the Sacro-Iliac Joint, Sacrum or Acetabulum.
c. Angiography with intervention/embolisation can be utilised for uncontrolled hemorrhage from pelvic vessels
d. An ipsilateral double pubic ramus fracture is a stable fracture
Ans. d

13. In spinal trauma it is true that:
a. The thoracolumbar junction is vulnerable due to its poor mobility
b. The lower cervical spine is particularly vulnerable in children
c. The dorsal column fibres decussate at the level of entry
d. Spinal cord injury most often occurs between C5 an C7
Ans. d

14. With regard to facial trauma you would usually expect to find:
a. An adjoining wound in mandibular fractures
b. A hanging teardrop sign of orbital floor fracture on CT
c. Maxillary fractures in children under 6 years old
d. A Le Fort type 2 fracture when the eyes are mobile with maxillary traction
Ans. a

15. Which of the following is correct with regards to blunt abdominal injury?
   a. Microscopic hematuria always needs further investigation
   b. Anterior urethral injuries are associated with pelvic fractures
   c. In a stable patient with extravasation of contrast from the spleen or splenic artery, if available, angio-embolisation is the treatment of choice
   d. Free air on CXR is not an indication for laparotomy

   Ans. c

16. With regards to spinal cord injuries, which of the following is correct?
   a. Brown-Sequard syndrome manifests as loss of motor function and position sense on the same side, and loss of pain and temperature on the opposite side
   b. Transverse spinal cord syndrome has sparing of the dorsal columns
   c. Cervical spine injuries occur most commonly at C4/5
   d. In patients with a cervical spine fracture, it is unnecessary to look for further fractures elsewhere

   Ans. a

17. Which of the following is true of Renal injuries?
   a. Microscopic hematuria in the trauma patient is an indication for renal tract imaging
   b. IVP is the investigation of choice in the stable patient
   c. Renal injuries are more common in the paediatric abdo trauma patient than the adult patient
   d. All clinically significant renal injuries are associated with hematuria

   Ans. c

18. Which of the following is not a complication of crush injury?
   a. Hyperkalemia
   b. Hypercalcemia
   c. Coagulopathy
   d. Hyperphosphatemia

   Ans. b

19. Regarding urogenital trauma which is TRUE?
   a. Ureteric injuries are common in blunt trauma
   b. Bladder dome injuries require conservative treatment
   c. Bladder body injuries require immediate surgical repair
   d. Absence of displaced pelvic ring # nearly always exclude urethral injury

   Ans. d

20. Which is true regarding trauma in the elderly?
   a. Spine injuries are commonest in mid to lower
   b. Spine levels B 10% of patients hospitalised for falls die within 1 year
   c. Patient medications rarely affect management of injuries
   d. Most deaths from trauma result from motor vehicle crashes

   Ans. d

21. Which of the following is TRUE regarding splenic injuries?
   a. Ultrasound is the definitive investigation of choice in stable patients
   b. A fracture of the left 8th–10th ribs is associated with a~5% risk of splenic injury
   c. Grades I and II splenic injuries should always be conservatively managed
   d. Traumatic splenectomy patients have a lower risk of infections than non traumatic splenectomy patients

   Ans. d

22. Regarding blunt abdominal trauma, which statement is TRUE?
   a. The finding of free intra-peritoneal gas on CT is pathognomonic for hollow viscus perforation
   b. Oral contrast greatly enhances the correct interpretation of CT findings
   c. Trendelenburg positioning usually decreases the sensitivity of a FAST scan
   d. Abase excess of -6 or more negative is a good predictor of the need for early blood transfusion

   Ans. d

23. Regarding spinal injuries, which is TRUE?
   a. The most commonly fractured cervical vertebra is C4
   b. The use of steroids in spinal injuries greatly improves long-term motor function
   c. Big toe flexion is classically preserved in central cord syndrome
   d. Anterior cord syndrome typically results from a hyperextension mechanism
   Ans. c

24. Central cord syndrome:
   a. Is usually seen in older patients who sustain a hyperflexion injury of their neck
   b. Affects laterally placed nerve fibres of the lower extremity
   c. Prognosis for recovery of function is good
   d. The dorsal columns are affected
   Ans. c

25. The NEXUS criteria includes all of the following except:
   a. No painful distracting injury
   b. Normal level of alertness
   c. No evidence of intoxication
   d. The patient is able to actively rotate their neck 45 degrees left and right
   Ans. d

26. Regarding abdominal trauma, which of the following is TRUE?
   a. A gunshot wound seen to pass extra peritoneally on CT reliably predicts successful non operative management
   b. In blunt trauma, children are more likely to incur solid organ damage compared with adults but are more often treated conservatively
   c. At least 800 mL must be drained after DPL to accurately diagnose hemoperitoneum as the red cell count increased with volume drained
   d. Serial abdominal examinations should be done for up to 8 hours, or overnight, with blunt abdominal trauma
   Ans. b

27. Unstable cervical spine injuries include all of the following except:
   a. Anterior tear drop fracture
   b. Extension tear drop fracture
   c. Bilateral facet joint dislocation
   d. Anterior wedge fracture
   Ans. d

28. In renal trauma all of the following are true except:
   a. Hematuria in the paediatric population correlates well with the degree of injury
   b. Radiographic studies reveal a normal functioning kidney in renal pelvic rupture
   c. Bladder rupture can be intraperitoneal or extra peritoneal
   d. Kehr sign suggests extra peritoneal bladder rupture
   Ans. d

29. With regards to genitourinary trauma which is false?
   a. In blunt abdominal trauma the kidney is involved more frequently in children than in adults
   b. The absence of hematuria does not exclude significant genitourinary injury
   c. Intraperitoneal bladder rupture needs to be repaired surgically
   d. Retrograde cystogram may show a false negative in extra peritoneal bladder rupture if a wash out film is not preformed
   Ans. d

30. **With regards to the spinal cord – which is false?**
    a. Posterior columns contain vibration and proprioception fibres
    b. Up to 10% of motor fibres run in the contralateral anterior corticospinal tract
    c. Fibres for pain and temperature typically ascend 1–2 levels before crossing
    d. Fibres for the upper limbs are more medial than those for the lower limbs in the corticospinal tract
    Ans. b
31. **With regard to trauma in pregnancy which of the following is TRUE?**
    a. Diagnostic peritoneal lavage is contraindicated
    b. Uterine rupture only occasionally results in foetal mortality
    c. The most common source of abdominal hemorrhage is splenic injury
    d. The foetus is unlikely to be compromised if the mother does not appear hypovolaemic
    Ans. c
32. **Which of the following is TRUE?**
    a. At least 300mL of contrast is required for adequate cystography
    b. DPL is less sensitive than CT for small bowel injury
    c. A negative FAST scan obviates the need for a CT scan
    d. A positive DPL necessitates laparotomy
    Ans. a
33. **With regards to scrotal trauma, which is FALSE?**
    a. Testicular rupture is bilateral in 2% of blunt trauma
    b. Testicular rupture is bilateral in 30% of penetrating trauma
    c. USS gives excellent indication of injury severity
    d. Immediate surgical exploration of intra testicular hematoma has an orchidectomy rate of 5%
    Ans. c
34. **With regards to Bowel injury, which is FALSE?**
    a. It is present in 5% of blunt abdominal trauma
    b. CT is highly sensitive for mesenteric injury
    c. Chance fracture of the lumbar vertebrae has a 90% incidence of small bowel injury
    d. Free intra-abdominal gas is seen on CT in 60% of cases of small bowel rupture
    Ans. d
35. **With regard to Anterior Spinal Cord injury which of the following is INCORRECT:**
    a. Results from either direct blunt injury to the cord itself or compression of the anterior spinal artery by disc, bone or hematoma causing is chemic damage to the anterior cord
    b. Patient presents with loss of motor and pain sensation bilaterally below the level of the lesion
    c. Posterior cord function is tested with a tuning fork for vibratory sensation or by testing of proprioception using dorsi and plantar flexion of the great toe
    d. Prognosis after this injury is good
    Ans. d
36. **With regard to Cauda Equina Syndrome which is INCORRECT:**
    a. Involves injury to the lumbosacral nerve roots
    b. Characterized by an are flexic bowel and/or bladder
    c. Motor and sensory loss is predictable
    d. The affected limbs are flexic
    Ans. c
37. **In regards to trauma in pregnancy:**
    a. Lack of PV bleeding excludes the diagnosis of placental abruption
    b. A non reactive CTG confirms foetal distress at 30/40
    c. Tocolytics are generally contra-indicated if labour is established post abruption at 34/40
    d. Lack of maternally felt foetal movements correlates well with foetal distress in the 2nd trimester
    Ans. c

38. **Which of the following is FALSE?**
    a. Ultrasound is useful in determining specific renal injuries
    b. Lumbar vertebral fractures are associated with renal tract injuries
    c. CT is particularly useful in children where non renal injuries are more likely
    d. Contrast CT is better than IVP at diagnosing ureteral injury
    Ans. a
39. **Which of the following with regards a DPL, is FALSE?**
    a. Is positive if more than 10 mls blood is drained straight away
    b. The procedure itself can give a false positive test
    c. Is positive if more than 1 × 105 RBC/microlitre are seen
    d. Is performed without surgical dissection of rectus fascia when a pelvic fracture is suspected
    Ans. d
40. **With regard to compartment syndromes, which symptom or examination finding is reliable in making the diagnosis?**
    a. Pain on passive stretch
    b. Tight compartments
    c. Pain out of proportion to injury
    d. There is no one finding that is reliable
    Ans. d
41. **Complications of spinal cord injury include:**
    a. Autonomic Instability
    b. Neurogenic shock
    c. Pulmonary Oedema
    d. All of the above
    Ans. d
42. **With respect to cervical spine injuries:**
    a. Clay shoveller's # classically involves the upper thoracic spine
    b. Jefferson's # is a hyper extension injury
    c. Regarding odontoid fractures, type 2 is the most common
    d. Predental space should be less than 3 mm in children
    Ans. c
43. **Which of the following is used in the Injury Severity Score:**
    a. GCS
    b. Anatomical region injured
    c. Heart rate
    d. Blood pressure
    Ans. b
44. **The following is TRUE with regards to abdominal trauma:**
    a. In blunt abdominal trauma, liver injuries are more common than splenic injuries
    b. In stabbing injuries of the abdomen, liver injuries are more common than splenic injuries
    c. In gunshot injuries of the abdomen, splenic injuries are more common than liver injuries
    d. Diaphragmatic injuries are common in blunt abdominal trauma
    Ans. b
45. **The following is TRUE with regards to hepatic injuries:**
    a. It is the most common cause of death in abdominal trauma
    b. Hepatic injuries are proportionately more common in adults (when similar trauma is sustained by adults and children)
    c. It is rare to have an associated splenic injury
    d. Gallbladder injury is commonly associated
    Ans. a

Perio Innovations

PERIOAID: Toothpick holder which is one of the most effective aids available for cleaning exposed furcation after periodontal therapy
PERIOCARE: Zinc Oxide Non Eugenol periodontal dressing in the form of paste-gel
PERIODEX: 0.12 % Chlorhexidine gluconate
PERIODONTOMETER: Instrument used for measuring tooth mobility
PERIOGARD: Rapid chairside test kit for Aspartate aminotransferase
PERIOGUARD: 0.12 % Chlorhexidine gluconate
PERIOPAPER: Blotter on which GCF is collected
PERIOALERT: Immunoassay to detect serum antibodies to specific bacterial pathogens
PERIOCHECK: Rapid chair side test kit developed to detect neutral proteases in GCF
PERIOCHIP: Pale orange chip of 4 mm × 5 mm × 350 micrometer size, weighing 7.4 mg which contains 2.5 mg chlorhexidine gluconate
PERIOCLINE: Subgingival delivery of 2% Minocycline hydrochloride
PERIOGRAFT: Non porous hydroxyl apatite alloplast
PERIOGLASS: Bioactive glass alloplast with Sodium and Calcium salts, phoshphates, silicon dioxide of irregular particles of 90-170 micrometer.
PERIOPAC: Premixed Zinc oxide Non Eugenol dressings
PERIOPIK: Tip used for subgingival irrigation
PERIOSCAN: Chairside diagnostic kit using BANA Reaction to identify Tannerella forsythia, P.gingivalis, Treponema denticola and Capnocytophaga species
PERIOPROBE: Electronic probe with a tip diameter of 0.5 mm and standardised probing force of 0.3-0.4 N
PERIOPLANER/PERIOPOLISHER: Powered devices for the removal of plaque and calculus with reciprocating motion
PERIOSCOPY: It is 0.99 mm diameter reusable fibreoptic endoscope with 24–46 power magnification and fibreoptic illumination
PERIOSTAT: Subantimcrobial dose of doxycycline hyclate 20 mg for chronic periodontitis twice daily
PERIOTEST: For determining tooth mobility. Scale ranges from -8 to + 50
-8 to 9 – clinicaly firm teeth
10–19 first distinguishable sign of movement
20–29 crown deviates within 1 mm of normal position
30–50 mobility is readily observed
PERIO-TOR: Instrument tips for scaling and root planning causing minimal removal of tooth structures
PERIOTRON: Electronic machine used for measuring the amount of GCF
PERIOTRIEVER: Highly magnetised instrument for retrieving broken instrument tips from the periodontal pocket
PERIO 2000 SYSTEM: Diamond Probe which combines the feature of periodontal probe with silver sulphide sensor for the detection of volatile sulphur compounds
PERIOWAVE: Photodynamic disinfection system using low intensity lasers
PERIOSIM: Haptics developed at the University of Illinois Chicago for training soft skills to students
PERIOPREDICT: Measures variations in the genes for Interleukin-1 (IL-1), a key mediator of inflammation, and identifies individuals who are at an increased risk for more severe periodontal (gum) disease
PERIOTEMP: Detects pocket temperature differences of 0.1 degree Celsius from a refererred subgingival temperature.

OMFS SR Paper (Jan 2015)

1. **Best approach for infraorbital fracture:**
   a. Transconjunctival b. Subciliary
   c. Subsphenoidal d. Midtarsal
   Ans. b

Ref: Journal of Maxillofacial and Oral Surgery June 2009, Volume 8, Issue 2, pp 99–102

We conclude by saying that transconjunctival approach provides an excellent aesthetic result when done meticulously. However the subciliary and the subtarsal incisions provide a more rapid, direct approach to the orbital floor and infraorbital rim with minimal morbidity and an aesthetically acceptable scar. The infraorbital incision is the least acceptable aesthetically.

2. **Postoperative hematoma in TMJ ankylosis is managed by:**
   a. Vacuum drain b. Physiotherapy
   c. Sternoclavicular graft d. Arthroplasty
   Ans. a
3. **Treatment of medially displaced subcondylar fracture:**
   Ans. Open Reduction
4. **Extension of parotid gland is till:**
   a. Masseteric fascia b. Pretracheal fascia
   c. Prevertebral fascia d. All
   Ans. a
5. **The principle of distraction osteosynthesis is:**
   a. Traction b. Tension
   Ans. b
6. **The protocol for distraction osteosynthesis is:**
   Ans. 0.5 mm per turn.
7. **Most important step in vestibular incision is:**
   a. Suturing of periosteum at base towards chin
   b. Suturing of mucosa
   c. Suturing away from chin
   d. Suturing to adjacent mucosa
   Ans. a
8. **A 75-year-old male who is diabetic and osteopetrotic mandibular fracture is treated by?**
   a. Gunning splints b. 2 mini plates
   Ans. a
9. **Bacteria responsible for dry socket according to Nitzin's theory is:**
   a. Treponema denticola b. Borrelia
   c. Prevotella d. Tannerella
   Ans. a
10. **Regarding transbuccal approach which is correct?**
    a. Inferior border plating
    b. Superior border plating
    c. A single stab incision
    Ans. b

11. The most commom form of OKC:

a. Orthokeratinised b. Parakeratinised

Ans. b

Ref: Archives of Oral Sciences and Research Orthokeratinized Odontogenic Cyst: A Case Report S Hemavathy, Sahana NS*, D Vinay Kumar*, Suresh T*, Chandrakala J*, Mohammed Asif*.*

The orthokeratinized OKC was more often associated with an impacted tooth (75.7%), as compared with 47.8% for the parakeratinized OKC. Recurrence rate in parakeratinised OKCs is at least 42.6% of the cases, compared with only 2.2% for orthokeratinized OKCs. But due to the less aggressive clinical behavior and recurrence pattern of the orthokeratinized variant ultimately warranted the designation of the orthokeratinized variant as a separate entity, "Orthokeratinized Odontogenic Cyst".

12. Best approach for condylar fracture:

a. Transparotid
b. Preauricular
c. Hinds

Ans. a

Ref: Acta Otorhinolaryngol Ital. Dec 2010; 30(6): 303.

The Transparotid approaches with partial parotidectomy permits very good anatomical repositioning of the displaced condylar or subcondylar osseous segments in all cases, since isolation of the facial nerve branches and removal of a limited part of the parotid gland tissue overlying the lesion allow perfect exposure of the fracture site. The wide operation field allows the facial nerve to be preserved and permits easy internal rigid fixation with plates, as the drill, screws and screwdriver can be positioned exactly perpendicular to the bone surface instead of obliquely, as occurs with many different approaches.

13. A child has brown teeth, chipped enamel and obliterated canal, diagnosis is:

a. Amelogenesis imperfecta b. Dentinogenesis imperfecta
c. Regional odontodysplasia d. Dentin dysplasia

Ans. b

14. BSSO for mandibular facial deformity, planning needed is:

a. CBCT b. Face bow transfer
c. Bone Scan d. MRI

Ans. b

15. Heterotopic bone formation is seen in:

a. Costochondral graft b. Sternoclavicular graft
c. Silastic d. Cadaveric graft

Ans. c

The problem of heterotopic calcification is frequently seen after placement of alloplastic materials in the TMJ, particularly when alloplasts of Proplast/Tefon (Vitek Inc., Houston, TX) or Silastic (Dow-Corning, Midland, MO) have been previously implanted. Heterotopic bone can also result from trauma, reactive arthritis, osteoarthritis, sepsis, inflammation, and connective tissue/autoimmune diseases such as rheumatoid arthritis, psoriatic arthritis, ankylosing spondylitis, and scleroderma. These calcifications can cause continued worsening pain and a progressive decrease in range of motion that may lead to bony ankylosis. A variable amount of fibrosis and possibly reactive tissue are commonly associated with the heterotopic bone, thereby worsening the effect.

16. Type II NOE fracture refers to:

a. Attached canthus to central segment b. Unattached canthus
c. Involves one portion of medial rim d. Comminution of central fragment

Ans. a

Ref: fonseca 3/e vol 2 p663

Type I: Naso-Orbital-Ethmoid fractures: The simplest form of NOE fracture involves only one portion of the medial orbital rim with its attached medial canthal tendon. It may occur in a bilateral or unilateral form. When bilateral type fracture occurs, there is no medial canthal tendon displacement, and transnasal wiring is not required.

Type II NOE fracture: It may occur in a bilateral or unilateral form and may be large segments or comminuted. Most commonly the canthus remains attached to a large central segment. Reduction is usually best accompalished by control of the specific segment of the bone that is that is associated woth canthal tendon.

TYPE III NOE fractures: This fracture includes comminution involving the central fragment of the bone where the medial canthal tendon attaches. The canthus is rarely avulsed completely, but on occasion the fragments of bone are so small that reconstruction is not possible. In this circumstance, transnasal wiring of the canthus is required, as is osseous reconstruction.

17. Best access to isolated nasal bone fracture is by:

a. Conical　　b. Linear

c. Elliptical　　d. Circular

Ans. a

Transconjunctival approach is usually used.

18. As per recent study TMJ ankylosis can be due to:

a. Hypercoagulablity of blood　　b. Medially displaced fracture of condyle

c. Burst condyle　　d. Middle ear infection

Ans. a

Ref: Medical hypothesis 81 (2013) 561–63

Temporomandibular joint (TMJ) ankylosis is often described as either fibrous or bony, and, in traditional opinion, fibrous ankylosis can progress into bony ankylosis. The most common aetiology of TMJ ankylosis is trauma, mainly condylar fracture.

19. Orbital reconstruction is best done by:

a. Bone graft　　b. Titanium mesh

c. Resorbable plate　　d. All of the above

Ans. b

Ref: Fonseca 3/e Vol 2 p673

Autologous grafts are perhaps the most favored for significant floor defects. The donor sites that are usually harvested have been the inner aspect of the anterior iliac crest and the posterior iliac crest.

20. Carrol Girard screw is used for:

a. Lefort II　　b. Zygomatic arch reduction

c. Mandibular fracture reduction　　d. Nasal fracture

Ans. b

21. Longest acting LA:

Ans. Bupivacaine + Etidocaine

22. In PPF, bony buttress are intact, the first plating is done at:

a. Frontozygomatic suture　　b. Zygomatic buttress

c. Infraorbital area

Ans. b

23. For telecanthal surgery the best approach is:

Ans. Bicoronal

24. In successful Lefort I surgery minimum bone involvement is:

Ans. 4

25. The treatment modality used in Sinus lift procedure these days is:

Ans. direct one step or two step Antrostomy.

26. The principle of lag screw is:

Ans. Dynamic compression

27. Best graft for reconstruction of mandible is:

a. Vascularised fibula　　b. Anterior pedicled graft

c. Iliac crest　　d. Rib

Ans. a

Ref: Reconstruction of mandible with free fibular vascular graftmedind.nic.in/ibd/t03/i1/ibdt03i1p49g.pd

Free fibular graft is the best choice because it gives the contour of the mandible and it withstands multiple osteotomies due to its dual blood supply (periosteal & end artery).It is the standard and mainstay for mandibular bony reconstruction. Non-vascularised autogenous bone grafts can be harvested from local and/or distant sites. If the defect size is small, local or intra-oral donor sites may be sufficient. For larger defects and when a moderate amount of bone is required, distant or extraoral sites are preferably employed. All other reconstruction options could be worth mentioning only in terms of simplicity, lack of the requirement for elaborate equipment, technical capability and longer operating room time and resources. Simplicity does not, however, always bring desirable outcome, particularly as mandibular defects become more centrally placed. Then, these conservative endeavours bring more unpredictable results and often greater or more protracted complications. Free bone grafts have been used frequently for mandibular reconstruction. Autogenous bone grafts from the calvarium, rib, ilium, tibia, fibula, scapula, and radius have been used. New novel developments and techniques are tested to eliminate need for bone harvesting from a donor site; these include transport disc distraction osteogenesis (TDDO), tissue-engineering and modular endoprosthesis for mandibular reconstruction.

28. In costochondral graft the chondral part length is safe when it is?

a. 1–2 mm
b. 2–4 mm
c. 4–6 mm
d. 7–9 mm

Ans. b

Ref: Robert E Marx: Atlas of ORAL and EXTRAORAL BONE HARVESTING p70

After completing the periosteal elevation, transsect through the cartilage, leaving 3 mm of cartilage on the rib in adults and children.

29. Bench compression test in mandible angle fracture when force applied on 38 region?

a. Superior border will show tension
b. Superior border will show compression
c. Superior border will show torsion

Ans. a

30. Which loading is done at 2nd& 3rd molar region which is present at superior border?

a. Tensile stress
b. Torsional stress
c. Compressive stress

Ans. a

31. In case of pterygoid buttress fracture plating is done by using:

a. 1.5 mm plate
b. 2 mm plate
c. 2.4 mm plate

Ans. b

Four holed straight plate without gap or an L shaped plate is fixed using 5 mm screws
Textbook of Oral and Maxillofacial Surgery
edited by Rajiv M. Borle

32. In BSSO artery and vein are not injured using:

a. Piezoelectric handpiece
b. Surgical bur

Ans. a

33. After BSSO Osteotomy alone is done in which segment?

a. Distal
b. Proximal
c. Lateral

Ans. a

34. In Costochondral grafting, the chondral part is taken using

a. Rib shearer
b. Rib cutter
c. 701 bur
d. No.11 Blade

Ans. d

No.11 blade is the preferred answer even though rib cutter has been used too. The periosteum over the rib is incised, either with the use of electrocautery or sharply with a scalpel, and a periosteal elevator is used to subperiosteally strip the superficial portion of the rib. A rib stripper is then used to completely subperiosteally strip the pleural surface of the rib. This maneuver is performed all the way to the vertebral and sternal ends of the ribs. ***A rib cutter is then used*** to excise the rib at its costochondral and costovertebral junctions.

Once the periosteal dissection is complete, the bony portion of the rib can be osteotomized or the cartilage harvested to its desired dimensions. The osteotomy can be accomplished with a saw or rib cutter forceps. A malleable retractor is placed behind the rib or cartilage to protect the periosteum and prevent an inadvertent pleural injury. Cartilage-only grafts can be procured with a scalpel, but great care is needed to avoid perforating the pleura.

35. **Storiform appearance is seen in:**

    Ans. Fibrous histiocytoma

36. **Alcoholic patient came in casuality, C.T scan is normal, what should be avoided in management:**

    a. NSAIDS　　b. Tramadol

    c. IMF + reduction　　d. Local block

    Ans. b

Drinking alcohol while taking Tramadol may increase your risk of certain tramadol side effects, such as:

Seizures

Unusual behavior

Memory problems

Drowsiness

Dizziness

Problems with coordination

Shallow or infrequent breathing

Passing out.

You may also be more sensitive to the effects of alcohol if you are taking tramadol. You may not be able to safely drink as much alcohol as you are used to drinking. According to the prescribing information for this medication, people who are intoxicated with alcohol should not take tramadol.

37. **In complicated fracture treatment the primary healing step is:**

    a. Debridement　　b. Simplification

    c. Reconstruction plating

    Ans. b

38. **True about contact healing and gap healing is:**

    a. Callus not formed in contact healing　　b. Callus not formed in gap healing

    c. Both are types of primary healing　　d. None of the above

    Ans. a

This type of bone healing is termed primary or direct bone union, and it requires absolute immobilization between the osseous fragments, that is, rigid fixation, and minimal distance (gap)between them.

39. **Coin shaped lesion in lungs is diagnosed as malignant Ameloblastoma histopathologically appeared as:**

    a. Ameloblastoma　　b. Increased mitosis

    c. Pleomorphism

    Ans. c

40. **TMJ develops at around:**

    Ans. 10 weeks

41. **Total joint prosthesis replacement is not done in:**

    a. Tumour of condyle　　b. Recurrent dislocation

    c. Avascular necrosis　　d. Osteoarthritis

    Ans. b

Biomet Total TMJ Replacement System

Indications
- Arthritic conditions: Osteoarthritis, traumatic arthritis, rheumatoid arthritis
- Ankylosis, including but not limited to recurrent ankylosis with excessive heterotopic bone formation
- Revision procedures where other treatments have failed (e.g. alloplastic reconstruction, autogenous grafts)
- Avascular necrosis
- Joints that have undergone multiple operations
- Fracture
- Functional deformity
- Benign neoplasms
- Malignancy (e.g. posttumor excision)
- Degenerated or resorbed joints with severe anatomic discrepancies
- Developmental abnormality

General contraindications to using the total TMJ replacement system, as well as any other system, include the following:
- Active or chronic infection
- Conditions in which there is insufficient quantity or quality of bone to support the components
- Systemic disease with increased susceptibility to infection
- Patients with extensive perforations in the mandibular fossa and/or bony deficiencies in the articular eminence or zygomatic arch that would severely compromise support for the artificial fossa component
- Partial TMJ joint reconstruction
- Known allergic reaction to any materials used in the components (Note: Patients with known or suspected nickel sensitivity should not have Co-Cr-Mo devices implanted since this material contains nickel.)
- Patients with mental or neurological conditions who are unwilling or unable to follow postoperative care instructions
- Skeletally immature patients
- Patients with severe hyperfunctional habits (e.g. clenching, grinding)
- Patients with a foreign body reaction due to previous implants.

TMJ Concepts Patient-Fitted TMJ Reconstruction Prosthesis System

Indications for using TMJ Concepts Patient-Fitted TMJ Reconstruction Prosthesis System include the following:
- Inflammatory arthritis involving the TMJ that is not responsive to other treatment options
- Recurrent fibrous and/or bony ankylosis that is not responsive to other treatment options
- Failed tissue graft
- Failed alloplastic joint reconstruction
- Loss of vertical mandibular height and/or occlusal relationship due to bone resorption, trauma, developmental abnormality, or pathologic lesion

Contraindications to using TMJ Concepts Patient-Fitted Temporomandibular Joint Reconstruction Prosthesis include the following:
- Active or suspected infections in or around the TMJ site
- Uncontrollable masticatory muscle hyperfunction (clenching or grinding) which could cause joint overloading and loosening of prosthesis screws
- Known allergy to material components of the prosthesis.

42. Pedicled BFP (Buccal Fat Pad) is done in all except:

a. TMJ ankylosis b. OSMF
c. OAF d. Defects of hard palate

Ans. a

The buccal fat pad has been used to reconstruct defects in the hard palate, the soft palate (up to midline), the retromolar trigone, the buccal mucosa, the anterior tonsillar pillar, the superior alveolar ridge (up to the canine region), and the superior buccal sulcus. It can be used alone or in combination with other flaps such as the pedicled temporalis muscle myocutaneous flap (Samman *et al.*) or the pectoralis major myocutaneous flap, where the posterior portion of the defects (palatal region and tonsillar pillar) were reconstructed by the buccal fat pad, leaving the anterior and inferior portion to be covered by myocutaneous flaps.

The pedicled buccal fat pad flap has also been used to close oroantral and oronasal fistula and to cover the nasal or antral surface of bone grafts used for maxillary reconstruction.

43. Le-Measurier technique is related with:

a. Cleft lip
b. Disc displacement
c. Disimpaction of the maxilla

Ans. a

Le-Clarke Method is related to Option B

44. True about orbital apex injury:

a. Rarely occurs in children
b. Vision is not hampered
c. Corticosteroids are contraindicated
d. More common in adults

Ans. c

45. If impacted 3rd molar is to be extracted in patient planned for bilateral sagittal split osteotomy then, osteotomy should be done:

a. At the time of surgery
b. 1 month prior to surgery
c. 6 months prior to surgery
d. After surgery

Ans. c

Repeat Nov AIIMS 2013

46. Equipoise is:

a. True certainity in RCT
b. False certainity in RCT
c. True uncertainity in RCT
d. False uncertainity in RCT

Ans. c

47. CHARGE includes all except:

a. Coloboma
b. Hyperthyroidism
c. Cardiac disease
d. Ear deformities

Ans. b

48. SMAS encompasses all except:

a. Platysma
b. Buccinator
c. Risorius
d. Triangularis

Ans. b

49. Submucosal plating is indicated in:

a. Pediatric mandible
b. Midpalatal fracture
c. Atrophic mandible
d. C shaped septal fracture

Ans. d

50. Which of the following autogenous graft is not preferred for grafting?

a. Sternal
b. Parietal
c. Temporal
d. Costochondral

Ans. c

51. Velopharyngeal closure can be all except:

a. Sagittal
b. Central
c. Bow-tie
d. Axial

Ans. d

52. Best method to restore midfacial fracture:
Ans. Dividing face into equal thirds.

53. Incision given in BSSO Surgery is:
Ans. Above the lingula.

54. Simplification of fracture is associated with:

a. Comminuted #
b. Simple linear angle #
c. Symphyseal #
d. Parasymphyseal #

Ans. a

55. To avoid heterotopic bone formation best protocol is to use:

a. Masseter
b. Buccinator
c. Pterygoids
d. Temporalis

Ans. a

56. Sign and symptoms of Unilateral and bilateral TMJ ankylosis is:

Ans. class 2 malocclusion on the affected part.

57. Most important thing to be done at the operated area of costochondral graft is:

a. Saline irrigation at the area of operation
b. Closure in layer and drain
c. Intercostal block
d. Immobilisation of chest

Ans. a

Once the graft is removed, ***the wound should be irrigated thoroughly*** and checked for the presence of a pleural injury. This examination can be performed by asking the anesthesiologist to inflate the lung maximally while the wound is irrigated with saline. Bubbles may be seen in the presence of a pleural tear, although false-negative results can be seen with this maneuver. If no tear is visualized, the wound is closed in anatomic layers, beginning with the periosteal sheath. Special care should be taken to avoid pleural perforation and injury to the intercostal nerve during suturing. Well-placed dermal sutures are particularly useful for taking tension off the skin closure to allow for optimal healing.

58. Line of management in anterior table & posterior table frontal sinus # is:

Ans. Autogenous cancellous material.

Ref: Peter Ward Booth

59. AO System 3D distraction one turn will give a separation of:

a. 0.25 mm
b. 0.55 mm
c. 0.35 mm
d. 1 mm

Ans. c

Per day distraction is 1.05 mm in three times one turn per time corresponds to 0.35 mm.

60. Reidel procedure is associated with:

a. Maxillary sinus
b. Frontal sinus
c. Sphenoidal sinus
d. Ethmoidal sinus

Ans. b

61. 8-year-old child with unilateral TMJ Ankylosis, the graft preferred is:

Ans. Gap arthroplasty with interpostional costochondral.

62. The width suggestive of traumatic telecanthus is:

Ans. More than 38 mm.

63. Treatment of angle fracture:

Ans. One plate at upper border.

64. Champy's osteosynthesis line for angle fracture passes through:

Ans. External Oblique Ridge.

65. A 6-year-old child with parasyphyseal fracture is best treated with:

a. ORIF with physiotherapy
b. IMF for 4 weeks
c. ORIF for 1 week
d. ORIF for 3 weeks

Ans. b

66. Midfacial fractures are related to:

a. Vertical buttress
b. Horizontal buttress

Ans. b

67. Ellis maneuver is used for:
a. To reduce parasymphyseal fracture
b. To reduce symphyseal fracture
c. To reduce bilateral condylar fracture
d. To reduce maxilla
Ans. a

68. Incision used in NOE # treatment is:
Ans. Maxillary vestibular approach with Extended Glabellar approach

69. Atrophic mandible is best treated with:
a. Reconstruction plate
b. Mini plate
Ans. a

70. Ideal length of condylar segment in Costochondral graft is:
Ans. 5 mm

71. Surgical approach to TMJ associated complication is:
Ans. Facial Nerve damage

72. The recently suggested fourth pillar of face is:
a. Vomero-nasal
b. Ethmoido-zygomatic
c. Fronto-occipital
d. Ethmoido-vomerian
Ans. d

73. The complication of Malignant ameloblastoma is:
a. Hypocalcemia
b. Hypokalemia
c. Hypercalcemia
d. Hyperkalemia
Ans. c

74. Litchenstein theory is associated with:
a. Osteosarcoma
b. Osteochondroma
c. Leiomyoma
d. Chondroblastoma
Ans. b

75. Stereolithography uses which laser?
a. CO_2
b. Argon
c. Hol-YAG
d. YAGG
Ans. b

76. The regime used in trismus with Trismus screw at 2nd-4th day is:
a. 10–15 × 5–6 insertions
b. 20–25 × 8–10 insertions
c. 50–60 × 10–12 insertions
d. 20–25 × 3 insertions
Ans. b

77. Kent Vitek Prosthesis is:
Ans. Teflon coated flourethyl polyethylene used in TMJ Reconstruction.

78. The most ideal posterior tooth to replace with an implant is:
a. First molar
b. Second molar
c. First premolar
d. Second premolar
Ans. c

79. Which drug can cause false ankylosis?
a. Bismuth poisoning
b. Aspirin toxicity
c. Tetracycline toxicity
d. Styrchnine poisoning
Ans. d

80. Cleft of hard and soft palate till the incisive foramen according to Veau is grouped as:
a. Group I
b. Group II
c. Group III
d. Group IV
Ans. b

81. In class II div 1 malocclusion for advancement of 16 mm of mandible, technique:

a. Distraction
b. Inverted L osteotomy
c. BSSO
d. Lower total subapical osteotomy

Ans. b

82. In Bi jaw surgery how to proceed:

a. Done in 4 week stage
b. IMF require
c. BSSO proceed Le-Fort I
d. Rigid fixation is necessary

Ans. c

Ref: Fonseca's orthognathic surgery pg 428

In most cases of 2 jaw surgeries, the mandibular osteotomies are performed first. The reason for this is that if the maxilla were repositioned and stabilized before the mandible was sectioned, the drill or saw used on the mandible could displace the repositioned maxillary segments. Also by oosteotomizing the mandible before maxillary surgery, the total amount of time that the maxillary soft tissues remain detached is shortened.

83. Not true about frontal sinus fracture:

a. Least common in children
b. More common in adult
c. Posterior table injuries are more
d. Anterior table injuries are more

Ans. c

Ref: Fonseca 3/e Vol 2 p772

Frontal sinus fractures are rare in children and uncommon in adolescents. The majority of the patients are males (66% to 91%) and between 20 to 30 years of age.

Frontal sinus injuries are frequently associated with blunt trauma secondary to motor vehicle accident.

Overall, frontal sinus injuries involving the anterior table alone range from 43 to 61%, isolated posterior table fractures range from 0.6 to 6%, and injuries involving both the tables range from 19 to 51%.

Peterson's: Most victims are male (66–91%) and young (usually 20–30 yr of age, range 6–72 yr), and most frontal sinus and NOE injuries are sustained in motor vehicle or motorcycle collisions (44–85%). NOE fractures can occur in isolation, but they most often occur in association with other midface fractures. As many as 60% of patients with NOE fractures have associated non facial injuries. 43 to 61% of reported patients had anterior table fractures only, 19 to 51% had anterior and posterior table fractures, 2.5 to 25% had injuries to the nasofrontal duct, and 0.6 to 6% had posterior fractures only.

84. Obliteration of frontal sinus is done when?

a. Anterior table is fracture
b. Posterior table is fractured
c. Anterior table fracture involving nasofrontal duct
d. Sinus lining

Option A& D are not the Answer, confusion is between option B & C

If option C is sinus floor fracture involving the nasofrontal duct then it will be the Answer otherwise posterior table is the Answer.

Ref: Fonseca 3/e vol 2 p729–30

Management of Anterior Table Fractures:

Simple green stick or non displaced anterior table fractures requires no surgical management. Recent case reports have indicated that minimally displaced and non comminuted fractures may be addressed via an endoscopic or insufflation approach when no stabilization is necessary. Displaced and multifragmented fractures requires operative intervention to address contour deformity and possibly to reduce the risk for mucocele development.

Management of Sinus Floor Fractures Involving the Nasolacrimal Duct:

Fractures of the NOE complex, supraorbital rim, and frontal sinus floor may obstruct the nasofrontal duct. Generally if the nasofrontal duct is damaged, ductal repair is not feasible and ductal obstruction and sinus obliteration is the recommended management strategy.

Management of Posterior Table Fractures:

Some clinicians may recommend that with a large patent duct, and with no concurrent dural tears or brain injury exist, any amount of posterior table displacement is inconsequential and may be managed with observation. Other

suggests that nasofrontal duct obstruction and sinus obliteration is the recommended treatment strategy.
If the nasofrontal ducts are injured, obstructed and cannot be repaired, then the ducts should be obstructed and the sinus obliterated regardless of the condition of the posterior table.

Sinus Obliteration

Nasofrontal duct obstruction is necessary to seal off the frontal sinus from nasal contaminants. Sinus obliteration adds one more layer to the seal but also eliminates the dead space or air within the sinus that may permit fluids to accumulate, thus causing a seroma or a hematoma. Furthermore, after cranialization, sinus obliteration cushions and protects the brain. Historically, sinus obliteration has been accomplished in a number of ways, including inserting no substance or object (theoretically permitting bone fill after curettage) or hydroxylapatite, glass wool, bone, cartilage, muscle, absorbable gelatin sponge, absorbable knitted fabric, acrylic, or fat. The use of fat has been reported most frequently, and this method historically has provided the most desirable results.

85. Transnasal wiring is done:

a. Posterior to lacrimal crest
b. Ethmoid bone
c. Nasal bone
d. Medial canthal ligament

Ans. a

Ref: Fonseca 3/e Vol 2

Transnasal wiring technique:a 2 cm incision is made approximately 10mm medial to the insertion of medial canthus. By following the anterior lacrimal crest in a superinferior direction, the bone bearing the medial canthal ligament is exposed.
Peterson's: For NOE fractures including avulsion of the MCT or in which the MCT is attached to a small bone segment, transnasal wiring should be considered. The point of fixation of the wires should be directed posterior and superior to the lacrimal fossa so that the medial canthal distance is decreased and widening of the nasal bones and blunting of the medial canthal area can be avoided. Wires must be passed through the medial orbital bone and the superior nasal septum or the perpendicular plate of the ethmoid. Their passage can be facilitated with the use of a spinal needle or a wire-passing awl.

86. Hypothyroid in children shows:

a. Myxedema
b. Cretinism
c. Gigantism
d. Acromegaly

Ans. b

87. Prolotherapy makes use of:

a. Distilled water
b. Blood
c. Steroid
d. Sodium morrhuate

Ans. d

Prolotherapy involves the injection of an irritant solution into a joint space, weakened ligament, or tendon insertion to relieve pain.Most commonly, hyperosmolar dextrose (a sugar) is the solution used; glycerine, lidocaine (a commonly used local anesthetic), phenol, and sodium morrhuate (a derivative of cod liver oil extract) are other commonly used agents. The injection is administered at joints or at tendons where they connect to bone.
Prolotherapy treatment sessions are generally given every two to six weeks for several months in a series ranging from 3 to 6 or more treatments. Many patients receive treatment at less frequent intervals until treatments are rarely required, if at all.

88. Facial nerve paralysis is most commonly seen in:

a. Warthin's tumor
b. Mucoepidermoid carcinoma of parotid
c. Pleomorphic adenoma.

Ans. b

89. Incorrect regarding trocar:

a. Check retractor is optional
b. Upper border plating iis optional
c. Lower border plating is optional
d. Single stab incision is used.

Ans. b

90. In dentinogenesis imperfecta, the defective gene is:

a. Chromosome 4
b. Chromosome 6
c. Chromosome 8
d. Chromosome 21

Ans. a

Dentinogenes is Imperfecta is commonly known as hereditary opalescent dentin or Capdepont dysplasia. It is a localized mesodermal dysplasia affecting both primary and permanent dentition and is a genetic disorder of tooth development inherited in an autosomal dominant pattern caused by mutations in the Dentin Sialophosphoprotein (DSPP) gene (cytogenetic location of 4q21.3). The term 'dentinogenesis imperfecta' was coined by Robert and Schour in 1939 and probably first recognized by Barret in 1882.

Mutations in the DSPP gene lead to the production of abnormal DSPP-derived proteins or reduce the amount of these proteins in developing teeth. As a result, teeth have abnormally soft dentin. Teeth with defective dentin are discolored, weak, and prone to breakage and decay.

91. Minimally displaced zygoma fracture first point of fixation is:

a. Sphenozygomatic
b. Infrazygomatic
c. Infraorbital
d. Zygomatic buttress.

Ans. d

Ref: peterson's p 451

Low-Energy Zygomatic Complex Fractures

Low-energy, nondisplaced or minimally displaced zygomatic complex fractures may require no operative correction. Tarabichi treated consecutive low velocity ZMC fractures by a transoral open reduction and internal bone plate fixation of the zygomaticomaxillary buttress with excellent results in all but two patients, who had comminution of the orbital rim.

Middle-Energy Zygomatic Complex Fractures

The zygomaticomaxillary buttress is exposed first and stabilized with a plate if necessary. The zygomaticofrontal buttress is exposed next and also stabilized with a plate if required. This method requires proper patient selection, experience, and meticulous technique to ensure accurate reduction and stabilization. Other authors recommend routine exposure of two or more of the three anterior buttresses for middle-energy injuries: the zyomaticomaxillary buttress, zygomaticofrontal buttress, and the infraorbital rim. In this manner, multiple buttresses are visualized and the three-dimensional accuracy of the reduction can be confirmed.

High-Energy Zygomatic Complex Fractures

To restore proper projection, facial width, and orbital volume, exposure of the zygomatic arch and orbital floor is often required in addition to exposure of the anterior buttresses. A coronal flap is used to gain access to the zygomatic arch.

92. In Gun shot injury, Management is:

a. Reconstruction plate
b. IMF
c. Defragmentation
d. Bag of bones

Ans. d

An operative plan for a gunshot injury to the face is best formulated after characterization of the wound as low or high energy. The surgeon facing a gunshot injury should consider the concept introduced by Manson for evaluation of four components: soft tissue injury, bone injury, soft tissues loss (true avulsion), and bone loss. After evaluation of the wound, a decision is made regarding early definitive repair versus the need for delayed repair. The majority of civilian gunshot wounds resulting from assaults can be managed with early definitive repair because these injuries usually result in injury to the soft tissue and bone but rarely loss of these tissues. Impressive soft tissue injuries are usually not avulsive, and most can be closed primarily. Extensive débridement of soft tissue is not indicated.

93. In symphyseal fracture with lag screw fixation:

a. Load bearing
b. Load sharing

Ans. b

Ref: Peterson p 375

Lag screw techniques are also load-sharing in that the bone that is compressed is sharing the functional loads with the screws.

Load-Bearing versus Load-Sharing Fixation

The most simplistic way to discuss fixation schemes for fractures is to break them down into those fixation devices that are load-bearing and those that share the loads with the bone on each side of the fracture (load-sharing). Load-bearing fixation is a device that is of sufficient strength and rigidity that it can bear the entire load applied to the mandible during functional activities. Injuries that require load-bearing fixation are comminuted fractures of the mandible, those fractures where there is very little bony interface because of atrophy, or those injuries that have resulted in a loss of a portion of the mandible (defect fractures). In such cases the fixation device must bridge the area of comminution, minimal bone contact, or bone loss, and bear all of the forces transmitted across the injured area that are generated by the masticatory system. Load bearing fixation is sometimes called bridging fixation because it bridges areas of comminution or bone loss. The most commonly used load-bearing device is a mandibular reconstruction bone plate. Such plates are relatively large, thick, and stiff. They use screws that are generally greater than 2.0 mm in diameter (most commonly 2.3 mm, 2.4 mm, or 2.7 mm).

Load-sharing fixation is any form of internal fixation that is of *in*sufficient stability to bear all of the functional loads applied across the fracture by the masticatory system. Such a fixation device(s) requires solid bony fragments on each side of the fracture that can bear some of the functional loads. Fractures that can be stabilized adequately with load-sharing fixation devices are simple linear fractures, and constitute the majority of mandibular fractures. Fixation devices that are considered load-sharing include the variety of 2.0 mm miniplating systems that are available from a number of manufacturers.

Examples of rigid fixation in the mandible are the use of two lag screws or bone plates across a fracture, the use of a reconstruction bone plate with at least three screws on each side of the fracture, and the use of a large compression plate across a fracture. Properly applied, these fixation schemes are of sufficient rigidity to prevent interfragmentary mobility during the healing period.

94. Most important indication of airway obstruction:

a. Sternous breathing
b. Low BP
c. Increased heartrate

Ans. a

95. In mandible fracture with gonial flaring plating should be (best location):

a. Lower border plating
b. Buccal surface plating
c. Lingual surface reduction/plating

Ans. c

Classification of Medial Canthal Tendon Injuries

Medial canthal tendon injuries are classified according to three types:

Type I: Single-fragment bone segment with intact canthal tendon insertions

Type II: Comminuted central bone segment with fractures remaining external to the medial canthal tendon insertion

Type III: Comminuted single fragment with fractures extending into bone bearing the canthal insertion.

Orthodontics SR Paper (Jan 2015)

1. **Analysis gives vertical facial height in degree:**
   a. Sassouni
   b. Upper: lower facial height
   c. Jaraback
   d. Ricketts
   Ans. d

Ref: Kharbanda 2/e p238

2. **Dimensions of Ricket utility arch is:**
   a. 016 × 0.016 blue elgiloy
   b. 016 × 0.022 blue elgiloy
   c. 016 × 0.022 SS wire
   d. 016 × 0.022 TMA wire
   Ans. a

Ref: Kharbanda 2/e p398

3. **DICOM is:**
   a. Digital imaging and communication in medicine
   b. Direct imaging and communication in medicine
   c. Dental imaging and communication in medicine
   d. Digital ion complementary oxide metal
   Ans. a

Ref: Kharbanda 2/e p195

Digital Imaging and Communications in Medicine (**DICOM**) is a standard for handling, storing, printing, and transmitting information in medical imaging. It includes a file format definition and a network communications protocol.

4. **Upper molar position in Rickett analysis measures from:**
   a. Occlusal plane
   b. Palatal plane
   c. PTV
   d. Perpendicular to nasion
   Ans. c

Ref: OP Kharbanda 2/e p239

5. **CMOS is:**
   a. Complimentary metal oxide semiconductor
   b. Complimentary mineral oxide semiconductor
   c. Connective metal oxide semiconductor
   d. Complimentary mechanical oriented semiconductor
   Ans. a *Ref: Kharbanda 2/e p269*

Complementary metal-oxide semiconductor, or **CMOS**, typically refers to a battery-powered memory chip in your computer that stores startup information. Your computer's basic input/output system (BIOS) uses this information when starting your computer.

6. **MRI used for TMJ effusion:**
   a. T2W
   b. T1W
   c. Protein density
   d. Spinning property
   Ans. a

Ref: Kharbanda 2/e p202

Joint effusion and marrow edema—These are best evaluated on T2-weighted or STIR images in the sagittal or oblique sagittal plane. A joint effusion may be confined to either the superior or inferior joint compartment, or may involve both. It has been postulated that marrow signal abnormalities may reflect marrow edema, osteonecrosis, or may be related to osteoarthrosis. Sano et al. reported that joints with bone marrow signal alterations were more painful than joints with normal marrow signal.

7. Step bend placed between two incisors produce movement in:

a. Equal and same direction
b. Equal and opposite
c. Unequal and same
d. Unequal and opposite

Ans. a

Ref: Profitt 4/e p387, 388 Fig 10.39
Ref: OP Kharbanda p 363

8. Facial axis angle of Rickets:

a. Posterior angle between Ba-N & Pt-Gn
b. Anterior angle between Ba-N & Pt-Gn
c. Inferior angle between Ba-N & Pt-Gn
d. Superior angle between Ba-N & Pt-Gn

Ans. a

Ref: OP Kharbanda 2/e p238

9. William Down had classified facial forms into:

a. Hypodivergent and hyperdivergent
b. Vertical, horizontal, average grower
c. Forward and backward rotator
d. Retrognathic, mesognathic, prognathic

Ans. d

Ref: OP Kharbanda 2/e p156

10. In the field of orthodontics the first MRI study of TMJ in 1998 done in:

a. Imaging of TM Joint
b. Herbst appliance imaging for TMJ
c. Bionator study of TMJ
d. For Forsus study

Ans. b

Ref: OP Kharbanda 2/e p202

11. Trifocal ellipse arch forms are

a. Braider's arch form
b. Rickets arch form
c. Mushroom shaped form
d. Bonwill Hawley form

Ans. a

Ref: OP Kharbanda 2/e p251
***McConaill & Scher**-*Catenary curve*
Ricketts & Eugel-Pentamorphic arches*
***Bonwill Hawley**-*Equilateral triangle*
Fujita-Mushroom arch wires*
***James Currier**-*Computerised polynomial least square fitting programme*
***Begole**-*Cubic Interpolatory Spline*

12. For intrusion of lateral incisor:

a. 2 horizontal loops towards each other
b. 2 horizontal loops distally directed
c. 2 horizontal loops messily directed
d. 2 horizontal loops away from each other

Ans. c

Ref: Kharbanda 2/e p398

13. One couple system produced by:

a. Centred V bend
b. Off centred V bend
c. Step bend
d. Molar uprighting spring

Ans. d

Ref: Textbook of orthodontics by Bishara p214
Ref: OP Kharbanda 2/e p361

14. Not true about V bends:x

a. Bend towards gingival direction
b. Hook soldered on it
c. It delivers the torque
d. Neutralise anterior and posterior torque segments

Ans. c

Ref: Kharbanda 2/e p360-362

15. **When edgewise prescription used and 1st, 2nd and 3rd order bends given, additional bend needs?**
   a. Progressive lingual root torque
   b. Progressive buccal root torque
   c. Continous lingual root torque
   d. Continous buccal root torque

   Ans. a

16. **For vertical growth bite registration:**
   a. Bite beyond freeway space and little sagittal advancement
   b. Large advancement
   c. Bite registration within freeway space
   d. Same advancement for sagittal to vertical

   Ans. a

Ref: Kharbanda 2/e p479

17. **Which loop has greatest mechanical advantage of no residual movement?**
   a. Gjessing
   b. Mushroom
   c. Ricketts
   d. Opus

   Ans. a

Ref: Profitt 4/e p599, Kharbanda 2/e p406

18. **Prevalence of Class II malocclusion in Northern India:**
   a. 15%
   b. 22 %
   c. 32%
   d. 34%

   Ans. a

Ref: OP Kharbanda 2/e p26

19. **According to American Board of Orthodontics Discrepancy Index is calculated according to the trait of Class II malocclusion D1 with overbite 5–7 mm is:**
   a. 1 pts per side
   b. 2 pts per side
   c. 3 pts per side
   d. 4 pts per side

   Ans. c

Ref: Kharbanda 2/e p39

Overjet Measurements

- For ≥ 0 to < 1 mm, score 1 pt (edge-to-edge)
- For ≥ 1 to ≤ 3 mm, score 0 pts
- For > 3 to ≤ 5 mm, score 2 pts
- For > 5 to ≤ 7 mm, score 3 pts
- For > 7 to ≤ 9 mm, score 4 pts
- For > 9 mm, score 5 pts

Overbite is a measurement between two antagonistic teeth (lateral or central incisors) comprising the greatest overbite.

- For > 0 to < 3 mm, score 0 pts.
- For > 3 to < 5 mm, score 2 pts
- **For > 5 to < 7mm, score 3 pts**
- If any of the lower incisors are impinging on the palatal tissues (< 0.5 mm) or there is 100% overbite (a complete vertical overlap of antagonistic incisors, score 5 pts.

20. **In RME:**
   a. One quarter turn once daily
   b. Two quarter turns twice a day
   c. Two quarter turns once a day
   d. One quarter turn each in morning and evening

   Ans. d

Ref: OP Kharbanda 2/e p439

21. Type III Cu NiTi wire is used when?

a. Patient has low to normal pain threshold
b. More force required
c. Patient has good pain threshold
d. Where rapid tooth movement is required

Ans. a

Ref: OP Kharbanda 2/e p334

Type I- Limited clinical use
Type II- In patients with high pain threshold
Type IV- In patients who are sensitive to pain

22. A patient has Class II subdivision on left side, Katz Premolar classification shows:

a. 0 mm discrepancy at R & L sides
b. 0 mm on R & + 3 mm at L side
c. 0 mm on R & -3 mm at L side
d. 3 mm on R side & - 3 mm on L side

Ans. b

Ref: OP Kharbanda 2/e p53-54

23. Xi point is:

a. Geometric centre of maxilla
b. Geometric centre of condyle
c. Geometric centre of ramus
d. Geometric centre of symphysis

Ans. c

Ref: Kharbanda 2/e p237-238

24. Wits appraisal given by:

a. Wits
b. Merrifield
c. Down
d. Jacobson

Ans. d

Ref: Profitt 4/e p212

25. Drug for pain that does not affect the orthodontic movement is:

a. Aspirin
b. Acetaminophen
c. Diclofenac
d. Ibuprofen

Ans. b

Ref: Profitt 4/e p343

26. Prosthion is located in:

a. Mandible body
b. Maxilla
c. Ramus
d. Anterior cranial base

Ans. b

Ref: Kharbanda 2/c p221

27. Maxillary superimposition related to assess tooth movement by ABO:

a. Registration on palatal contour of palate
b. Registration on lingual curvature of palate
c. Registration along ANS and PNS plane registered at ANS
d. Superimposition along ANS and PNS plane registered at PNS

Ans. b

http://dent.umich.edu/sites/default/files/departments/opd/Gu%20cephalometric%20superimpositions%20216.pdf

28. I-point superimposition is standardisely registered at:

a. Sella
b. Nasion
c. Mandibular condyle
d. Occipital condyle

Ans. d

Ref: Kharbanda 2/e p281-282

29. In PA Cephalogram when maxillary constriction is present J:AG.AG ratio is less than:

a. 50% b. 60%
c. 70% d. 80%

Ans. d

Ref: Kharbanda 2/e p244-245

30. Titanium is not used for orthodontic purpose because:

a. Ti alloy only can give enough strength to implant
b. Ti alloy has more strength
c. Ti alloy has less strength
d. Biocompatibility is more for Ti

Ans. c *Ref: CRAIG 10/e p473*

31. In Burstone's T loop activation achieved is:

a. 3 mm b. 4 mm
c. 6 mm d. 8 mm

Ans. a *Ref: Kharbanda 2/e p404-405*

32. In Holdaway ratio analysis the ratio of 1:3 is:

a. Lower lip to lower incisor relation b. Upper lip to upper incisor relation
c. Upper lip to lower incisor relation d. Lower lip to upper incisor relation

Ans. d

Ref: Kharbanda 2/e p251

33. Centre of resistance of single rooted teeth is at:

a. 1/3rd length of root from alveolar crest b. 2/3rd length of root from alveolar crest
c. 3/4th length of root from alveolar crest d. 2/5th length of root from alveolar crest

Ans. a *Ref: Kharbanda 2/e p357*

34. A patient with OPG & cephalogram with condyle enlargement of right side, further needed is:

a. MRI b. CBCT
c. MDCT d. TC 99

Ans. d

Ref: OP Kharbanda 2/e p189

35. A patient came with lingually placed lateral incisor and retrognathic mandible and CVMI Stage III, the best treatment modality is:

a. Functional therapy followed by fixed therapy
b. Correction of incisors with removable appliance
c. Only fixed appliance therapy
d. Fixed therapy to correct lateral incisor followed by functional therapy

Ans. d

Ref: Kharbanda 2/e p187

36. Patient reports with retained deciduous canine, impacted permanent canine and retrognathic mandible. The X-rays best suited for diagnosis are:

I. Lateral Ceph II. OPG III. MDCD IV. CBCT

a. I only b. I, II
c. I, II, IV d. IV only

Ans. c

Ref: Kharbanda 2/e p195

37. Size of standard X-ray film:

a. 10 × 12 inch b. 8 × 12 inch
c. 12 × 8 inch d. 8 × 14 inch

Ans. a

Ref: Direct pick from AIIMS question bank

38. **Which is not used as flux?**
 a. Boric acid
 b. Borax
 c. HF
 d. KF
 Ans. c

Ref: Direct pick from AIIMS question bank

39. **Which of the following is used for etching porcelain?**
 a. 1.23% HF
 b. 4% HF
 c. 9.6% HF
 d. 37% HF
 Ans. c

Ref: Direct pick from AIIMS question bank

40. **Which is not true about orthodontic force:**
 a. Increased OPG
 b. Decreased OPG
 c. Decreased RANK
 d. Decreased RANK
 Ans. b

Ref: Kharbanda 2/e p71

41. **Maximum amount of retraction that can be achieved by orthodontic treatment alone is:**
 a. 7 mm
 b. 8 mm
 c. 17 mm
 d. 22 mm
 Ans. a

Ref: Kharbanda 2/e p14

42. **Which force is most physiological for tooth movement?**
 a. Intermittent
 b. Continous
 c. Interrupted
 d. Light and continuous
 Ans. d

Ref: Kharbanda 2/e p68-69

43. **All are true about CBCT except:**
 a. Less noise
 b. More noise
 c. Less soft tissue content
 d. Decreased exposure
 Ans. a

Ref: Kharbanda 2/e p195-198

44. **Which is not true about SABG?**
 a. Canine can erupt through graft
 b. Help in closure of fistula
 c. Orthognathic surgery can be done after SABG
 d. Grafted bone in case of lateral incisor missing not provided for side of implant
 Ans. d

Ref: Kharbanda p699-701

45. **MIP is a:**
 a. Medium intensity projection
 b. Maximum intensity projection
 c. Minimum intensity projection
 d. Maximum intensity production
 Ans. b

Ref: Direct pick from AIIMS question bank

In scientific visualization, a **maximum intensity projection (MIP)** is a volume rendering method for 3D data that projects in the visualization plane the voxels with maximum intensity that fall in the way of parallel rays traced from the viewpoint to the plane of projection. This implies that two MIP renderings from opposite viewpoints are symmetrical images if they are rendered using orthographic projection.

46. **MEAW technique is used for:**
 a. Class II with open bite
 b. Class II with retrognathism
 c. Class III with open bite
 d. Class III with deepbite
 Ans. c

Ref: Kharbanda 2/e p565

47. Activity index of GCF shows:
a. RANK/OPG
b. IL-1Beta/IL1-RA
c. IL- 1RA/IL-1Beta
d. OPG/RANK
Ans. b

Ref: Direct pick from AIIMS question bank

48. All are true about canine impaction except:
a. Canine impaction more common in females
b. Palatal impaction is more common than labial impaction
c. Labial impaction is more common than palatal impaction
d. Unilateral canine impaction is more common than bilateral
Ans. c

Ref: Kharbanda 2/e p621-624

49. Which statement is true?
a. Operating consistently locating the same cephalometric point located based on the judgement in different location in random error
b. Vertical deviation are more on landmarks which are on covered line point A*B
c. Both are true
d. Both are false
Ans. c
Ref: Kharbanda 2/e p219-221

50. All comes under IOTN except:
a. Cleft lip & Palate
b. BMP
c. Open bite
d. Crowding
Ans. b
Ref: Kharbanda 2/e p35-36

51. Most prevalent habit is:
a. Nail biting
b. Mouth breathing
c. Thumbsucking
d. Tongue thrusting
Ans. d
Ref: Kharbanda 2/e p135

52. For Type II backward rotation of mandible center of rotation lies at:
a. Incisal edge
b. Premolar
c. TMJ
d. Most distal occluding molar
Ans. d

Ref: Direct pick from AIIMS question bank

Forward Rotation of Mandible
Type I About the centre in the TMJ.
Type II. About the centre located at the incisal edges of the lower anterior teeth.
Type III. Centre of rotation to the of premolars region
Backward Rotation of Mandible
Type I Centre lies at the TMJ Openbite develops
TYPE II Centre is at the most distal occluding molars. This occurs in connection with growth in the sagittal direction at the condyles. The soft tissue of the chin may not follow this movement and a characteristic double chin may form. Difficulty in closing lips without strain.

53. Direct correlation between degree of injury and intensity of healing response:
a. Rapidly acquired phenomenon
b. Regionally acquired phenomenon
c. Regionally accelerated phenomenon
d. Rapid accelerated phenomenon
Ans. c
Ref: Kharbanda 2/e p601

54. SOX-9 is responsible for craniofacial growth and it shows:
a. Chondrocyte differentiation
b. Osteoblast differentiation

c. Cementoblast differentiation
d. Osteoclast differentiation
Ans. b

Ref: Kharbanda 2/e p516

55. Direction of force by Class III elastic in face mask:
a. 5–10 degrees downward from occlusion
b. 15–20 degrees downward from occlusion
c. 15–20 degrees upward from occlusion
d. 35–40 degrees downward from occlusion
Ans. b

Ref: Kharbanda 2/e p550

56. Most common malocclusion responsible for root resorption is:
a. Class III
b. Class II Dv 1
c. ClassII Dv 2
d. Class II with open bite
Ans. c *Ref: OP Kharbanda 2/e p539*

57. Most crucial in primary stability is:
a. Cortical bone thickness
b. Pitch
c. Diameter of tip
d. Length of implant
Ans. b *Ref: Kharbanda 2/e p595*

58. Stable element in Ti6Al4V in alpha phase is: *Ref: Direct pick from AIIMS question bank*
a. Al
b. Ti
c. Al, V
d. V
Ans. a

Types

The alloys of titanium can be classified into three main groups as follows:

- Alpha alloys: These are non-heat treatable and are generally very weldable. They have low to medium strength, good notch toughness, reasonably good ductility and have excellent properties at cryogenic temperatures. The more highly alpha or near alpha alloys offer high temperature creep strength and oxidation resistance.
- Alpha-Beta alloys: These are heat treatable to varying extents and most are weldable with the risk of some loss of ductility in the weld area. Their strength levels are medium to high. Hot forming qualities are good but cold forming often presents difficulties. Creep strength is not usually as good as in most alpha alloys.
- Beta alloys: Beta or near beta alloys are readily heat treatable, generally weldable, and offer high strength up to intermediate temperature levels. In the solution treated condition, cold formability is generally excellent.

Crystallographic Forms

The metallurgy of titanium is dominated by the crystallographic transformation which takes place in the pure metal at 882 C. Below this temperature, pure titanium has a hexagonal close packed structure known as alpha (α); above it, the structure is body centred cubic and termed beta (β). The fundamental effect of alloying additions to titanium is alteration of the transformation temperature and production of a two-phase field in which both alpha and beta phases are present. Elements having extensive solubility in the alpha-phase characteristically raise the transformation temperature and are called alpha stabilisers.

Alpha Stabilisers

Figure 1 typifies the binary phase diagram formed by addition of an alpha stabiliser (such as aluminium, oxygen, nitrogen or carbon) to titanium. Oxygen is added to pure titanium to produce a range of grades having increasing strength as the oxygen level is raised. Aluminium is the only other alpha stabiliser used commercially and is a major constituent of most commercial alloys. It is a very effective alpha-strengthening element at ambient and elevated temperatures up to about 550 C. The low density of aluminium is an additional advantageous feature but the amount that can be added is limited because of the formation of a brittle titanium-aluminium compound at aluminium contents exceeding about 8% by weight.

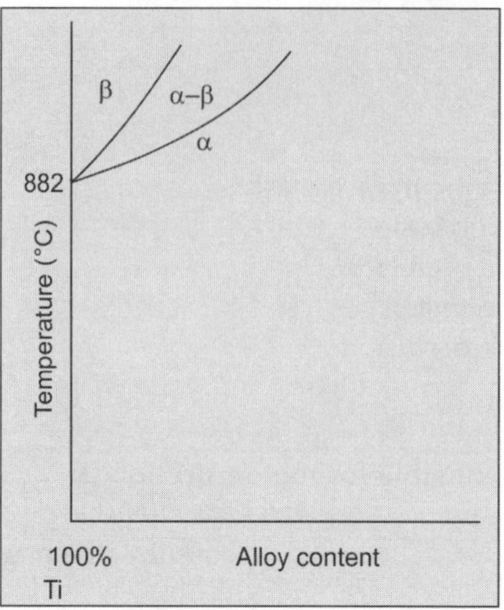

Fig. 1: Effect of alpha-stabilising elements on titanium

The alpha phase is also strengthened by the addition of tin or zirconium. These metals have appreciable solubility in both alpha and beta phases and as their addition does not markedly influence the transformation temperature they are normally classified as neutral additions. As with aluminium, the beneficial ambient temperature hardening effect of tin and zirconium is retained at elevated temperatures. **Figure 2** demonstrates schematically the phase diagram for titanium and a neutral element.

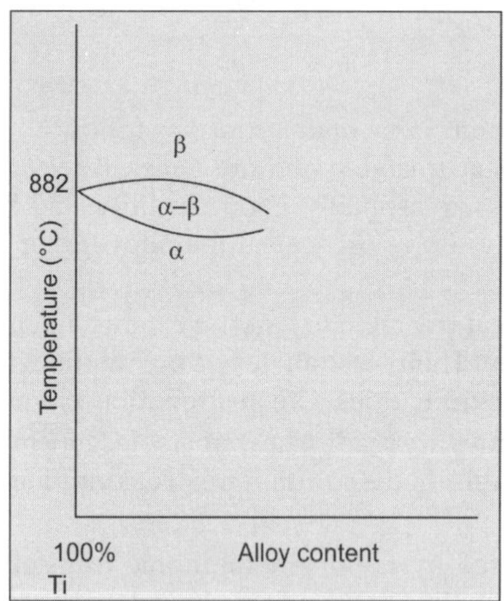

Fig. 2: Effect of neutral elements on titanium

Beta Stabilisers

Elements that depress the transformation temperature, readily dissolve in and strengthen the beta phase and exhibit low alpha phase solubility are known as beta stabilisers. They can be divided into two categories according to their constitutional behaviour with titanium:

- Beta-isomorphous elements
- Beta-eutectoid elements.

Beta-Isomorphous Elements

Beta-isomorphous elements exhibit complete mutual solubility with beta titanium. Increasing addition of the solute element progressively depresses the transformation temperature to give the characteristic phase diagram. Molybdenum and vanadium are the most important beta isomorphous elements, while niobium and tantalum have also found application in some alloys.

59. GOSLON index 5 for CLP shows:
   a. Describe only in sagittal plane
   b. Can be corrected by orthodontic and orthopaedic treatment
   c. 50 percent orthodontic surgery only treatment
   d. Can be treated by orthodontic treatment

   Ans. c *Ref: Kharbanda 2/e p696*

GOSLON Index-Great Ormond Street London

60. Dc point is located on:
   a. Centre of ramus
   b. Centre of mandible
   c. Centre of maxilla
   d. Centre of neck of condyle where bars Ba Na coincide

   Ans. d

Ref: Kharbanda 2/e p220

61. Malocclusion not needing retention is:
   a. Deepbite
   b. Open bite
   c. Anterior cross bite
   d. Rotation

   Ans. c

Ref: Kharbanda 2/e p752-753

62. Increased FOV of CBCT causes:
   a. Increased patient exposure
   b. Decreased contrast
   c. Decreased scanning time
   d. Increased noise

   Ans. a *Ref: Kharbanda 2/e p196-200*

For most applications, limited or focused
FOV CBCT is preferred over large volume CBCT for the following reasons:

- Increased resolution to improve the diagnostic accuracy of endodontic-specific tasks such as the visualization of small features including calcified/accessory canals, missed canals, etc.
- Highest possible resolution
- Decreased radiation exposure to the patient
- Time savings due to smaller volume to be interpreted
- Smaller area of responsibility
- Focus on anatomical area of interest

63. International Commission of radiation protection (ICRP) recent recommendation for radiation enforce is at:
   a. 1997
   b. 2003
   c. 2007
   d. 2013

   Ans. c

Ref: Direct pick from AIIMS question bank

The system of radiation protection that is used across Europe and worldwide is based on the recommendations of: the International Commission for Radiation Protection (ICRP); and the International Commission on Radiation Units and Measurements (ICRU). The conceptual framework adopted by the ICRP in its publication ICRP 60 (ICRP 1991) is one of a System of Radiological Protection and builds on the System of Dose Limitation central to earlier ICRP documents such as ICRP 26 (ICRP 1977). ICRP publication 60 (ICRP 1991) was substantially revised and updated in 2007 with the publication of ICRP 103 (ICRP 2007).

The ICRP system of radiation protection is based on three fundamental principles: justification, optimisation and dose limitation.

64. Muscles of facial expression are derivative of:
   a. 1st arch
   b. 2nd arch
   c. 3rd arch
   d. 4th arch

   Ans. b

65. Point showing high error possibility along X-axis is:
a. Orbitale
b. Condylion
c. Point A
d. Point B
Ans. a

Ref: Dental cocktail AIPG edition high yield facts

66. Most common complication of orthognathic surgery is:
a. Fracture
b. Erosion of condyle
c. Malunion
d. Loss of neurosensation due to injury to IAN
Ans. d

67. All are true about PA Ceph except:
a. Can be used for facial asymmetry
b. Grummon's analysis is not related to normative data
c. In upper facial asymmetry MSR can be drawn as a line from the midpoint of Z plane through the midpoint of Fr-Fr line
d. MSR has been selected as a pseudo vertical reference line
Ans. d

Ref: Kharbanda 2/e p215, OP Kharbanda p206–208

68. Maximum loading force for microimplants:
a. 150 gms
b. 300 gms
c. 400 gms
d. 500 gms
Ans. c

Ref: Kharbanda 2/e p596

69. Steiner's method for superimposition used:
a. Superimposition on SN plane registered at N
b. Superimposition on SN plane registered at Ba
c. Superimposition on Ba-N plane registered at N
d. Superimposition on SN plane registered at S
Ans. d

Ref: OP Kharbanda p176, Kharbanda 2/e p278

70. All are advantage of CBCT over MDCT except:
a. Less metal artefact
b. Less radiation exposure
c. Scan time is less
d. More soft tissue contrast
Ans. d

Ref: Kharbanda 2/e p196-200

71. Resistance to corrosion is due to:
a. TiO
b. Ti (OH) 2
c. Ti
d. Ti N
Ans. a

72. Nerve for first pharyngeal arch is:
a. Facial
b. Trigeminal
c. Vagus
d. Glossopharyngeal
Ans. b

73. Ti Graphite composite is usually:
a. Monophasic
b. Biphasic
c. Triphasic
d. Tetraphasic
Ans. c

74. Latency period of distraction osteogenesis is:
a. 5–7 days
b. 5–7 weeks
c. 2–3 days
d. 15–20 days
Ans. a

Ref: Kharbanda 2/e p672

75. Which arch is absent in human embryo development:
a. 4th
b. 5th
c. 6th
d. 7th
Ans. b

76. Gold Standard diagnosis for OSA is:
a. Rhinomanometry
b. Polysomnography
c. Neuroendoscopy
d. Cephalometry
Ans. b

Ref: Kharbanda 2/e p713

77. Least common impaction is:
a. Lateral incisor
b. Central incisor
c. Second premolar
d. Maxillary canine
Ans. b

Ref: Kharbanda 2/e p622

78. More chance of relapse is found in:
a. BSSO with prognathism
b. BSSO with retrognathism
c. Genioplasty with augmentation
d. Genioplasty with reduction
Ans. c

Ref: OP Kharbanda 2/e p659

79. Chemokines are formed in response to orthodontic force by:
a. Cell differentiation
b. Cell hypertrophy
c. Cell proliferation
d. Cell death
Ans. a

Ref: OP Kharbanda 2/e p70-75

80. Bird's eye view is taken at:
a. 15 degrees
b. 30 degrees
c. 45 degrees
d. 75 degrees
Ans. c

Ref: OP Kharbanda 1/e p141

Prosthodontics SR Paper (Jan 2015)

1. **Which full mouth technique is based on mathematical and anthropological techniques?**
   a. Younis
   b. Hobo and Takyoma
   c. Neymann
   d. Pankey Mann Schuyler
   Ans. b
2. **Hobo's Technique differs from Pankey Mann Schuyler in all except:**
   a. Teeth arrangement (Antero-posterior)
   b. Posterior first and anterior next
   c. Based on canine guided occlusion
   d. None
   Ans. c
3. **Pickling done with:**
   a. Nitric acid
   b. 20% HCL
   c. 50% HCL
   d. Phosphoric acid
   Ans. c
4. **Which cement is used for cementation of self–retained monolithic zirconia crown?**
   a. Conventional GIC
   b. Resin cement
   c. Dual core resin cement
   d. Resin modified GIC
   Ans. d
5. **Occusal morphology was advocated by?**
   a. Myeson
   b. Schuyler
   c. Siebert
   d. Okeson
   Ans. d
6. **Why TMJ called compound joint?**
   Ans. Because of the presence of 3 components (condyles, glenoid fossa and articular disk)
7. **Overextended dentures results in:**
   Ans. Epulis fissuratum
8. **Selective grinding is done in all of the following except:**
   Ans. Major corrections
9. **Collateral ligament is a part of:**
   Ans. TMJ
10. **When translational movement happens in TMJ then the condyle:**
    Ans. Moves along with the meniscus anteriorly beneath the articular eminence.

The temporomandibular joint contains 4 types of receptor nerve endings which have different functional characteristics.

These synovial receptors are located in the fibrous joint capsule, in the lateral ligaments, and in the retrodiscal pad. They are not contained in the central portion of the disc, nor in the synovial tissues. The temporal, masseter, and auriculotemporal nerves terminate on these synovial receptors

Type I receptors provide continuous movement and postural perception of the mandible. They also coordinate facilitory and inhibitory reflex effects of the masticatory muscles.

Type II receptors effects the masticatory muscles when mandibular movements are initiated.

Type III receptors are only active when excessive tension is developed in the temporomandibular joint's lateral ligament. Type III receptors are activated in pterygoid and mylohyoid muscle spasms as well as temporalis and masseter muscle inhibitions.

Type IV receptors are the pain receptors of the articular tissues, and in normal/healthy joints they are inactive. They become activated if the joint capsule, retrodiscal pad, and the temporomandibular joint ligament are subjected to marked mechanical deformation and tension, or with direct chemical irritation.

11. Movement in laterotrusive cusp:

Ans. Along inner and outer inclines.

12. A patient has pain during swallowing which muscle is being affected?

Ans. Superior constrictor

13. What type of reflex you will see when mandible is in the rest position

a. Flexor reflex with involvement of cortex
b. Flexor reflex without involvement of cortex
c. Mitotic reflex with involvement of cortex
d. Mitotic reflex without involvement of cortex

Ans. d

14. Patient not able to chew in centric ,the causes can be all except:

Ans. Decreased VDO

15. The thing to be considered in a diabetic patient before placing an implant is when HbA1c:

a. Less than 3
b. More than 3
c. Less than 7
d. More than 7

Ans. d

16. If the coefficient of thermal expansion of metal is lower in PFM then:

Ans. Failure of bonding between Metal and porcelain.

17. The pontic preferred for maxillary posterior region is:

Ans. Modified Ridge Lap

18. When will you do a tentative fabrication for RPD design?

a. After final surveying
b. After diagnostic surveying
c. Before diagnostic surveying
d. Before final surveying

Ans. b

19. Horizontal fulcrum line, in which plane movement will happen?

a. Transverse
b. Vertical
c. Horizontal
d. Axial

Ans. c

20. If eyeball is removed but eyelid and adjacent structures in eyes are preserved then it is called:

a. Exenteration
b. Occuloplasty
c. Enucleation
d. Evisceration

Ans. c

Evisceration, Enucleation, and Exenteration are the three main surgical techniques by which all or part of the orbital contents are removed. **Evisceration** is the removal of the contents of the globe while leaving the sclera and extraocular muscles intact. **Enucleation** is the removal of the eye from the orbit while preserving all other orbital structures.

Exenteration is the most radical of the three procedures and involves removal of the eye, adnexa, and part of the bony orbit.

Evisceration is usually indicated in cases of endophthalmitis unresponsive to antibiotics and for improvement of cosmesis in a blind eye. Enucleation is indicated for the above two conditions as well as for painful eyes with no useful vision, malignant intraocular tumors, in ocular trauma to avoid sympathetic ophthalmia in the second eye, in phthisis with degeneration, and in congenital anophthalmia or severe microphthalmia to enhance development of the bony orbit. Exenteration is indicated mainly for large orbital tumors or orbital extension of intraocular tumors.

21. **What is the surface in noble replace implant?**
 a. Titanium plasma spray
 b. Hydroxy apatite
 c. Nano particle
 d. Platinum reinforced
 Ans. C

22. **Bone tap is used in which condition?**
 a. D1 & D2 bone with tapered implant
 b. D3 & D4 bone with tapered implant
 c. D1 & D2 bone with square implant
 d. D3 & D4 bone with square implant
 Ans. c

23. **The main difference between major and minor diameter in implant is:**
 a. Thread length
 b. Thread form
 c. Thread width
 d. Thread depth
 Ans. d

24. **All are true about envelope of function except:**
 a. Less than envelope of motion
 b. More than envelope of motion
 Ans. b

25. **What is the maximum torque that is given for implant?**
 a. 50 N
 b. 60 N
 c. 70 N
 d. 100 N
 Ans. c

26. **IPS impress and IPS Emax contains mainly:**
 Ans. Lithium disilicate

27. **Unglazed and glazed porcelain has main difference in:**
 Ans. Strength

28. **What is the indication of cast circumferential clasp in Kennedy Class I RPD?**
 a. 0.01 inches
 b. 0.015 inches
 c. 0.02 inches
 d. 0.025 inches
 Ans. a

29. **Non rigid connector true is All except:**
 Ans. Not used in long span ridges

30. **Which type of occlusion will you assign for FPD?**
 a. Canine guided
 b. Reorganised
 c. Group functional
 d. Confirmative
 Ans. d

31. **What is the reason for shrinkspot porosity?**
 Ans. By shrinkage of a portion of metal as it solidifies from the molten state without flow of additional molten metal from surrounding areas.

32. **All are indications of basal implant except:**
 Ans. Will not be used in maxilla.

33. **Reasons for black casting are all except:**
 Ans. Overheating of the metal.

34. **What type of occlusion is preferred in posterior implant**
 a. Balanced
 b. Canine guided
 c. Group function
 d. Lingualised
 Ans. d

35. **What is A-P (Antero-posterior) spread in Implant?**
 a. Distance from the centre of anterior implant to the distal end of posterior implant
 b. Distance from the centre of posterior implant to the distal end of anterior implant

c. Distance from the centre of anterior implant to the mesial end of posterior implant
d. Distance from the centre of posterior implant to the mesial end of anterior implant
Ans. a

36. If a surgeon is doing a surgery to remove a soft palatal tumor what would you suggest?
a. Removal of entire soft palate for fabrication of speech appliance
b. Removal of Tsoft palate without compromising tumor margin, but leave a part of it
c. Remove entirely if 3/4th is to be removed
d. Excise only a half portion of the soft palate
Ans. b

37. Particle size of modern hybrid composite is:
Ans. 0.04–3.5 micrometres.

38. All of the following waxes are used for diagnostic waxup except
a. Ivory wax up
b. Blue inlay wax
c. Utility wax
d. Modelling wax
Ans. d

39. The cause of continuous pain after delivering a complete denture is mainly:
Ans. Defective registration of centric occlusion.

40. All are true about composite except:
a. The power of LED is more intense than QTH
b. Plasma arc can cure deeper areas
c. Conventional composite can be used in more depth
d. Microfilled composite cannot be used in all situations
Ans. b

41. Endodontically treated teeth should be restored with:
Ans. Posts

42. The occlusal scheme indicated in patients with neuromuscular incoordination is:
a. Lingualised arch with monoplane teeth
b. Lingualised arch with decreased vertical dimension
c. Bilateral balanced with monoplane teeth
d. Bilateral balanced with decreased vertical dimension
Ans. c

43. Resilient lining materials have ADA number:
a. 65
b. 75
c. 85
d. 95
Ans. b

44. What type of restoration is indicated to a patient underwent 50Gy Radiotherapy?
a. Implant supported
b. Acrylic RPD
c. Valplast
d. Cast Partial Denture
Ans. d

45. Continous defects of mandible which treatment is preferred?
a. Cast partial
b. Implant supported
c. Either A or B depending on the situation
d. Bone quality based
Ans. c

46. What type of final impression material is suggested for patient with Carcinoma of tongue?
a. Polyether
b. ZOE
c. Addition silicon
d. Alginate
Ans. a

47. **What type of occlusal scheme preferred for single complete dentures for making necessary alteration?**
   a. Before final impression
   b. After pickup impression
   c. During jaw relation records
   d. At laboratory remount
   Ans. c
48. **Wrought wire clasp has the following advantages except:**
   Ans. Decreased flexibility
49. **All are contraindications of Indirect sinus lift except:**
   a. Sinus infection
   b. Chronic topical steroid use
   c. Radiation therapy
   d. Bone height less than 4 mm
   Ans. d
50. **The anterior and lateral movements are called:**
   a. Posselt movement
   b. Hobo movement
   c. Bennet movement
   d. Pankey Mann movement
   Ans. c
51. **The height and width of cusp are affected by all except:**
   Ans. Intercondylar distance
52. **If there is acute curve of Spee then,what type of cusp form is used?**
   a. Steep
   b. Shallow
   c. Flat
   d. Broad
   Ans. b
53. **Which type of articulator is being used for FPD?**
   a. Semiadjustable
   b. Fully adjustable
   c. Non adjustable
   d. Any of the above
   Ans. a
54. **How much bone is required for direct sinus lift?**
   a. 0.5–1 mm
   b. 0.75–1.5 mm
   c. 3–5 mm
   d. 6–9 mm
   Ans. c
55. **If phosphoric acid level rises to more than 50%, it results in formation of:**
   Ans. Dicalcium phosphate monohydrate.
56. **Subperiosteal implant is indicated when the bone level is less than?**
   a. 4 mm
   b. 6 mm
   c. 9 mm
   d. 10 mm
   Ans. b
57. **FGP (Functional Generation Path) is used for recording:**
   a. Maxillary anteriors
   b. Mandibular anteriors
   c. Maxillary posteriors
   d. Mandibular posteriors
   Ans. c
58. **If anterior guidance is set as zero, the factors that affects disocclusion of condyle are all except:**
   Ans. Mediolateral curve
59. **If canine is replaced with implant prosthesis what type of occlusion you will prefer?**
   a. Canine guided
   b. Unilateral group function
   c. Bilateral balanced
   d. Lingualised
   Ans. b
60. **PM2 according to Carl Misch means:**
   a. Hinge movement
   b. Opening and closing movement
   c. Lateral movement
   d. None
   Ans. a

61. Complete denture with permanent soft liners are indicated in:
a. Epulis fissuratum
b. Thick mandibular ridge
c. Extremely atrophied ridge
d. Young patients
Ans. C

62. Chewing stroke begins from:
a. Centric relation
b. Centric relation or centric occlusion
c. Physiologic rest position
Ans. c

63. All are true about rest position except:
a. Remains unchanged
b. Not affected by gravity,head position
c. Habitual postural position
d. Strained position of condyles
Ans. d

64. Disocclusion of posterior components during lateral exertion against opposing natural teeth or fixed prosthesis is seen in:
Ans. Implant protective occlusion (IPO)

65. The problem in long standing case of Kennedy Class 1 situation is:
a. Atrophy of residual ridge
b. Resorption of ridge adjacent to abutment area
c. Decreased interocclusal space
d. Difficulty in adjustment of denture
Ans. b

66. Cast circumferential clasp in distal extension:
a. Should not be used
b. Should be used with caution
c. Retentive tip should engage more than 0.01 inch undercut
d. Retentive tip should engage more than 0.02 inch undercut
Ans. c

67. The undercut used for retention of maxillary obturator is:
a. Distolingual
b. Mesiolingual
c. Anterior
d. Posterior
Ans. b

68. When doing a casting pressure should be maintained for.... seconds?
a. 2
b. 3
c. 4
d. 5
Ans. c

69. Maximum acceptable abrasive value is:
a. 150
b. 250
c. 350
d. 450
Ans. b

70. Embedded fracture post was by:
a. Mccollum
b. Schuyler
c. Masserann
d. Jorgenson
Ans. c

71. The custom shaped fossa for condylar heads are being made by:
a. Cephalograms
b. Stereograms
c. Monograms
d. Normograms
Ans. b

72. In CIELAB system +a* usually corresponds to:
a. Red-green
b. Red-purple
c. Blue-green
d. Yellow-purple
Ans. b

73. All are female devices except:
a. Ceka
b. Zagg & Zest
c. Rotherman
d. Bonal ball
Ans. b

74. The cluster of neurons in the brainstem that drives the rhythmic chewing is termed as:
a. Peripheral pattern generator
b. Central pattern generator
c. Peripheral pattern scintillator
d. Central pattern scintillator
Ans. b

75. Kinoscope belongs to:
a. II A
b. II C
c. III A
d. III B
Ans. d

76. A modified method used with an U shaped metal occlusal template that is slightly convex on the lower surface:
a. Stansbury method
b. Swenson method
c. Yurkstas method
d. Vig method
Ans. c

77. Hex lock type implants are preferred in:
Ans. Cleft palate patients

78. The unit of surface energy is:
a. Erg/cm^2
b. Dyne/cm
c. Joule/m^3
d. Erg/m^3
Ans. b

79. All are true about mouth protectors except:
a. Made from laminate polymers are stronger than single material sheet
b. Thickness of sheet varies between 1.6–3 mm
c. They may be custom made or stock or fabricated inside the mouth
d. As the contact of ethylene increases, the hardness of polymer increases
Ans. a

80. Groper's appliance is:
a. Fixed anterior
b. Removable anterior
c. Fixed posterior
d. Removable posterior
Ans. a

81. A patient with carcinoma with chemotherapy the treatment of choice is:
Ans. Make RPD, No implant treatment required.

82. A carcinoma patient needs complete denture which mouth opening method is not indicated?
Ans. Trismus screw

83. False about soft splint:
Ans. It increases vertical dimension.

84. The diameter of anterior implants designated for use in narrow spaces is in the range of:
a. 2.25 mm
b. 3.25 mm
c. 4.25 mm
d. 5.25 mm
Ans. b

85. In long-term endosseous implants which is preferred:
a. SLA coated
b. Plasma sprayed
c. Hydroxy apatite
d. Laser
Ans. b

86. A Paget disease patient with impacted teeth, the preferred restoration is:
a. Complete denture with soft liner
b. Conventional complete denture
c. Extraction of all impacted teeth and then complete denture
d. Extraction of anterior impacted teeth followed by tooth tissue supported denture
Ans. A

87. American Heart Association Antibiotic Prophylaxis is indicated in all except:
Ans. Placement of orthodontic brackets

88. Contamination of casting occurs in all except:
a. Residual waxes
b. Prolonged heating of alloy
c. No use of flux
d. Gases in mould cavity
Ans. b

89. Skyfurcation is usually done in:
a. Maxillary anteriors
b. Maxillary molars
c. Mandibular anteriors
d. Mandibular posteriors
Ans. b

Ref: Shillingburg Dental Cocktail AIPG Edition High Yield Facts

90. Q 2 was repeated twice in the exam

AIIMS SRship Paper (July 2014)

1. **No mobility, no displacement is seen in:**
   a. Concussion
   b. Subluxation
   c. Luxation
   d. Intrusion
   Ans. a
2. **Cleft lip and palate is:**
   a. Monogenic
   b. Multifactorial
   c. Polygenic
   Ans. b
3. **Nitrous oxide is transported in:**
   a. Serum
   b. RBC
   c. Undissolved
   Ans. a
4. **Posterior border of tonsil is formed by:**
   a. Palatoglossal
   b. Palatopharyngeus
   c. Levatorvellipalatini
   Ans. b
5. **In a child with renal impairment which can be given:**
   a. Lidocaine
   b. Mepivacaine
   c. Articaine
   d. Benzocaine
   Ans. c
6. **Long acting LA:**
   a. Lidocaine
   b. Tetracaine
   C. Bupivacaine
   d. Dibucaine
   Ans. d
7. **Which is true?**
   a. Leeway space is more in maxilla is .....mm on each side
   b. Leeway space is more in mandible and is .....mm on each side
   Ans. b
8. **Acute fluoride toxic dose based on:**
   a. Age
   b. Weight
   Ans. b
9. **A child with red coloured urine, flourescent:**
   Ans. Porphyria
10. **Hyrax force is:**
    a. 100 gm/side
    b. 250 gm/side
    c. 250 gm on both sides
    Ans. c
11. **NiTi wires true is:**
    Ans. 1/3rd to 1/4 thmodulous of elasticity as compared to stainless steel
12. **1st tooth eruption is coincided with which milestone:**
    a. Rolling over stomach
    b. Walking
    c. Light fixation
    d. Speech
    Ans. a

13. Size of teeth affected in:

a. Morphodiffrentiation
b. Histodiffrentiation

Ans. a

14. Thumbsucking, child has open bite ,at what age t/t should be given:

a. 5 years
b. 10 years
c. 6 years
d. 12 years

Ans. b

15. Phentolamine in urine is seen in:

a. Odontodysplasia
b. Dentogenesisimpefecta
c. Amelogenesis imperfect
d. Osteogenesis imperfect

Ans. a

16. Midline diastema of 8 mm:

a. Wait till canine erupts
b. Frenectomy
c. Check for supernumerary teeth
d. Start orthodontic treatment

Ans. c

17. Fusion of palatal shelves with nasal bone occurs at:

a. 4 weeks
b. 8 weeks
c. 12 weeks
d. 30 weeks

Ans. c

18. Intermolar width increases till:

a. 9 years thereafter increases slowly
b. 12–13 years thereafter remains constant
c. 18 years of life

Ans. b

19. Greenish discharge from lesion on neck of children:

a. Brachial cyst
b. Mucocele
c. Thyroglossal cyst

Ans. a

20. Non trainable i.q when a child cannot learn tooth brushing is:

a. 38–50
b. < 20
c. 50–70

Ans. a

21. Dentin mineralisartion starts at:

a. Cuspal tips
b. Cervical area
c. DEJ

Ans. a

22. Diffrence in weight and frankel behavior modification is:

a. Frankel based on behavior shows at time of appointment while wright based on overall child behavior
b. Opposite of a Wright based on behavior shows at time of appointment while Frankel based on overall child behavior
c. Both
d. None

Ans. a

23. N_2O in environment is best recorded by:

a. Infrared spectrophotometer
b. Laminar flow

Ans. a

24. **Comprehensive school dental health care first adopted in:**
    a. New Zealand
    b. Sweden
    c. US
    d. France
    Ans. a
25. **Treatment time for pre-schoolers:**
    Ans. Morning
26. **Treatment time for older children:**
    Ans. Afternoon
27. **Calcification sequence of primary teeth:**
    Ans. ADBCE
28. **Which primary molar doesn't resemble any permanent teeth?**
    Ans. Primary mandibular first molar.
29. **Tell show do given in year?**
    Ans. 1959 Addleson (cornerstone of behavior guidance)
30. **Parents presence best benefit for child in age of:**
    Ans. 3.5 years – 4years
31. **If canines are not clinically palpable by age of 9 years then:**
    Ans. Take IOPA

(Canines which are impacted 85% are paltally impacted, and 15% are buccaly erupted, canine impacted palatally does not cause crowding and buccally impacted canine do crowding).

32. **Bitewing film used in smaller child:**
    Ans. Size 0
33. **Pediatric pt. which type of Digital X-ray system used:**
    Ans. Phosphor based
34. **Anterior mandibular occlusal technique:**
    Ans. Patients head is positioned so that occlusal plane is 45 degree to floor

Central X-ray -à -10 degrees to tip of chin, -55 degrees to plane of film.

Some Important High-yield Facts from OP Kharbanda

1. Stages of Development of Speech

STAGE	PERIOD	FEATURES
I	0–8 weeks	Reflexive crying and vegetative sounds
II	8–20 weeks	Cooing and laughter
III	16–30 weeks	Vocal play
IV	25–50 weeks	Reduplicated babbling: consonant-vowel syllabes
V	50 + weeks	Non-reduplicating babbling
VI	Around one year	First words

2. Morley's Ratio
   It depicts the percentage of incisor show on posed smile with respect to clinical crown height. Usually it is 75–100%
3. The total height of both casts in occlusion should be about 7–7.5 cm
4. Orthoproof of Holland uses 3D CT Technology
5. The base of nose has a Gull in flight contour
6. Burlington growth study conducted by Dr. Frank Popovich
7. Hellman introduced polygonal portrayal of Down's Analysis values in facial growth
8. Wylie and Johnson's method to determine any malformation of the mandible was incorporated and Riedel's Go-Gn plane was used to represent the body of the mandible
9. Sassouni analysis-Facial types

Type I	Anterior cranial base plane does not pass through O
Type II	Palatal plane does not pass through O
Type III	Occlusal plane does not pass through O
Type IV	Mandibular base plane does not pass through O

10. Facial height ratio is FHR = S-Go/N-Me
11. Merrifield profile line is also called Z angle ,average value is 80 +/- 9 degrees
12. DDR-Direct Digital Radiography
13. The greatest degree of certainity has been found for cephalometric landmarks Sella Turcica and Articulare
14. The greatest inaccuracy was seen for N-SS and N-SM ,while accuracy was greater for Me-Go and N-Me
15. Bracket customization was by Shetty and Malhotra
16. Self ligating brackets was by Stolzenberg
17. The corrosive behaviour is tested according to ISO 10271
18. TTR-Temperature Transition Range coined by Buehler
19. Supercable wire by Hanson
20. The corrosion which occurs in the area where wire and brackets contact each other is Fretting corrosion
21. Fiddler et al reported presence of N-Nitrosodibutylamine and N-Nitrosopiperidine from eight brands of elastic rubber bands used in orthodontics
22. Active stabilisation can overcome prolonged forces up to 5–10 gm/cm^2
23. Gianelly and Goldman suggested terms Maximum, Moderate and Minimum to indicate the extent to which the teeth of the active and reactive units should move when a force is applied

24. Nanda classified anchorage into

Group A Space Closure	100-75% from anteriors, 25% from posteriors
Group B Space Closure	Equal from anteriors and posteriors
Group C Space Closure	75-100% posterior protraction

25. CODIM-Computer Oriented Dental Irregularity Matrices
26. Clincheck is a part of Interactive Treatment Planning
27. Technique of IPR (InterProximal tooth Reduction) by Sheridan
28. Crysta growth technique was introduced by Maijer and Smith as an alternative to Acid etching for bonding brackets in 1979
29. 2 × 4 appliance is used for quick resolution of cross bite
30. Jones Jig appliance delivers 70–75 gm force
31. Insta Nance was developed by Hilgers
32. A projet bite guage is used in bite registration in Class II D1 cases
33. HERBST APPLIANCE

Type I	Fixing system to crown or bands
Type II	Fitting directly to archwire through screws
Type IV	Ball and socket system with special locking clasps

34. Forsus available in 5 lengths- 25 mm, 29 mm, 32 mm, 35 mm and 38 mm
35. Peck and Peck called Class II D2 "A heritable pattern of small teeth in well-developed jaws
36. Yunis Varon syndrome is associated with Canine impaction
37. Palatal canine impaction is mostly associated with Class II D2 cases
38. CANINE IMPACTION

FEATURE	PERCENTAGE
Incidence	0.8–2.8
Palatal : buccal	85:15
Bilateral:unilateral	8:92
Female:male ratio	2.3:1
Left: Right	5:2
Maxilla:Mandible	8:1

39. Sector Classification by Ercison and Kurol and modified by Lindauer
40. The angle suggested for canine impaction predictor is 31 degrees
41. TWEED GROWTH TRENDS

Type A	Both maxilla and mandible grow downward and forward but at the same pace
Type B	Both grow downward and forward but maxilla grows at greater pace than mandible resulting in vertical growth
Type C	Mandible grows at greater pace and are horizontal growers

42. Trutains are vacuum formed plastic retainers
43. The clefts of lip and alveolus may have bands of soft tissue bridging across the two sides called Simonnarts bands
44. Presurgical orthopaedics introduced by McNeil and popularised by Burstone
45. SABG was by Boyne and Sands 1972
46. Bergland Index to evaluate the success of grafted bone based on height of interdental septum

Type I	Normal
Type II	75% of normal bone height
Type III	Less than 75%
Type IV	No bony ridge

47. Goosecoid is another homeobox containing transcription factor which has an important role in craniofacial development
48. Aggrecan is a Cartilage-specific proteoglycan
49. Twist is a positive regulator of osteoblast differentiation
50. Osterix is required for osteogenic differentiation

Endodontics SR Questions

1. **Rate of flow of dentinal fluid is affected by all except:**
   a. Tubule diameter
   b. Tubule length
   c. Tubule direction
   Ans. c
2. **Endodontic panacea is:**
   a. Calcium hydroxide
   b. Formocresol
   c. Triple antibiotic paste
   Ans. a
3. **Stainless steel obeys the law:**
   a. Hookians elasticity
   b. Transformation law
   Ans. a
4. **Mineral phase of pulp stones:**
   a. Flourapetite
   b. Whitlokite
   c. Carbonated hydroxyapatite
   Ans. c

The mineral phase of pulp calcifications has been shown to consist of typical carbonated hydroxyapatite.

5. **Structure of pulp stones:**
   a. Arranged in concentric layers
   b. Have tubular structure like dentine
   Ans. b

Pulp stone
True: Made of dentine and lined by odontoblasts.
False: Formed from degenerating cells which mineralize.
Free Stone: Not related to pulp space wall, surrounded bynsoft tissue.
Adherent Stone: Attached to wall of pulp space, not fully enclosed by dentine.
Embedded Stone: Enclosed within canal wall, less attached than the above.
Denticle: An alternative term for pulp stone, more usually a calcification filled with epithelial remnants surrounded by odontoblasts.
Fibrodentine: Material produced by fibroblast-like cells against dentine prior to differentiation of a new generation of odontoblast-like cells.
Dystrophic calcification: Inappropriate biomineralization of the pulp in the absence of mineral imbalance.

6. **A crack is seen in the floor of endododontically treated mandibular molar. Treatment protocol is:**
   a. To extract it
   b. Seal the crack with biodentine
   c. Restore with composite
   Ans. a
7. **Orthodontic root extrusive force:**
   a. 75–100 gms
   b. 50–75 gms
   c. 25–50 gms
   Ans. c
8. **Exchange zone of instruments between operator and assistant:**
   Ans. Below chin
9. **Difference between stools used by operator and assistant:**
   Ans. Absence of foot rest

10. Distance of air abrasion source from surface:
a. 3–5 mm
b. 8–10 mm
c. Depends on the surface area
Ans. a

11. Predictor of post instrumentation pain. Or The patients with following had increased chances of pain after surgery:
a. Preoperative pain or mechanical allodynia
b. Necrotic pulp
c. Patency file
Ans. a

12. In a symptomatic tooth with apical periodontitis and tenderness on percussion after complete debridement:
a. Occlusal reduction is will not help to reduce postoperative
b. Occlusal reduction of functional cusp should be done
c. Reduction of tooth should be done
Ans. b

13. A patient with symptomatic pulp comes to a clinician without appointment. He has to adjust him between two patients. Treatment will be:
a. Perform pulpectomy and give calcium hydroxide dressing
b. Perform pulpectomy of largest canal and give cotton dressing
c. Give antibiotics and pain killers
Ans. b

14. Dentinal microcracks are maximum in:
a. Hand NiTi files
b. Wave one
c. Rotary Protaper
d. Hand protaper
Ans. c

Ref: Dentinal Microcrack Formation during Root Canal Preparations by Different NiTi Rotary Instruments and the Self-Adjusting File

15. 957, 557, 57 burs have common:
a. Head design
b. Taper
c. Are all end cutting burs
Ans. a

16. Best protocol to remove triple antibiotic paste:
a. PUI with NaOCl
b. 10% Citric acid
Ans. a

There were significant differences amongst the groups ($P < 0.001$). Passive ultrasonic irrigation (PUI) with 1% NaOCl removed significantly more TAP than the other irrigating solutions ($P < 0.05$). Distilled water, 1% NaOCl, ethanol and EDTA were associated with significantly more remaining TAP.

17. Butterfly effect:

The butterfly effect is an optical phenomenon seen in some sections of tooth roots. The aim of this work was to investigate the density of dentinal tubules in mesiodistal and buccolingual cross-sections of roots exhibiting the butterfly effect and to determine if the effect is featured throughout the length of roots and is age related.

18. Direction of Vertical root fractures in endodontically treated tooth:
a. Bucco lingual
b. Corono apical
c. Mesio distal
Ans. a

19. Best protocol for irrigation of immature teeth that will save SCAP and other stem cells:
a. 5.25% NaOCl and 2% CHX
b. 2.5% NaOCl and 17% EDTA
c. 0.5% NaOCl and 2% CHX
d. 6% NaOCl and 17% EDTA
Ans. d

Irrigation with 17% EDTA best supported cell survival (89% viability; $P < .001$ versus all other groups), followed by irrigation with 6% NaOCl/17% EDTA/6% NaOCl (74%; $P < .001$ versus the 2 groups containing 2% CHX). Conversely, protocols that included 2% CHX lacked any viable cells.

20. **Incidence of furcation canals in mandibular first molar according to Guttmann:**
    a. 29%
    b. 59%
    c. 71%
    Ans. A
21. **The success of orthograde retreatment in teeth with apical periodontitis:**
    a. More in anteriors and less in posteriors
    b. Less than teeth without apical periodontitis
    c. More than teeth without apical periodontitis
    d. equal
    Ans. b
22. **In a patient having high cholesterol, the factors affecting diet (a+b), fat(c) , ... (d). The combination of these factors, i.e. is example of:**
    a. Multiple linear regression
    b. Simple linear regression
    Ans. A
23. **The modification for a very dark tooth requiring porcelain veneer are all except:**
    a. Extend veneer 2–3 mm below gingival
    b. Increase thickness of resin
    c. Increase the opacity of porcelain by 5–10
    Ans. A
24. **Which was wrong statement?**
    Ans. Maximum time for heat testing 15 sec.
25. **Which test has least sensitivity?**
    a. Heat
    b. Cold
    c. EPT
    d. Test cavity
    Ans. c
26. **Main cause of NiTi instruments Fracture:**
    a. Torsonial and bending along with fatigue fracture
    b. Manufractures defects
    c. Operators use
    Ans. A
27. **McSpadden factor high it means:**
    Ans. Instrument will not fracture easily.
28. **Level of incidence in case studies regarding revascularization (repeat):**
    Ans. Class-II
29. **#35 file fractures below the curvature of root canal in the mesiobuccal root canal with PAI 4 in a symptomatic tooth. Line of treatment is:**
    a. To bypass the instrument
    b. To retrieve the instrument
    c. Periapical surgery
    Ans. c
30. **Amitryptaline contradiction:**
    Ans. Not used with vasoconstrictor.
31. **TNF alfa responsible for:**
    Ans. Bone resorption.
32. **Long term complication of intentional RCT:**
    Ans. Root resorption.

33. **Treponoma Denticola associated with:**
    Ans. Acute apical periodontitis.
34. **Obturation of vital tooth in multi visit procedure should be done**
    Ans. After 5–7 days.
35. **Maximum conduction velocity:**
    a. A alpha
    b. A beta
    c. A delta
    d. C fibres
    Ans. a
36. **White knuckle syndrome:**
    a. Tingling in hands and wrists
    b. General whiteness of fingers
    c. Pain and loss of sensation in fingers
    Ans. c
37. **Long standing perforations are sterilised by:**
    a. 2.5% NaoCl
    b. 2% CHX
    Ans. a
38. **Term Endodontics was coined by:**
    Ans. Dr Harry B Jhonston.
39. **AAE assessment difficulty scale:**

The AAE designed the Endodontic Case Difficulty Assessment Form for use in endodontic curricula. The Assessment Form makes case selection more efficient, more consistent and easier to document. Dentists may also choose to use the Assessment Form to help with referral decision making and record keeping.

Conditions listed in this form should be considered potential risk factors that may complicate treatment and adversely affect the outcome. Levels of difficulty are sets of conditions that may not be controllable by the dentist. Risk factors can influence the ability to provide care at a consistently predictable level and impact the appropriate provision of care and quality assurance.

The Assessment Form enables a practitioner to assign a level of difficulty to a particular case.

LEVELS OF DIFFICULTY

MINIMAL DIFFICULTY: Preoperative condition indicates routine complexity (uncomplicated). These types of cases would exhibit only those factors listed in the MINIMAL DIFFICULTY category. Achieving a predictable treatment outcome should be attainable by a competent practitioner with limited experience.

MODERATE DIFFICULTY: Preoperative condition is complicated, exhibiting one or more patient or treatment factors listed in the MODERATE DIFFICULTY category. Achieving a predictable treatment outcome will be challenging for a competent, experienced practitioner.

HIGH DIFFICULTY: Preoperative condition is exceptionally complicated, exhibiting several factors listed in the MODERATE DIFFICULTY category or at least one in the HIGH DIFFICULTY category. Achieving a predictable treatment outcome will be challenging for even the most experienced practitioner with an extensive history of favorable outcomes.

40. **Munsell color system:**
    Ans. Measures Color Quantitavely
    Note that qualitative measure is by CIELAB System
41. **Rubber dam on nose:**
    Ans. Due to off centric punching of holes.
42. **Halo effect in Composites:**

Bioactive glass fibers were investigated for use as a fixation vehicle between a low modulus, polymeric composite and bone tissue. In an initial pilot study, bioactive glass fiber/polysulfone composites and all-polysulfone control rods were implanted into the rabbit tibia; the study was subsequently expanded with implantation into the rabbit femur. Bone tissue exhibited direct contact with the glass fibers and adjacent polymer matrix and displayed a mechanical bond between the composite and bone tissue after six weeks implantation. Interfacial bond strengths after six weeks implantation averaged 12.4 MPa, significantly higher than those of the all-polymer controls. Failure sites for the composite at six weeks generally occurred in the bone tissue or composite, whereas the failure site for the polymer implants occurred exclusively at the implant/tissue interface. The bioactive glass fiber/polysulfone composite achieved fixation to bone tissue through a triple mechanism: a bond to the bioactive glass fiber, mechanical interlocking between the tissue and glass fibers, and close apposition and possible chemical bond between the portions of the polymer and bone tissue. This last mechanism resulted from an overspill of bioactivity reactions from the fibers onto the surface of the surrounding polymer which we call the halo effect.

43. **Halo effect is seen in all except:**
    Ans. Improper shade selection.
44. **Polymerisation shrinkage of siloranes:**
    a. 1% b. 2%
    c. 3% d. 4%
    Ans. a
45. **Wedge placement site for composites:**
    Ans. Below gingival crest.
46. **Acc to ALARA:**
    Ans. Leaded aprons are not necessary but thyroid collars are must.
47. **Safety limits of Hg in clinic:**
    Ans. 50 microgm/mm^3
48. **Triangular wedges are indicated in:**
    Ans. Deep gingival embrasures.
49. **Automatrix:**
    Ans. No wedge is required.
50. **Pin failure most common type is:**
    a. Pin tooth b. Pin restorative
    c. Pin fracture d. Tooth fracture
    Ans. a
51. **Classification of instrument fracture - type VI complete instrument #:**
    Ans. Full fracture
52. **Acc. to SOTOKOWA's classification class IV type of fracture is:**
    Ans. Partial clockwise twist
53. **Type IV isthumus means:**
    Ans. Complete or incomplete communication between 3 or more canals
54. **Endodontically treated tooth is:**
    Ans. More susceptible to caries.
55. **Two canal in mandibular premolar is more common in:**
    Ans. Afro-Americans
56. **Protaper treatment files are used at speed of:**
    Ans. 500–700 rpm
57. **A working length measured by gen3 apex locator is smaller by 3–4 mm when confirmed radiographically because:**
    a. Fluid in canal
    b. Lateral canal
    Ans. b
58. **Component of EndosolvR:**
    Ans. Formamide

59. **Rubber dam recommendation for endodontic purpose is:**
    Ans. Medium
60. **A 63-year-old patient have pain on biting. Radiograph shows asymmetric enlargement of distal canal in comparison to mesial canal. The reason can be:**
    Ans. Internal resorption
61. **Pt. having sensitivity after a class II amalgam restoration. Thus probable reason could be:**
    Ans. Poor condensation in proximal box.
62. **All are Ca(OH)2 based sealers except:**
    a. Apexit
    b. Sealapex
    c. Vitapex
    d. Tubliseal
    Ans. d
63. **In a patient with separated instrument beyond the confines of root canal. Treatment protocol would be:**
    Ans. Periapical surgery with apicectomy.
64. **While resecting the tooth, minimum amount of resection will be?**
    Ans. 3 mm
65. **LA of choice in hot tooth anaesthesia is:**
    Ans. Articaine
66. **Finger spreader is different from hand spreader in:**
    Ans. Can result in excessive stress
67. **Which solvent has been shown to be more efficient, (fastest) in softening GP?**
    Ans. Chloroform
68. **Old patients have increased chances of what condition after oral surgery?**
    Ans. Ecchymosis
69. **In concept of ALARA, max. permissible dose of radiation for dental tea in one year is:**
    Ans. 50 milisieverts
70. **Highest level of evidence is seen in:**
    Ans. Metaanalysis
71. **In a fully formed tooth has suffered an intrusive injury and the crown is partially exposed. The recommended treatment is:**
    a. No treatment
    b. Splint for 7–10 days
    c. Endodontically repositioning in to correct alignment in 3–4 weeks
    d. Repositioning with force
    Ans. c
72. **Ratio measurement method associated with which generation of apex locators:**
    a. First
    b. Second
    c. Third
    d. Fourth
    Ans. c
73. **Fan's Classification is used for:**
    Ans. C-shaped canals
74. **Acc. to IADT, no. of radiographs intrauma cases:**
    Ans. 4
75. **A patient presents for a post treatment examination after 3 yrs with no complaint of symptoms except apical radiolucency that was not before treatment. Treatment of this patient can be classified as which of the following?**
    Ans. Healing

76. Incisal edges of Access cavity of max. anterior teeth:
Ans. Should not be bevelled.

77. The purpose of wedging a matrix at gingival area of dental amalgam restoration of class II cavity is to achieve all except:
a. Displace gingival tissues
b. Prevent/minimize excess of amalgam at gingiva
c. Assist in establishing proximal contour
Ans. a

78. Ideally control tooth when testing a pulpally involved tooth is:
Ans. Adjacent and contralateral

79. False among finger and hand spreader:
Ans. Hand spreaders are associated with less chances of tooth fractures.

80. What is dentin blushing?
Ans. Vascular Haemorrhage or pulp tissue during the crown preparation.

81. Using the case difficulty, assessment symptom developed by American association of endodontics, in which any factor score is 3. treatment is done by?
Ans. Endodontist

82. For irrigating solution to reach effectively in apical 1/3rd of canal.canal should be enlarged to what size?
Ans. 35–40

83. Which type of external resorption has not been identified with replanted avulsed teeth?
a. Surface
b. Inflammatory
c. Refractory
d. Replacement
Ans. c

84. Which of the followin`g prescribed a buccomarginal flap design?
Ans. Associated with less gingival recession.

85. Which of the following is not an indication or periapical surgery?
a. Non- negotiable or blocked canal associated with symptomatic periradicular prosthesis.
b. Gross over obturating of obturating material
c. Obtain biopsy
d. To resolve any endodontic treatment failure
Ans. d

86. Which of the following occurs after minor extrusion of obturating material into periradicular tissues?
a. Swelling
b. Significant symptoms
c. Some tissue inflammation
d. More apical leakage
Ans. c

87. Which of the following is not a common cause of file separation?
a. Limited flexibility
b. Manufacturing defects
c. Amount of force applied
Ans. b

88. Which of the following describes lateral compaction GP?
a. Indicated for cases with internal resorption
b. Involves multiple steps
c. May manages length control well
d. It is difficult to retreat
Ans. c

Additional Questions of Periodontics SRship (July 2014)

1. **Ist formed bone of in an extraction socket:**
   Ans. Woven bone
2. **Minimum bone loss per implant annually:**
   a. 0.2 mm
   b. 0.4 mm
   c. 0.6 mm
   d. 0.8 mm
   Ans. a
3. **Minimum implant diameter to resist greaterocclusal loads in posterior area:**
   a. 4 mm
   b. 6 mm
   c. 7 mm
   d. 8 mm
   Ans. a
4. **After supracrestal fibrotomy, what is true minimum time for retraction?**
   a. 10 weeks
   b. 12 weeks
   c. 14 weeks
   d. 16 weeks
   Ans. 12 weeks
5. **Category A of biomedical waste is disposed in which bags?**
   Ans. Black
6. **Particle size of Biogvain is:**
   Ans. 300–375 micron
7. **Motrin is brand name for:**
   Ans. Ibuprofen
8. **Which of the following agent is not used for conditioning?**
   Ans. Chlorhexidine
9. **Which of the following is true for gingival enlargement?**
   a. Prevalence in patients taking dilitazem is less than 5%
   b. Seen more in patients taking tacrolimus than cyclosporine
   c. More in pt. taking cyclosporine than tacrolimus
   Ans. c
10. **Observers assessment of alterness, sedation scale does not include:**
    Ans. Color
11. **Pt. report having experienced a washing out weekend failure far about 24 hrs after surgery, due to:**
    Ans. Transient bacteremia induced by surgical procedure.
12. **First sign of lignocaine toxicity?**
    Ans. Tachycardia
13. **Which is not a side effect of placing a fresh autogenous graft in infrabony pocket?**
    a. Arthusrxn
    b. Cell mediated rxn
    c. Root resorption
    d. Rejection
    Ans. c
14. **After completion of orthodontic t/t in a hemiseptal defect, the tooth should be stabilised for?**
    Ans. At least 6 months
15. **Subclassification 'C' in furcation classification of furcation involvement is:**
    a. Probable vertical depth of 1–3 mm
    b. Probable vertical depth of 4–6 mm

c. 7 mm or more probable depth from roof apically
d. Radiographically in floor
Ans. c

16. **What is periostat?**
Ans. 20 mg doxycycline

17. **Which of the following not included in mucogingival procedure?**
Ans. Intrabony reconstructive therapy.

18. **Which of the following means is utilized in retraction of periodontal coe-pack?**
a. Mechanical b. Chemical
c. Both d. None
Ans. a

19. **Which of the following syndrome is not associated with periodontitis?**
a. Histiocytosis b. Ehlerdanlos syndrome
c. Mafans syndrome d. Cohen syndrome
Ans. c

20. **Which of the following is not associated with early loss of deciduous dentition?**
Ans. Steven Johnson syndrome.

21. **PHP index is given by?**
Ans. Podshadley

22. **Which of the following takes into account the thickness of plaque?**
Ans. Plaque index

23. **Preferred flap for reconstructive surgery:**
Ans. Papilla preservation flap.

24. **In GTR margins of membrane removed after?**
a. 2–3 weeks b. 4–6 weeks
c. Never
Ans. b

25. **Plaque formation rate at night:**
Ans. Decreased by 50%

26. **Who invented first commercial silk floss?**
Ans. Levi Spear Parmley

27. **Osse us reshaping that would not involve the overall result k/as:**
Ans. Compromised osseous reshaping.

28. **Fibroblast in healing would will have?**
a. More nucleoli b. More RER
c. More SER
Ans. b

29. **Which of the following fibre loss is needed for apical migration of junctional epithelium?**
a. Transseptal b. Circular
c. Horizontal d. Dentogingival
Ans. d

30. **Bacterial products that initiate the inflammatory process are:**
Ans. Proteases, hyaluronidase, endotoxin

Medical AIIMS (May 2015)

OPHTHALMOLOGY

1. **When compared to blood vitreous humor has high concentration of:**
   a. Pottasium
   b. Ascorbate
   c. Sodium
   d. Glucose
   Ans. b

   Ref: Duane Ophthalmology ch 38

   The potential spaces for blood to accumulate in vitreous humor are:
   1. The canal of Petit
   2. The cloquet canal
2. **Universal marker of limbal stem cells:**
   a. Elastin
   b. Keratin
   c. ABCG2
   d. Collagen
   Ans. c

   Ref: Limbal stem cells in Review J.Ophthal 2009

   ABCG2
   Also known as BRCP1 (Breast Cancer Resistant Protein 1)
   It is ATP binding cassette group
   If question asks about corneal stem cells select KERATIN as answer
3. **Painful loss of vision in one eye, deranged reflex and increase in dark adaptation time is seen in:**
   a. CRAO
   b. CRVO
   c. Retrobulbar neuritis
   d. Ocular Ischemic Syndrome
   Ans. c

   Ref: Duane Opthalmology 2/e p729

   Hereditary optic neuritis (Leber's disease)
   Impaired depth perception (Pulfrich Phenomenon)
   Episodic or transient loss of vision on moving away from heat (Uhtoff's symptom)
4. **The most common mode of spread of retinoblastoma is:**
   a. Vascular
   b. Direct invasion
   c. Lymphatics
   d. Optic nerve
   Ans. d

   Ref: Pediatric Ophthalmology by Craig. S.Hyott 3/e p453
5. **Multifocal ERG is very useful because:**
   a. Can assess macula
   b. Can assess rods
   c. Can assess RPE
   d. Can assess function of ganglion layer
   Ans. d

   Ref: Walsh and Hoyt Clinical Neuroophthalmology 2/e p1132

6. **Evisceration of eye is not done in:**
   a. Expulsive hemorrhage
   b. Severe globe trauma
   c. Malignancy
   d. Panophthalmitis
   Ans. c

Ref: Duane ophthalmology 3/e ch 82

7. **High molecular weight proteins in cataractous lens seen only in humans:**
   a. HM 2 and 4
   b. HM 3 and 4
   c. HM 2 and 3
   d. HM 1 and 2
   Ans. b

Ref: Biochemistry of eye by David RP 3/e p28

HM 1	Large isolate from alpha crystalline preparations of gel chromatography
HM 2	Directly isolated from total soluble fractions
HM 3	Disulphide bonded aggregate
HM 4	Aggregates held together by divalent bonds

8. **Right Trochlear Nerve palsy can lead to all except:**
   a. Hypertropia
   b. Right head tilt
   c. Esotropia
   d. Vertical diplopia
   Ans. b

Ref: Paralytic Strabismus Prasad and Volpe 2/e p221

9. **Sensory nerve supply of cornea is by:**
   a. Infraorbital
   b. Nasociliary
   c. Infratrochlear
   d. Supraorbital
   Ans. b

Ref: Basic Anatomy O Rabilli 2/e ch 46

Termination of Descemet's membrane is called ring of Schwalbe
Pigment deposition on cornea is by chloroquine and amiodarone
Drug causing circular deposits in cornea is Amiodarone
Black cornea is associated with epinephrine
Pigment deposition anterior to Schwalbe line is Sampaolesi line

10. **Drugs causing amorphous whorl like corneal opacity are all except:**
    a. Amiodarone
    b. Quinine
    c. Chlorpromazine
    d. Indomethacin
    Ans. b

Ref: Kanski Ophthalmology review 2/e p231

11. **True statements regarding direct ophthalmoscopy are all except:**
    a. 2 disc diameter field of vision
    b. Self illuminated device
    c. Image is virtual and erect
    d. Magnification is 5 times
    Ans. c

Ref: Duane ophthalmology 3/e ch 63

12. Cherry Red spot after trauma is due to:

a. Pigment deposition
b. Berlin's edema
c. CRVO
d. CRAO

Ans. c

Ref: Duane ophthalmology 3/e ch 55

13. Cherry red spot and Hollenharst plaque are seen in:

a. CRAO
b. CRVO
c. Branch RVO
d. Branch RAO

Ans. a

Ref: Duane ophthalmology 3/e ch 45

PHYSIOLOGY

14. Which of these is secreted by beta cells of pancreas along with insulin?

a. Glucagon like peptide
b. Amylin
c. IGF
d. Somatostatin

Ans. b

Ref: Ganong 23/e ch 17

15. In the following figure wave B represents EEG shows high amplitude, low frequency waves as compared to waves A and C and EOG and EMG are nearly flat when compared to A in C also they are flat:

	Awake	REM	NREM
EEG			
EMG			
EOG			

a. REM
b. NREM
c. Quiet wakefulness
d. Awake

Ans. b

Ref: Ganong 23/e p234

16. In a study mannitol 10 g is injected IV and the concentration measured after some time is 50 mg/100 ml in this time 10 % of mannitol is excreted. What is the volume of the ECF?

a. 18 L
b. 14 L
c. 42 L
d. 38 L

Ans. a

Ref: Ganong 23/e p2-6

If 10 % was excreted that means 9 gm is still in the body and if we use the equation for Vd then we get
Vd = Dose/Plasma concentration
So Vd (ECF) is 9/50 * 100 = 18 L

17. Which is true regarding alpha and gamma neurons during voluntary movements?

a. Only gamma acts
b. Gamma acts first
c. Alpha acts first
d. Both act together

Ans. d

Ref: Neurosciences fundamentals Laurie Lundy 4/e p192

18. **The clot formed is not stable unless extensive cross linking occurs.This is done by:**
   a. Thrombin
   b. Plasmin
   c. Factor XIII
   d. HMWK
   Ans. c

Ref: Ganong 23/e p531

19. **If the interstitial hydrostatic pressure is 2mm Hg, the interstitial oncotic pressure is 7 mm Hg and capillary hydrostatic pressure is 25 mm Hg. What should be the capillary oncotic pressure to allow a net filtration pressure of 3 mm Hg**
   a. 21
   b. 25
   c. 27
   d. 29
   Ans. c
   Fluid movement =k (Pc-Pi)–(pc-pi)
   Insering scores 3=(25-2)–(x-7)
   That gives x = 27

Ref: Ganong 23/e p548

20. **A 50% increase in radius of vessel will cause rise in blood flow by:**
   a. 5 times
   b. 8 times
   c. 12 times
   d. 14 times
   Ans. a

Ref: Ganong 23/e p541

R = 8 L * Blood viscosity/r4
In the above question radius increased by 50%, so flow = (1.5)4 = 5.02

21. **In the following diagram left ventricular pressure is nearly equal to diastolic BP at which number**

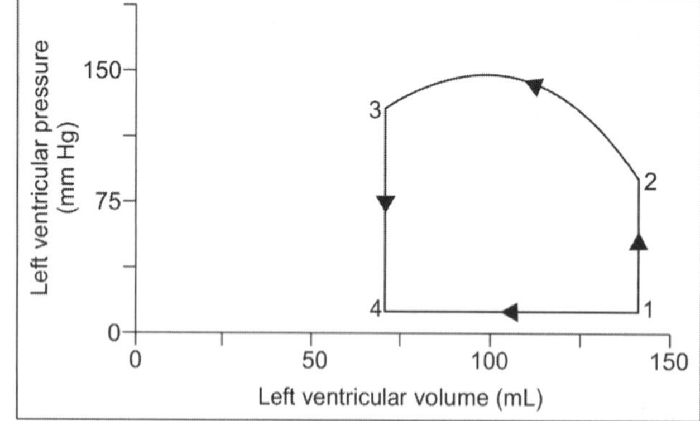

   a. 2
   b. 3
   c. 4
   d. 5
   Ans. a

Ref: Cardiovascular Physiology Richard Klabunde 2/e p227

ANATOMY

22. Muscle not inserted on greater tuberosity:

a. Teres minor
b. Supraspinatus
c. Infraspinatus
d. Subscapularis

Ans. d

Ref: Grays Anatomy 40/e p777

23. Card test done for:

a. Lumbricals
b. Palmar interossei
c. Dorsal interossei
d. Adductor pollicis

Ans. b

Ref: Grays Anatomy 40/e p782

24. Which nerve does not have a general visceral efferent?

a. Olfactory
b. Facial
c. Oculomotor
d. Glossopharyngeal

Ans. a

25. Cranial nerve nucleus lying beneath the facial colliculus is:

a. Facial
b. Abducens
c. Glossopharyngeal
d. Trigeminal

Ans. b

Ref: Grays Anatomy 40/e p240

26. Mesorectal fascia does not contain which of the following?

a. Inferior rectal vein
b. Parirectal node
c. Superior rectal vein
d. Inferior mesenteric vein

Ans. a

Ref: Grays Anatomy 40/e p1046

27. Which of these is not a support of the uterus?

a. Urogenital diaphragm
b. Pelvic diaphragm
c. Perineal body
d. Rectovaginal septum

Ans. d

Ref: Grays Anatomy 40/e p876

28. Reticular framework is present in all tissues except:

a. Thymus
b. Bone marrow
c. Spleen
d. Lymph node

Ans. a

Ref: Grays Anatomy 40/e p1194

29. What is the stage present in the oogonia at birth?

a. Telophase I
b. Prophase I
c. MetaphaseI
d. Anaphase I

Ans. b

Ref: Langman Embryology 4/e p58

30. At which stage of maturation of the spermatocyte the assortment of maternal and paternal chromosomes takes place?

a. Spermatogonia to primary spermatocyte
b. Primary to secondary spermatocyte
c. Secondary spermatocyte to spermatids
d. Spermatids to spermatozoa

Ans. b

Ref: Langman Medical Embrology 4/e 556

31. Not a branch of external carotid artery:
  a. Transverse cervical artery
  b. Lingual artery
  c. Superior thyroid artery
  d. Ascending pharyngeal artery
  Ans. a

Ref: Student Grays 32/e p911

32. All are derived from Mesonephros except:
  a. Glomerulus
  b. Paroophoron
  c. Vas deferens
  d. Epididymis
  Ans. b

Ref: Langman Medical Embrology 8/e p322

33. Microvilli are not present in:
  a. Duodenum
  b. Gallbladder
  c. PCT
  d. Collecting duct
  Ans. d

Ref: Grays Anatomy 40/e p17-19

34. Brown adipose tissue is present in all except:
  a. Around blood vessels
  b. Subcutaneous tissue
  c. Adrenal cortex
  d. Scapula
  Ans. b

Ref: Grays Anatomy 40/e p675

BIOCHEMISTRY

35. A 7-year-old boy presents with severe abdominal pain. On examination he has xanthomas. Blood drawn for work up has milky appearance of plasma. Which lipoprotein is increased?
  a. Chylomicron
  b. Chylomicron remnants
  c. LDL
  d. HDL
  Ans. a

Ref: Harrison 19/e p3176 http://www.rxpgonline.com/modules.php?name=usertoolsandfile=redirectandurl=http:// usmle. biochemistryformedics.com/milky-plasma-your-diagnosis/

36. If in a person, Total Cholesterol = 300mg/dL, HDL = 25mg/dL and TAG=150mg/dL, find out the value of LDL:
  a. 245
  b. 125
  c. 95
  d. 55
  Ans. a

Ref: NCEP Expert Panel Guidelines

37. In a person, LDL is highly elevated but the level of LDL receptors is normal. What could be the cause?
  a. Phosphorylation of LDL receptors
  b. ApoB100 mutation
  c. Lipoprotein lipase deficiency
  d. Cholesterol Acyl CoA transferase deficiency
  Ans. b

Ref: Harrison 19/e p3176

38. An infant at 7 months with history of vomiting and failure to thrive. Patient improved with IV glucose. After one month returns with same complaints. On evaluation found to have high glutamine and uracil. Which is the likely enzyme defect?

a. CPS1
b. Ornithine transcarbamoylase
c. Arginase
d. Argininosuecinase

Ans. b

Ref: Harper 27/e ch 28

39. A child was found to have hypoglycemia, hepatomegaly and accumulation of highly branched glycogen called limit dextrins. He is likely to be suffering from:

a. Cori's Disease
b. Von Gierke's Disease
c. Anderson's Disease
d. McArdle's Disease

Ans. a

Ref: Harper 27/e ch 28

40. A 48-year-old lady presented with Anemia and hepatosplenomegaly. On examination of crumpled tissue paper appearance is seen. Which is the product likely to have accumulated?

a. Glucocerebroside
b. Sphingomyelin
c. Sulfatide
d. Ganglioside

Ans. a

Ref: Harper 27/e ch 24

41. A child comes with coarse facial features, big tongue, hepatosplenomegaly, mucous discharge from nose. Diagnosis is:

a. Hurler's syndrome
b. Beckwith Wiedemann Syndrome
c. Hypothyroidism
d. Proteus syndrome

Ans. a

Ref: Harper 27/e ch 47

42. Thiamine deficiency can cause lactic acidosis due to which enzyme dysfunction:

a. PEP carboxykinase
b. PDH
c. Pyruvate carboxylase
d. Pyruvate kinase

Ans. b

Ref: Harper 27/e ch 18

43. Enzyme used for both glycogenesis and glycogenolysis is:

a. Glycogen synthase
b. Phosphoglucomutase
c. Glycogen transferase
d. Glucose transferase

Ans. b

Ref: Harper 27/e ch 14

44. In fasting states RBC use:

a. Glucose
b. Alanine
c. Ketone body
d. Fatty acid

Ans. a

Ref: Harper 27/e ch 11

45. **RNAi can cause the following in a gene:**
    a. Knock in
    b. Knock out
    c. Knock down
    d. Knock up
    Ans. c

Ref: RNA Technology by RK Guar 4/e p328

PATHOLOGY

46. **Specific site to which the CRE recombinase binds:**
    a. RE site
    b. Lox P site
    c. Sigma site
    d. LAC site
    Ans. b

Ref: Molecular pathology manual 3/e p332

47. **A 10 year old boy with muscle weakness and fatigue with increased lead in blood. Which of following enzyme production in the liver is increased:**
    a. ALA synthase
    b. Ferrochetalase
    c. PBG deaminase
    d. Heme oxygenase
    Ans. d

Ref: Robbins 5/e p1156

48. **In granular dystrophy of cornea which stain is used:**
    a. Masson trichrome
    b. Congo Red
    c. Colloidal iron
    d. PAS
    Ans. a

Ref: Foundations of ophthalmic pathology 5/e p111

49. **Oil red stain is used for:**
    a. Frozen specimen
    b. Glutaraldehyde fixed specimen
    c. Alcohol fixed specimen
    d. Formalin fixed specimen
    Ans. a

Ref: Rosai and Ackerman 10/e p534

50. **In the following karyotype what is the abnormality seen. (Picture) Shows 2 X-chromosomes and 1 Y-chromosome.:**

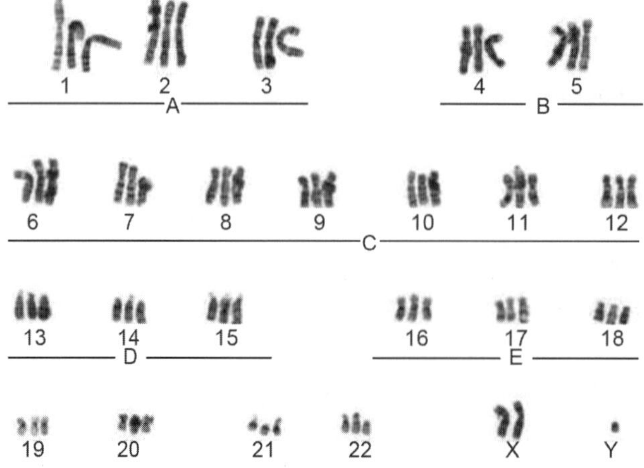

a. Gynecomastia with long thin limbs
b. Short stature with polydactyly
c. High pitched crying
d. Loose connective tissue at the nape of the neck

Ans. a

Ref: Shaw Gynecology 4/e p242

51. Immunofluorescence study. This photo was taken by attaching the camera to the microscope. What is the requirement for such a microscope?

a. Dark field condenser
b. Phase shifter
c. Dichroic mirror
d. Cathode ray tube

Ans. c

Ref: Fundamentals of light microscopy and electronic imaging

52. A 10-year-old boy with mass in the abdomen. On imaging the paraaortic lymph node is enlarged on biopsy starry sky appearance is seen. What is the underlying abnormality:

a. p53 gene mutation
b. RB gene mutation
c. Translocation involving BCR-ABL genes
d. Translocation involving MYC gene

Ans. d

Ref: Robbins pathology 9/e p597

53. A child with edema and decreased urine output. On evaluation, serum albumin is 2.5 g/dL, S. creatinine is 0.5 mg/dL, urine protein is 3+ with no RBC casts:

Pathological change expected is

a. Minimal change disease
b. Interstitial nephritis
c. IgA nephropathy A
d. Post-streptococcal glomerulonephritis

Ans. a

Ref: Robbins 9/e p917

54. Most common nephropathy associated with malignancy:

a. Membranous
b. MCD
c. IgA
d. FSGS

Ans. a

Ref: Robbins 9/e p914

55. The phenomenon where subsequent generations are at risk of earlier and more severe disease is known as

a. Anticipation
b. Mosaicism
c. Nonpenetrance
d. Atavism

Ans. a

Ref: Robbins 9/e p168

56. In Langerhans cell histiocytosis, the characteristic abnormality seen is:

a. Birbecks granules
b. Lipschut bodies
c. Langhans giant cell
d. Touton giant cell

Ans. a

Ref: Robbins 9/e p622

57. **A 45-year-old patient presents with fever, night sweats, weight loss. On X-ray a mass in apical lobe of lung is seen. On histopathology found to have caseous necrosis. What is the underlying process?**
   a. Enzymatic degeneration
   b. Hypersensitivity reaction with modified macrophages, lymphocytes and giant cells
   c. Acute decrease in blood supply
   d. Fibrinoid necrosis
   Ans. b

Ref: Robbins 9/e p370

58. **Forward scatter in flow cytometry is used to assess:**
   a. Cell death
   b. Cell size
   c. Cell granules
   d. Cell Fluorescence
   Ans. c

Ref: Wintrobes hematology 13/e ch 2

59. **Collagen typical of basement membrane:**
   a. Type I
   b. Type V
   c. Type IV
   d. Type III
   Ans. c

Ref: Robbins 9/e p44

PHARMACOLOGY

60. **Best hypertensive drug in pulmonary hypertension:**
   a. Bosentan
   b. Amlodipine
   c. Beta blockers
   d. Nitrates
   Ans. b

Ref: Katzung 9/e p984

61. **Antihypertensive not used in pregnancy:**
   a. Enalapril
   b. Nifedipine
   c. Methyl dopa
   d. Labetalol
   Ans. a

Ref: Chesely hypertensive disorders in pregnancy 7/e p444

62. **DOC for hypertension in pregnancy:**
   a. Enalapril
   b. Verapamil
   c. Alpha Methyldopa
   d. Diazoxide
   Ans. c

Ref: Chesely hypertensive disorders in pregnancy 7/e p441

63. **Heterochromia iridis is caused by:**
   a. Latanoprost
   b. Prednisolone
   c. Timolol
   d. Olapatadine
   Ans. a

Ref: Katzung 9/e p545

64. Adrenergic beta receptor having lipolysis property in fat cells:

a. Beta 1
b. Alpha 2
c. Beta 3
d. Alpha 1

Ans. c

Ref: Katzung 9/e p324

65. Diuretic which can be given in mild to moderate hypertension:

a. Loop diuretic
b. Thiazide
c. Osmotic diuretic
d. Potassium sparing diuretic

Ans. b

Ref: Katzung 9/e p675

66. All of these drugs can cause hearing loss except:

a. Metronidazole
b. Vancomycin
c. Kanamycin
d. Quinine

Ans. a

Ref: KDT 5/e p721

67. Which of the following is a protease inhibitor?

a. Saquinavir
b. Nevirapine
c. Abacavir
d. Enfuvirtide

Ans. a

Ref: KDT 5/e p770

68. What is the type of inhibition of acetylcholinesterase caused by organophosphates

a. Competitive
b. Non-competitive
c. Uncompetitve
d. Suicidal

Ans. a

Ref: Katzung 9/e p765

69. Which does not act by increasing insulin secretion for its action?

a. Exenatide
b. Sitagliptin
c. Rosiglitazone
d. Repaglinide

Ans. c

Ref: Katzung 9/e p982

70. Nitroglycerine is effective as sublingual medication because:

a. Non ionic, highly lipid soluble
b. Ionic, lipid soluble
c. Ionic, less lipid soluble
d. Non ionic, less lip soluble

Ans. a

Ref: Katzung 9/e p30

71. **In a child admitted with H influenza meningitis, cefotaxime was started instead of ampicillin. Which of these is the likely reason for this?**
   a. H influenza stains known to produce β-lactamase
   b. H influenza stains known to have altered pencillin binding protein
   c. More easier to administer
   d. Can be used in case of renal failure
   Ans. a

Ref: Katzung 9/e p643

MICROBIOLOGY

72. **Antibiotics and supportive care reverse transcriptase is a RNA dependent DNA polymerase. Which of these use it?**
   a. Hepatitis A virus
   b. Hepatitis B virus
   c. Hepatitis E virus
   d. Hepatitis C virus
   Ans. b

Ref: CDC Guidelines

73. **A vesicle on skin microscopy on Tzank smear showed giant cells. Causative agents is:**
   a. Vaccinia virus
   b. Varicella zoster
   c. Tuberculous
   d. Molluscum contagiosum
   Ans. b

Ref: Barr cutaneous cytology 6/e p326

74. **Vibrio cholerae acts by disrupting which of the following:**
   a. Hemidesmosome
   b. Gap junctions
   c. Anchoring junctions
   d. Tight junctions
   Ans. d

Ref: Bacterial Infections by Evans 4/e p239

75. **Filarial stage of adult worms responsible for diseases in all of the following except:**
   a. Onchocerca volvulus
   b. Brugia malayi
   c. Wuchereria bancrofti
   d. Mansonella ozzardi
   Ans. a

Ref: Baron Microbiology 4/e p623

76. **IgE receptor present on:**
   a. Mast cell
   b. NK cell
   c. B cell
   d. Promonocyte
   Ans. a

Ref: Robbins pathology 7/e p725

FORENSIC MEDICINE

77. **Two bodies are found outside the car following an accident. The doctor conducting the autopsy was able to decide who was driver and who was passenger based on all of these features except:**
   a. Sparrow foot mark
   b. Seat belt abrasion over left shoulder
   c. Steering wheel imprint
   d. Whiplash injury
   Ans. a > d

Ref: Forensic Medicine and Toxixology by Gautam Viswas

78. Lower two parts of the sternum fuses with its body by age:
a. 12 years
b. 14 years
c. 8 years
d. 10 years
Ans. b

Ref: Grays Anatomy 38/e p559

79. Mr X fired his gun at Mr Y who moved and escaped with the bullet only grazing his thigh. There was only a little bleeding and no other significant injury. Mr X is liable for arrest under which section of IPC?
a. 302
b. 304
c. 324
d. 326
Ans. c

Ref: Indian Penal Codes, Govt of India Gazette

80. High court has the power to stay the execution of a pregnant woman according to section:
a. 416 Cr. PC
b. 417 Cr. PC
c. 418 Cr. PC
d. 419 Cr. PC
Ans. a

Ref: Indian Penal Codes, Govt of India Gazette

81. A person was advised by his orthopedician to get regular dressing of his wound done, but the patient did not give much care. The patient visited after some time at which time the orthopedician again advised regular dressing but did not do the dressing himself as he said he was busy. Finally the wound enlarged and the underlying bone developed osteomyelitis. Which statement is true?
a. Doctor not guilty under contributory negligence
b. Doctor guilty under 'Last clear chance' doctrine
c. Doctor partly guilty under contributory negligence
d. Doctor partly guilty under 'Last clear chance' doctrine
Ans. d
Fee splitting-dichotomy
Contributory negligence by-both doctor and patient
Onus of proof in civil negligence is in–patient
The thing or fact that speaks for itself–res ipsa loquitur
Penal erasure done for-serious professional misconduct

Ref: Indian Penal Codes, Govt of India Gazette

82. Rat hole tear is associated with which injury?
a. Postmortem artefact
b. Firearm
c. Razor blade
d. Assault
Ans. b

Ref: Forensic Medicine by Rao 2/e p127

83. Segmented of blood in blood vessel after death is called:
a. Kevorkian sign
b. Rokitansky sign
c. Tache noir
d. Carvallo's sign
Ans. a

Ref: Forensic Medicine by Rao 2/e p432

Yellow triangles on sclera which change to brownish black 3–4 hours after death is called as tache noir

84. Acrid (pear like) smell is seen in:
a. Ether
b. Paraldehyde
c. Phenol
d. Nitrobenzene
Ans. b

Ref: Forensic Medicine by Rao 2/e 708

85. A man fell from 35 feet height. Eyewitnesses say that he landed on his feet. Which of the following injuries is possible
a. Ring fracture of foramen magnum + Lumbar spine injury
b. Pond fracture skull + Cervical spine injury
c. Gutter fracture skull + Cervical spine injury
d. Depressed fracture skull + Cervical spine injury
Ans. a

Ref: Forensic Medicine by Rao 2/e 336

86. The 'knot' in judicial hanging is placed at:
a. The back of the neck
b. The angle of jaw
c. Below the chin
d. Choice of hangman
Ans. c

Ref: Forensic Medicine by Rao 2/e 389

87. A bomb blast took place in Delhi following which 2 persons died. All of the following are true about their injuries except:
a. Injuries due to burns or air blast
b. Force of explosion
c. Injury to internal organs
d. Bruise, laceration, fractures are triad of main injuries seen
Ans. a

Ref: Forensic Medicine by Rajesh Barade Ref: Forensic Medicine by Rao 2/e p217

88. After an incised wound new collagen fibrils are seen along with growing epithelium. The age of the wound is:
a. 4–5 days
b. About 1 week
c. 12–24 hours
d. 24–72 hours
Ans. a

Ref: Robbins p 563

89. Sweating is absent in:
a. Heat stroke
b. Heat syncope
c. Heat exhaustion
d. Miner's cramps
Ans. a

Ref: KS Reddy 21/e p97

90. According to the 2013 amendment the age for sexual consent is:
a. 16 years
b. 18 years
c. 20 years
d. 15 years
Ans. b

91. HPV can cause all of these cancers except:
   a. Base of tongue carcinoma
   b. Nasopharyngeal carcinoma
   c. Ca cervix
   d. Tonsillar carcinoma
   Ans. b

Ref: Robbins 7/e p1163

ENT

92. Kashima operation done for:
   a. Vocal cord
   b. Recurrent Cholesteatoma
   c. Atrophic rhinitis
   d. Industrial injury
   Ans. a

Ref: Dhingra 3/e p442

93. The main vessel involved in bleeding from JNA:
   a. Internal maxillary artery
   b. Ascending pharyngeal artery
   c. Facial artery
   d. Ascending palatine artery
   Ans. a

Ref: Scott and Brown 3/e p2098

94. Eustachian tube function is best assessed by:
   a. Politzer test
   b. VEMP
   c. Rhinomanometry
   d. Tympanometry
   Ans. d

Ref: Cummings otorhinolaryngology 2/e p2202

95. Topical treatment for recurrent respiratory papillomatosis includes:
   a. Acyclovir
   b. Cidofovir
   c. Ranitidine
   d. Zinc
   Ans. b

Ref: Cummings otorhinolaryngology p 878

PSM

96. In a group of 100 people, the average GFR is 85 ml/min with a standard deviation of 25. What is the range for 90% confidence interval?
   a. 80–90
   b. 81–89
   c. 75–95
   d. 70–100
   Ans. b

Ref: Medical statistics by Aviva 1/e p34

97. 'Nikshay' is a newly launched central government software. It is used for tracking:
   a. TB cases
   b. High risk pregnancies
   c. High risk new borns
   d. Cases with malaria
   Ans. a

Ref: RNTCP Guidelines

98. Sensitivity measures:
a. True positive
b. True negative
c. False positive
d. False negative
Ans. a

Ref: Park 23/e p125

99. In a survey the highest sample of 58 was entered by mistake as 85. This will lead to:
a. Increased mean, increased median
b. Increased mean, no change in median
c. No change in mean, increased median
d. Increased mean, decreased median
Ans. b

Ref: Park 23/e p847

100. Immunization statistical data of the community can be found by:
a. Sample registration system
b. District level household survey
c. Rural health statistics
d. Annual Health Survey
Ans. b

Ref: Park 23/e p765

101. Tuberculin test is a cheap and logistically simple test. But it leads to confusion because of:
a. High percentage of immunized people
b. HIV cases are less
c. Infection prevalence is more
d. Inadequate interpretation skills
Ans. c

Ref: CDC Guidelines

102. Food safety and standards authority of India comes under which ministry?
a. Rural statistics
b. Ministry of Health and Family Welfare
c. District level
d. Ministry of Agriculture
Ans. b

Ref: Park 23/e p548

103. The Haddon matrix is used for assessing the interventions for the prevention of:
a. Injury
b. Water pollution
c. Air pollution
d. Radiation exposure
Ans. a

Ref: Trauma contemporary principles and therapy 1/e p107

104. Increasing number of non-communicable disease when compared to previous years is a trend called as:
a. Cyclical
b. Periodical
c. Secular
d. Seasonal
Ans. c

Ref: Park 23/e p66

105. In a study two groups of newborns are checked for their weights based on whether their mothers received food supplements or not. The appropriate test which is can be used for comparing the data is:

a. Fischer's exact test
b. Student T-test
c. Paired T-test
d. Chi-square test

Ans. b

Ref: Park 23/e p852

106. A researcher wants to do a study of plasma lipids among people who jog and those who do not. But he is now concerned that the joggers might differ from the others in their diet, etc as well. This concern is known as:

a. Recall bias
b. Interviewer bias
c. Selection bias
d. Confounding bias

Ans. d

Ref: Park 23/e p72

107. Human Developmental Index is a composite measure which uses:

a. Life expectancy at age one, standard of living
b. Freedom, space and all things nice
c. Life expectancy at birth, knowledge, and income
d. Life expectancy at age one, knowledge and standard of living

Ans. c

Ref: Park 23/e p17

108. Window period is defined as the time taken from:

a. Entry of pathogen to appearance of first clinical symptoms
b. Exposure to laboratorial detection of disease
c. Entry of pathogen to cure of the disease
d. First clinical manifestation to cure of the disease

Ans. b

Ref: Park 23/e p92

109. Screening is not useful in which carcinoma?

a. Ca Prostate
b. Ca Colon
c. Ca Breast
d. Ca Testis

Ans. d

Ref: Park 23/e p855

110. A 10-year-old boy with dog bite comes to you. Appropriate action is:

a. Give CCDV
b. Withhold vaccine and observe dog for 10 days
c. Kill dog and send brain for biopsy
d. Wound dressing only

Ans. a

Ref: Park 23/e p1022

MEDICINE

111. Tropical spastic paraparesis is caused by:

a. HTLV
b. Hep B virus
c. HIV
d. HPV

Ans. a

Ref: Harrison 19/e ch 225

112. A person is HBsAg positive, but anti–HBc ab is negative. What should be the next step?
a. Repeat test after 6 months
b. Check HBeAg, if positive start treatment
c. Check HBV DNA load
d. Reassurance
Ans. b

Ref: Harrison 19/e p2031

113. In a female who had Steroid Resistant ITP it was decided to perform splenectomy. On day 3 post laparoscopic surgery patient had fever. Which of the following scenarios is likely?
a. Left lower lobe consolidation
b. Port site infection
c. Intraabdominal collection
d. Urine for pus should be sent
Ans. b

Ref: Harrison 19/e p557

114. Which of the following is not an autoimmune disorder?
a. Ulcerative colitis
b. Grave's disease
c. Rheumatoid arthritis
d. SLE
Ans. None > A

Ref: Robbins Pathology 7/e ch.6

115. Which of the following is false about TRALI?
a. Develops within 24 hours
b. Mostly seen after sepsis and cardiac surgeries
c. It is a cause of noncardiogenic pulmonary edema
d. Plasma is more likely to cause it than whole blood
Ans. a

Ref: Harrison 19/e ch 138

116. Best product to be given in multiple clotting factor deficiency and active bleeding:
a. FFP
b. Whole blood
c. Packed RBC
d. Cryoprecipitate
Ans. a

Ref: Wintrobe Hematology ch 57

117. A girl comes with Sydenhams chorea and acute rheumatic fever is suspected. Other major criteria of Rheumatic fever (arthritis, skin rashes, subcut nodules and carditis) are absent. No evidence of sore throat? Best investigation to prove rheumatic etiology is:
a. Brain biopsy
b. ASL O
c. Throat culture
d. Antihyaluronidase
Ans. b

Ref: Harrison 19/e p2149

118. Best non invasive investigation to check for viable myocardium is:
a. Echocardiogram
b. FDG-18

c. PET CT
d. MRI

Ans. b

Ref: Harrison 19/e ch 65

119. Which of the following statements is not true regarding H1N1:
a. Pregnant woman with sore throat can be treated without diagnostic test under category B
b. People on long term steroids cant receive Oseltamivir
c. Category B concerns with suspected H1N1 cases
d. Category C-H1NI may be needed

Ans. b

Ref: Harrison 19/e ch 178

120. Hypertensive hemorrhage most commonly affects:
a. Basal ganglion
b. Thalamus
c. Brain stem
d. Cerebrum

Ans. a

Ref: Harrison 19/e ch 330

121. A man comes with aphasia. He is unable to name things and repetition is poor. However comprehension, fluency and is unaffected. He is probably suffering from:
a. Anomic aphasia
b. Transcortical sensory aphasia
c. Conduction aphasia
d. Broca aphasia

Ans. c

Ref: Harrison 19/e p176

122. A young lady with C/F of hyperthyroidism with elevated T4 and TSH= 8.5. Further examination reveals bitemporal hemianopia. Next step of management:
a. Start antithyroid drugs, and do urgent MRI brain
b. Start antithyroid drugs, check TRH
c. Start antithyroid drugs, check repeat thyroid hormones
d. Start antithyroid drugs, check beta-HCG

Ans. a

Ref: Harrison 19/e p2304

123. Hyperdynamic state includes all except:
a. Anemia
b. Beri beri
c. Cor pulmonale
d. AV fistula

Ans. c

Ref: Harrison 19/e ch 117

124. Which of the following is not a part of Duke Criteria for infective endocarditis?
a. Splenomegaly
b. Fever >100.4 Celsius
c. IV drug user
d. Blood culture positive

Ans. a

Ref: Harrison 19/e p822

125. Which of the following cannot cause reduced DLCO?

a. Emphysema
b. Asthma
c. Pulmonary thromboembolism
d. Pneumonia

Ans. b

Ref: Harrison 19/e ch 239

126. Lymphatic spread most commonly seen in which type of thyroid carcinoma:

a. Papillary
b. Medullary
c. Follicular
d. Lymphoma

Ans. a

Ref: Harrison 19/e ch 324

GENERAL SURGERY

127. A young girl with a mass in lower abdomen involving umbilical and hypogastric regions. On examination it is cystic and mobile and the examiner is unable to insinuate fingers between the mass and the pelvic bone. Likely diagnosis:

a. Duplication of intestine
b. Mesenteric cyst
c. Omental cyst
d. Ovarian cyst

Ans. d

Ref: Harrison 19/e p2304

128. Mallory-Weiss syndrome mainly affects which vessel:

a. Left gastric artery
b. Right gastric artery
c. Phrenic vein
d. Coronary vein

Ans. a

Ref: Harrison 19/e p1345

129. Incision preferred for diaphragmatic surgery:

a. Circumferential
b. Radial
c. Vertical
d. Transverse

Ans. a

Ref: Adult Chest Surgery by David Sugarbaker

130. Which is not true regarding the basis of functional division of Liver?

a. Based on portal vein and hepatic vein
b. Divided into 8 segments
c. Three major and three minor fissures
d. 4 sectors

Ans. a

Ref: Harrison 19/e p2765

131. A pregnant lady was stabbed in the right side of the chest. She is yelling for help on entering the casualty. On examination she has tachycardia and BP was 90/60 mm Hg, breath sounds are decreased on the right side. What is the first consideration for her?

a. Intubate her
b. Establish IV line and start saline
c. Needle decompression in 2nd intercostal space
d. Oropharyngeal airway

Ans. b > c

Ref: Harison 19/e p1719

As mention in scenario the pt is talking so the air way (a) is patent. Breathing (b) is effect cause she has dec. Breath sound so possibiligy hemothorax with wide bore prompt action. Once decompressed, insert an intercostal chest drain under waterseal.

132. A 3-year-old child comes with hydrocoele of the hernia sac. Management will:
include

a. Herniotomy
b. Herniorrhapy
c. Hernioplasty
d. Wait for 5 years

Ans. b

Ref: Sabiston ch 71

133. In a patient with thrombocytopenia, what is the target platelet count after platelet transfusion to perform an invasive procedure?

a. 40, 000
b. 50, 000
c. 30, 000
d. 60, 000

Ans. b

Ref: Harrison 19/e p54

134. In the case of esophageal cancer prognosis is best determined by:

a. Age of patient
b. Cellular differentiation
c. Length of involvement
d. T stage

Ans. d

Ref: Schwartz surgery 5/e ch 24

135. MC and acceptable method of bariatric surgery is:

a. Biliopancreatic division
b. Biliopancreatic division with ileostomy
c. Laparoscopic gastric banding
d. Roux–en–Y procedure

Ans. d

Ref: Bariatric Surgery manual

136. A 60-year-old lady with family history of breast cancer comes with blood stained discharge from nipple. Next best step:

a. Ductoscopy
b. Nipple discharge cytology
c. Sono-mammogram
d. MRI

Ans. c

Ref: Harrison 19/e ch 55

137. Most common shunt for hydrocephalus is:
a. Ventriculoperitoneal
b. Ventriculopericardial
c. Ventriculopleural
d. Lumboperitoneal
Ans. a

Ref: AIIMS Manual

138. Oncotype dx test is done to check the usefulness of the following in breast cancer:
a. Chemotherapy in ER -ve
b. Hormone therapy in ER +ve
c. Herceptin in HER2 +ve
d. Chemotherapy in ER +ve
Ans. d

Ref: NCCN Guidelines

139. During laparoscopic inguinal hernia repair a tacker was place below and lateral to the iliopubic tract. Postoperatively the patient complained of pain. This is due to the involvement of:
a. Lateral cutaneous nerve of thigh
b. Ilioinguinal nerve
c. Genitofemoral nerve
d. Obturator nerve
Ans. a

Ref: Schwartz surgery 5/e ch 36

140. A middle aged man with RTA and bleeding from scalp. He is unconcious. A card in his pocket reveals that he is known diabetic on glimepiride+metformin, two tablets daily. What should be the next step?
a. Send blood for tests, start IV glucose and send pateint for CT scan
b. Start normal saline and send for CT
c. Send blood for test, wait for report and if hypoglycemic start glucose
d. Secure bleeeding first then send for CT scan
Ans. a

Ref: The unconscious diabetic manual by Green

141. According to the 2010 WHO criteria what are the characteristics of normal semen analysis?
a. Volume 1.5ml, count 15 million, morphology 4% progressive motility 32%
b. Volume 2.0ml, count 20 million, morphology 4% progressive motility 32%
c. Volume 1.5ml, count 20 million, morphology 4% progressive motility 32%
d. Volume 2.0ml, count 15 million, morphology 40% progressive motility 32%
Ans. a

Ref: WHO Manual 5/e p309

OBG

142. What is the level of proteinuria to diagnose the lady to have severe preeclampsia?
a. 20 mg
b. 200 mg
c. 300 mg
d. 3000 mg
Ans. c

Ref: ACOG Guidelines

143. Carbetocin dosage during labor is:
a. Single 100 microgram dose over 1 minute
b. Single 100 microgram dose over 10 minutes
c. Single 10 microgram dose over 1 minute
d. Single 10 microgram dose over 10 minutes
Ans. a

Ref: ACOI Guidelines

144. Dose of dexamethasone to prevent RDS in newborn is:
a. 12 mg 12 hourly 2 doses
b. 12 mg 24 hourly 2 doses
c. 6 mg 24 hourly 4 doses
d. 6 mg 12 hourly 4 doses
Ans. d

Ref: IAP Guidelines

145. A 32-year-old P2L2 lady comes 5 days after unprotected sexual intercourse. Best management for contraception is Levonorgestrel:
a. Levonorgestrol 0.75mg
b. Copper IUCD
c. 2 tablets of high dose OCP, repeated after 24 hours
d. Laparoscopic tubectomy
Ans. b

Ref: WHO Guidelines

146. A G6+0+0 lady with h/o recurrent missed abortions at 14-16 weeks comes to you with abortion. Which of the following tests is not warranted?
a. Lupus anticoagulant
b. Anticardiolipin antibody
c. VDRL for wife and husband
d. Fetal karyotype
Ans. c

Ref: Shaw Gynecology 2/e p310

147. In galactorrhea–amenorrhea syndromes, which is the investigation you should advise (apart from serum prolactin):
a. TSH
b. LH
c. Urinary ketosteroids
d. HCG
Ans. b

Ref: Shaw Gynecology 2/e p564

148. Drug not given in PCOD:
a. Tamoxifen
b. Clomiphene
c. Oral contraceptive
d. Metformin
Ans. a

Ref: Shaw Gynecology 2/e p431

149. A lady underwent vaginal hysterectomy for Ca cervix. Following the surgery after her urethral catheter was removed, she complained of urinary incontinence. On examination she had normal voiding as well as continuous incontinence. Methylene blue dye was instilled in her bladder through her urethra and she

was given oral phenazopyridine. After some time her pad was checked and it showed yellow staining at the top portion, but not the middle or bottom portions. She is likely to have:

a. Ureterovaginal fistula
b. Vesicovaginal fistula
c. Urethrovaginal fistula
d. Vesicouterine fistula

Ans. a

Ref: Shaw Gynecology 2/e p221

150. A 16-year-old girl was brought with primary amenorrhea. Her mother mentioned that she started developing breast at the age of 12. She was prescribed OCPs 2-years-back by a doctor with no effect. She was having normal stature and was a football player. On examination breast was well developed (Tanner's stage 5) and pubic hair was minimal (Tanner's stage 1) What is the diagnosis?

a. Premature ovarian failure
b. Turner's syndrome
c. Total androgen resistance
d. Mullerian agenesis

Ans. d

Ref: Shaw Gynecology 2/e p743

151. A young lady with 6 weeks amenorrhea had nausea and vomiting with severe abdominal pain. Her BP was100/80 mmHg. Examination revealed a 5 × 5cm adnexal mass. What is the plan of management?

a. Plan for immediate laparoscopic surgery
b. USG
c. Give IV fluids, keep NPO and observe for 4–5 days
d. Beta HCG

Ans. b > d

Ref: Shaw Gynecology 2/e p798

152. A lady with abdominal mass was investigated. She was found to have b/l ovarian masses with smooth surface. On microscopy they revealed clear cells with signet ring shapes. Diagnosis is:

a. Dysgerminoma
b. Krukenberg tumor
c. Primary adenocarcinoma of the ovaries
d. Mucinous cystadenoma

Ans. b

Ref: Shaw Gynecology 2/e p1310

153. What are the cut off values in 2 hour OGTT for FBS, PP1 hr and PP 2 hours respectively:

a. 92, 182, 153
b. 90, 180, 153
c. 95, 180, 155
d. 92, 180, 153

Ans. c

Ref: High risk pregnancies by Hemant Deshpande 2/e p61

PEDIATRICS

154. In a child surgery was done for EHBO with hepaticojejunal anastomosis. Post operative bilirubin level after 2 weeks was 6 mg/dl from a preoperative level 12mg/dl. The reason for this could be:

a. Normal lowering of bilirubin takes time
b. Delta bilirubin
c. Anastomotic stricture
d. Surgical failure

Ans. c

Ref: OP Ghai 3/e ch 34

155. **Fluid of choice in diarrhea in an infant:**
   a. ORS
   b. Salt water
   c. Sugar water
   d. Dextrose
   Ans. a

Ref: WHO Guidelines

156. **A mother comes with history of neural tube defect in first child. What is the amount of folic acid you will prescribe during preconceptional counseling (In micrograms/day)?**
   a. 4
   b. 40
   c. 400
   d. 4000
   Ans. c

Ref: OP Ghai 3/e ch 31

157. **Regarding Japanese encephalitis vaccine, what is not true?**
   a. Not given for infants less than 6 months
   b. 2 primary doses given to children in the 1–3 years age group
   c. Immunity starts two weeks after vaccination
   d. Booster doses are given after 1 year and repeated every 3 years
   Ans. a

Ref: OP Ghai 3/e ch 28

158. **A 1-month-old child with conjugated bilirubinemia and intrahepatic cholestasis. On liver biopsy and staining with PAS red colored granules were seen inside the hepatocytes. Probable diagnosis is:**
   a. Alpha1 antitrypsin deficiency
   b. Congenital hepatic fibrosis
   c. Crigler-Najjar syndrome
   d. Dubin-Johnson syndrome
   Ans. a

Ref: Robbins 9/e p815

DERMATOLOGY

159. **26-year-old man from Bihar comes with juicy looking papules over face and back of neck which were hypopigmented and normoaesthetic with no nerve thickening. History of prolonged fever in childhood was present. Diagnosis:**
   a. Tuberculoid leprosy
   b. Post-kala-azar dermal leishmaniasis
   c. Lepromatous leprosy
   d. Lupus vulgaris

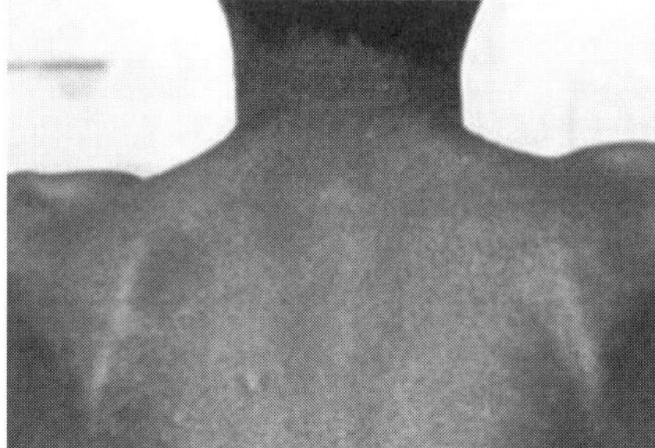

   Ans. b

Ref: Neena Khanna 1/e p347

160. A lady came with unilateral white skin lesions with leukotrichia. Shows 2 white spots 1 × 1 cm each over left side of chin and neck. Diagnosis:

a. Segmental vitiligo
b. Piebaldism
c. Nevus achromicus
d. Albinism

Ans. a

Ref: Neena Khanna 1/e p159

161. A lady came with complaints of a bluish lesion over left side of forehead and left eye. Shows irregular bluish lesion in left superior conjunctiva and forehead. Diagnosis is:

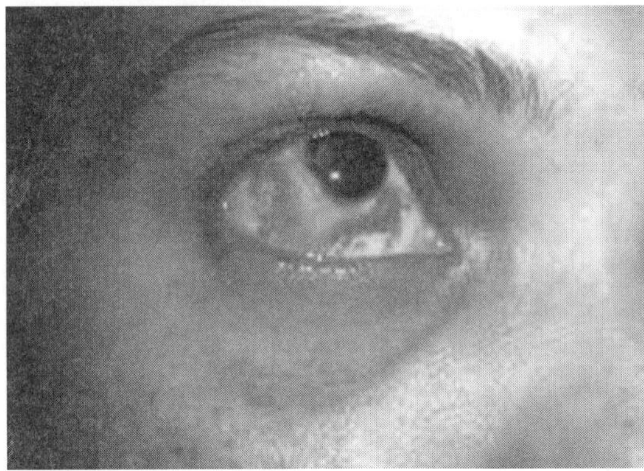

a. Nevus of Ota
b. Nevus of Ito
c. Becker's nevus
d. Mongolian spot

Ans. a

162. The patient came with h/o bullae involving >30 % body surface area and erosions of the lips for the past 7 days. It shows forearm with extensive reddish bullae. What is probable regarding the etiology?

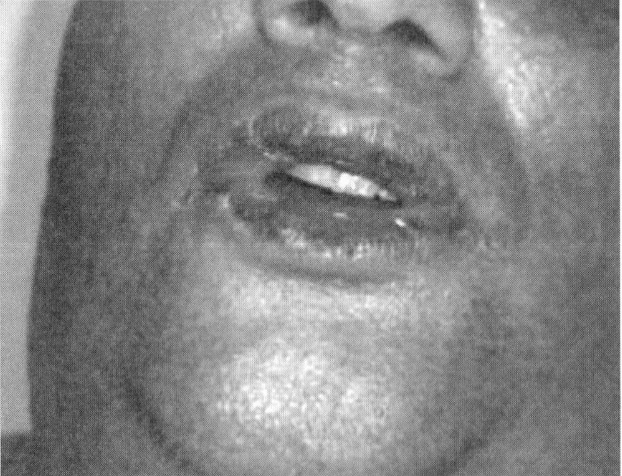

a. Drugs
b. Bacterial infection
c. Viral infection
d. Fungal infection

Ans. a

Ref: Neena Khanna 1/e p84

163. A patient came with h/o itchy tense blisters whose roof settled as above shows big blisters on forearm which have subsided with the roof sticking to the floor without much damage. Diagnosis:

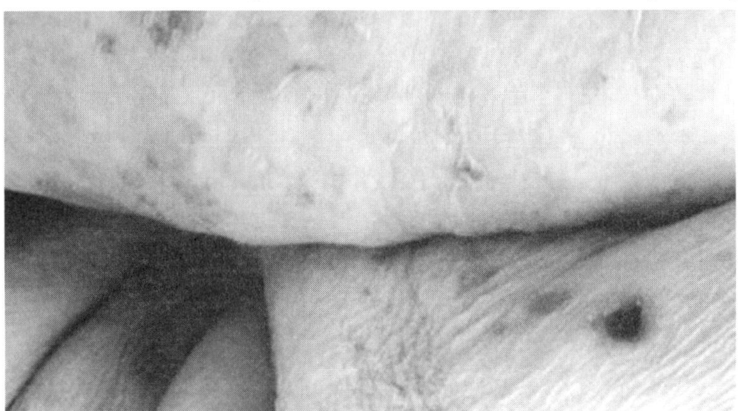

a. Bullous pemphigoid
b. Pemphigus vulgaris
c. IgA disease
d. Psoriasis

Ans. a

Ref: Neena Khanna 1/e p654

Bullous pemphigoid (BP) is the most common autoimmune disease that results in subepidermal blistering. This condition typically presents with generalized itchy eruptions with blisters and can be associated with significant morbidity. In the early stages, the blisters can have quite a polymorphic clinical appearance in the absence of vesicles and bullae.

Considered a disease of the elderly, BP usually does not develop until after age 60 years.1, 2 Each year, approximately 6 to 13 new diagnoses of BP are made per 1 million people.1 Interestingly, patients older than age 90 years are at an approximately 300-fold greater risk for developing BP than are patients younger than age 60 years.1 There also appears to be a higher predominance of the disease in men than in women.

164. A child came with similar lesions over elbows, shaft of penis and shows pinhead papules over right elbow. Diagnosis:

a. Lichen nitidus
b. Lichen planus
c. Scabies
d. Molluscum contagiosum

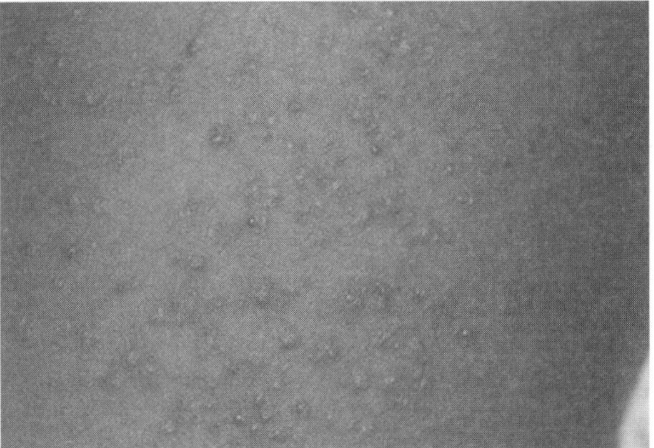

Ans. a

Ref: Neena Khanna 1/e p654

165. A man with Leprosy came with the following lesion. Picture shows a single target lesion of about 7 cm diameter over forearm. Diagnosis:

a. LL
b. BL
c. BT
d. BB

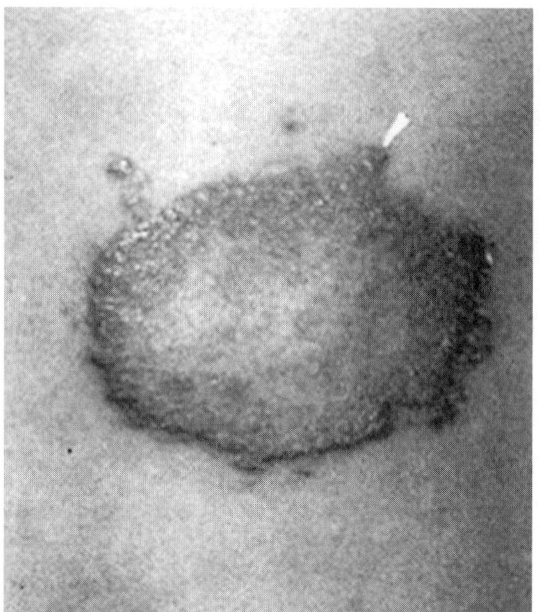

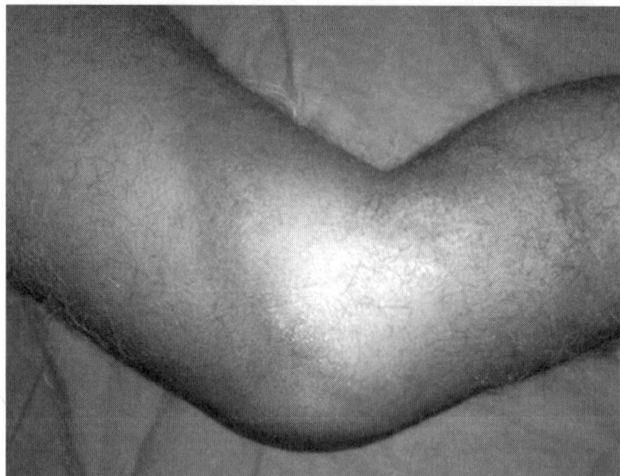

Ans. c > d

Ref: Neena Khanna 1/e p259

Target lesions can be observed in the BB form of leprosy.

Ref: Leprosy: A Practical Guide

Enrico Nunzi, Cesare Massone

166. A 7-month-pregnant lady comes with the following lesions all over the body. Shows multiple small pustules over skin. Which of these drugs is the appropriate treatment?

a. Cyclosporine
b. Azathioprine
c. Methotrexate
d. Retinoids

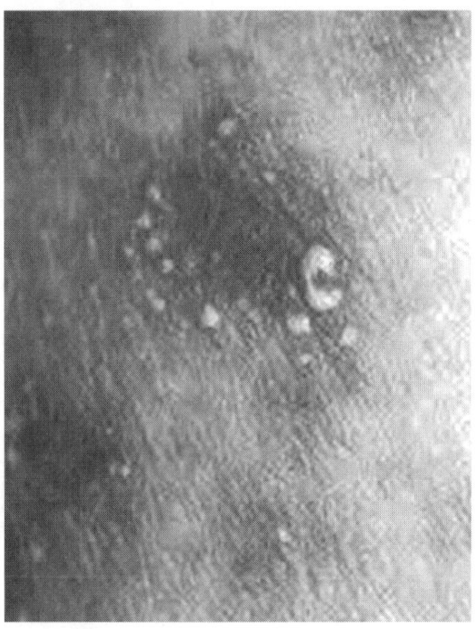

Ans. a

Ref: Neena Khanna 1/e p50

ANESTHESIA

167. Which anesthetic agent can cause pain on IV administration?

a. Thiopentone
b. Propofol
c. Ketamine
d. Midazolam

Ans. b

Ref: Ajay Yadav 5/e p57

168. Which of the following combinations can be used for day care surgery?

a. Remifentanil, Midazolam, Propofol
b. Fentanyl, Midazolam, Thiopental sodium
c. Morphine, Midazolam, Propofol
d. Remifentanil, Ketamine, Propofol

Ans. a

Ref: AIIMS Anaesthesia Division Protocol

169. Muscle relaxant that can be used in a patient with high S. Bilirubin value and S.Creatinine of 4.5mg/dL:

a. Vecuronium
b. Atracurium
c. Pancuronium
d. Rocuronium

Ans. b

Ref: AIIMS Anaesthesia Division Protocol

170. In a patient with coronary artery disease with pulse rate of 48/min and low BP. Which of these anesthetic agent is contraindicated?

a. Ketamine
b. Dexmedetomidine
c. Etomidate
d. Pentacozine

Ans. b

Ref: KDT 5/e p375

RADIOLOGY

171. Judet view of X-ray is for
   a. Pelvis
   b. Calcaneus
   c. Scaphoid
   d. Shoulder
   Ans. a

Ref: Turek's Orthopedics 2/e p542

172. Shenton line is seen in X-ray of:
   a. Knee
   b. Shoulder
   c. Elbow
   d. Hip
   Ans. d

Ref: Turek's Orthopedics 2/e p542

173. IOC for acute appendicitis in children:
   a. USG
   b. MRI
   c. CECT
   d. X ray
   Ans. a

Ref: Schwartz surgery 5/e p2981

174. Investigation of choice in stress fracture:
   a. MRI
   b. CT
   c. Bone scan
   d. X-ray
   Ans. a

Ref: Evidence Based sports medicine 1/e p539

Nuclear Medicine and Radiologic Imaging in Sports Injuries edited by Andor WJM. Glaudemans, Rudi AJO Dierckx, Jan L. Gielen, Johannes Zwerve More recently MRI has replaced scintigraphy as the investigation of choice for stress fracture

175. Investigation of choice for biliary atresia in a 2-month-old is:
   a. Hepatic scintigraphy
   b. ERCP
   c. USG
   d. Intraoperative cholangiography
   Ans. a > d

Ref: Liver disease in Newborn by Friedrick
http://www.jneonatalsurg.com/.../index..../jns/article/view/7/43

176. Patient with h/o tachyarrhythmias is on implantable cardioverter defibrillator. He develops shock. Best method to know the integrity of ICD is to do:
   a. Contrast CT
   b. MRI
   c. USG
   d. Plain radiograph
   Ans. d

Ref: Cardiac Pacing by David

177. Expansion of the space is seen in:
a. Intramedullary tumor
b. Intradural tumor
c. Intraparenchymal tumor
d. Extradural tumor
Ans. b

Ref: Tumors of brain by Franco

178. Earliest diagnosis of pregnancy can be established by:
a. USG of fetal cardiac activity
b. Fetal cardiac Doppler study
c. HCG levels
d. Urine pregnancy test
Ans. c

Ref: Dutta Obstretics 2/e p307

PSYCHIATRY

179. A smoker is worried about the side effects of smoking. But he does not stop smoking thinking that he smokes less and takes a good diet. This thinking is called as:
a. Self exemption
b. Contemplation
c. Self-protection
d. Distortion
Ans. b

Ref: Prochaska model 3/e p119

180. A woman comes to the psychiatrist with history of spending a lot of time in washing her hands. She is distressed about it but says that she cannot stop the practice and spends a lot of time on it. This has started affecting her social life as well. What is the best mode of treatment in her?
a. Cognitive behavioral therapy
b. Exposure and response prevention
c. Systematic desensitization
d. Flooding
Ans. b

Ref: DSM 3/e p237

181. Which of these is not a part of catatonia?
a. Akathisia
b. Ambivalence
c. Ambitendency
d. Akinesia
Ans. b

Ref: DSM 3/e p253

182. Key symptom for alcohol withdrawal syndrome is:
a. Visual hallucinations
b. Sleep disturbance
c. Tremors
d. Diarrhea
Ans. c

Ref: Kaplan and Saddock 3/e p96
Emergencies in Adult Nursing by Philip Downing 1/e p80

183. A person with histrionic, shy, avoidant personality comes under which cluster:
  a. A
  b. B
  c. C
  d. D
  Ans. b

Ref: Oxford textbook of Psychiatry 6/e p140

184. Uncertainty and excessive sense of responsibility seen in:
  a. Generalized anxiety disorder
  b. OCD
  c. Depression
  d. Personality disorder
  Ans. b

Ref: DSM 3/e p437

185. A person was diagnosed to have schizophrenia and for that was receiving antipsychotic medications. Following this he developed rigidity and inability to move his eyes. But he was able to respond to which of the following drugs should be given IV for this condition?
  a. Promethazine
  b. Haloperidol
  c. Risperidone
  d. Diazepam
  Ans. a

Ref: DSM 3/e p455

186. A man comes with history of abnormal excessive blinking and grunting. He says he has no control over his symptoms which have risen in frequency of late. This has started affecting his social life making him depressed.Which of the following medications should be used in him?
  a. Carbamazepine
  b. SSRIs
  c. Risperidone
  d. Oral medications for treatment of blepharospasm and other cranial dystonias
  Ans. b

Ref: DSM 3/e p65

ORTHOPEDICS

187. Jersey finger is caused by rupture of:
  a. Flexor digitorum profundus
  b. Extensor digiti minimi
  c. Flexor digitorum superficialis
  d. Extensor indicis
  Ans. a

Ref: Oxford textbook of orthopaedics 1/e p624

188. Most metabolically active part in the bone is:
  a. Periosteum
  b. Endosteum
  c. Cancellous
  d. Cortical
  Ans. b

Ref: Gray's Anatomy 40/e p91

189. Removal of vertebral disc is by all these methods except:
a. Laminotomy
b. Laminectomy
c. Laminoplasty
d. Hemilaminectomy
Ans. c

Ref: Lumbar disc herniation by Postachini 3/e p419

190. In Osteoporosis which of these is seen:
a. Normal calcium, decreased ALP
b. Decreased calcium, increased ALP
c. Normal calcium, normal ALP
d. Decreased calcium, decreased ALP
Ans. c

Ref: Harrison 18/e ch 354

191. Traction not used in lower limb:
a. Gallows
b. Bryant
c. Dunlop
d. Perkin
Ans. c

Ref: Smart study orthopaedics 4/e p128

192. A 42-year-old man is diagnosed to have irreparable tear of the rotator cuff. Treatment of choice will be:
a. Tendon transfer
b. Total shoulder replacement
c. Reverse shoulder replacement
d. Acromioplasty
Ans. a

Ref: AOO Manual

MISCELLANEOUS

193. Methacholine has main agonist action at:
a. M2
b. M3
c. M4
d. M1
Ans. a

Ref: Goodman and Gilman 11/e p127

194. ABO Blood group is an example of:
a. Codominance
b. X linked recessive trait
c. Autosomal dominant
d. Autosomal recessive
Ans. a

Ref: Ganong 23/e p527

195. A 20-year-old lady presented with photosensitive rash, erythema and telengectasia in the midfacial region increased with exposure of light. The most probable diagnosis is:
a. SLE
b. Acne Vulgaris
c. Atopic dermatitis
d. Acne rosacea
Ans. d

Ref: Rooks Dermatology 8/e p432

196. All are true regarding SIRS except:
   a. Respiratory rate more than 24/minute
   b. Heart rate -90/min
   c. Urine flow of 0.5 ml/kg/hr
   d. Oral temperature more than 38°C
   Ans. c

Ref: Harrison 18/e ch 271

197. A lady who is 9 weeks pregnant comes with a 2.5 cm mass in the upper and outer quadrant of left breast USG failed to show any abnormality. The ideal management would be:
   a. Reassurance
   b. Work up after pregnancy completed
   c. Aspirate the cyst and reassure
   d. Finger guided core biopsy
   Ans. d

Ref: Management of Breast diseases by Ismail Jatoi

198. ABO Blood group is an example of:
   a. Co dominance
   b. Autosomal dominant
   c. Autosomal recessive
   d. X linked recessive
   Ans. a

Ref: Ganong 23/e p527

199. Patient with history of tachyarrhythmias is on implantable cardioverter defibrillator. He develops shock. Best method to know the integrity of ICD is:
   a. Contrast CT
   b. USG
   c. MRI
   d. Plain radiograph
   Ans. d

Ref: Cardiac pacing by David

AIPG 2015

1. **Total cholesterol is 300. LDL is 25 mg/dl, TG is 150mg/dl What would be HDL?**
   a. 125 mg/dl
   b. 85 mg/dl
   c. 95 mg/dl
   d. 245 mg/dl
   Ans. d

   Ref: International Journal of Life Science and Medical Research April 2014 Vol 4 Issue 2 p 25-31

2. **Maternal antibodies are transferred to child in all except:**
   a. Chicken pox
   b. Measles
   c. Pertussis
   d. Rubella
   Ans. c

   Ref: Park 22/e p114

3. **Quality of X-ray is increased by:**
   a. Increased mA
   b. Decreased mA
   c. Increased kVp
   d. Increased mas
   Ans. c

   Ref: White and Pharaoh 5/e p11

4. **Which is avoided in parotid fistula?**
   a. Atropine
   b. Aspiration and dressing
   c. Pilocarpine
   d. Propantheline
   Ans. d

   Ref: Peterson OMFS 2/e p522

5. **Anterior choroidal artery is a branch of:**
   a. Middle meningeal artery
   b. External carotid
   c. Internal carotid
   d. Anterior communicating
   Ans. c

   Ref: BD Chaurasia 4/e p103

6. **The tendon of Sartorius gracilis and semitendinosus muscles forms a pes anserinus at the neck of tibia Similar kind of structure is also seen in:**
   a. Submandibular gland
   b. Parotid gland
   c. Cheek
   d. TMJ
   Ans. b

   Ref: Advanced therapy in Facial Plastic and Reconstructive surgery by Regan Thomas

7. **Which nerve is compressed by aneurysm of posterior communicating artery of circle of Willis?**
   a. Trochlear
   b. Optic
   c. Oculomotor
   d. Hypophysis cerebri
   Ans. c

Ref: Snell 7/e p906

8. **Premaxillary part of maxilla develop from:**
   a. Frontonasal process
   b. Lateral nasal processes
   c. Medial nasal processes
   d. Maxillary and mandibular process
   Ans. a

Ref: Human Embryology IB Singh 8/e p136

9. **Schwannoma of 8th cranial nerve site is:**
   a. Intracanalicular
   b. Cisternal
   c. Parotid
   d. Intrapetrous
   Ans. b

Ref: Snell 8/e p776

10. **Which cranial nucleus underlies the facial colliculus?**
    a. Sixth
    b. Seventh
    c. Ninth
    d. Twelfth
    Ans. a

Ref: Grays Anatomy 40/e p242

11. **General visceral efferent component is found in all except:**
    a. Facial
    b. Glossopharyngeal
    c. Olfactory
    d. Oculomotor
    Ans. c

Ref: BD Chaurasia 4/e p335

12. **All are true about superior laryngeal nerve except:**
    a. It passes from thyrohyoid membrane
    b. It supply larynx below the vocal cord
    c. It anaesthetize the internal laryngeal nerve
    d. It passes between thyroid cartilage and hyoid bone
    Ans. b

Ref: BD Chaurasia 4/e p223

13. **Which of the following structures pass through the area marked in the diagram?**
    a. Maxillary nerve
    b. Lesser petrosal nerve
    c. Sensory branch of mandibular nerve
    d. Motor root of trigeminal nerve
    Ans. a

Ref: BD Chaurasia 4/e p321

14. Epidural hematoma is due to involvement of:
   a. Superficial temporal
   b. Middle meningeal
   c. Cavernous sinus
   d. Maxillary artery
   Ans. b

Ref: BD Chaurasia 4/e p101

15. All forms boundary of facial recess except:
   a. Incus
   b. Tendon of stapedius
   c. Chorda tympani
   d. Facial nerve
   Ans. b

Ref: Cummins 5th ed ch 142 page 332

16. House Brackmann scale is for which nerve:
   a. Optic
   b. Trigeminal
   c. Hypoglossal
   d. Facial
   Ans. d

Ref: Peter Ward Booth Maxillofacial Trauma 2/e p295

17. False about hypoglossal nerve paralysis is:
   a. Loss of tactile sensation over the tongue
   b. Atrophy of the tongue on involved side
   c. Deviation of tongue to affected side on protrusion
   d. Deviation of uvula to same side
   Ans. a

Ref: Human Anatomy Gray e book page 540

18. Which is not a part of Waldeyer's lymphatic ring?
   a. Pharyngeal tonsil
   b. Tubal tonsil
   c. Palatine tonsil
   d. Submandibular nodes
   Ans. d

Ref: B D Chaurasia 4/e p321

19. In mechanical trituration of amalgam what is adversely affected:
   a. Tarnish resistance
   b. Hardness of the filling
   c. Final gloss of the filling
   d. Working time
   Ans. d

Ref: Skinners 10/e p523

20. Temperature used in glass bead sterilizer is:
   a. 100–150 degree F
   b. 425–475 degree F
   c. 345–375 degree F
   d. 225–275 degree F
   Ans. b

Ref: Ingle 5/e p86

21. Main drawback of esthetic fiber reinforced post over metallic post is:
a. Better esthetics
b. Bonding to dentin
c. Technique sensitive and expensive
d. Modulus of elasticity near to dentin
Ans. c

Ref: Cohen 10/e p783-784

22. Necrosis and degeneration in short time is seen with:
a. Avulsion
b. Intrusion
c. Extrusion
d. Lateral luxation
Ans. a

Ref: Cohens 10/e p621

23. False about sodium hypochlorite:
a. Antimicrobial effect
b. Tissue dissolving property
c. Chelation
d. Can stain dentin
Ans. c

Ref: Cohen 10/e p312

24. False positive electric pulp test is due to all except:
a. Anxiety
b. Intake of analgesics the previous night
c. Liquefactive necrosis of pulp
d. Tooth wet by saliva and surrounding tissues
Ans. b

Ref: Cohens 10/e p17

25. The local anesthetic to be given in apicectomy surgery of maxillary incisors is:
a. Bilateral infraorbital
b. Bilateral PSA
c. Bilateral maxillary and greater palatine
d. Bilateral ASA and nasopalatine
Ans. d

Ref: Grays Anatomy 40/e p890

26. Floor of the mouth is measured by:
a. Perio probe
b. Custom tray
c. Both A and B
d. Straight probe
Ans. c

Ref: McCracken 11/e p40

27. In making complete denture for maxillary:
a. Relief is not required
b. Relief is provided when there is compression of nasopalatine vessels
c. Relief given when foramen approaches the crest of the bone
d. Relief is given for incisive foramen in all cases
Ans. d

Ref: Nallaswamy 1/e p54

28. Pre carve burnishing is used for all except:
a. Initiates carving
b. Removes excess mercury
c. Margin of amalgam well condensed
d. Increase setting time
Ans. a

Ref: Sturdevant 4/e p682

29. Sharp stabbing pain from anterior teeth conducted to brain by:
a. A delta fibers
b. C fibers
c. Beta fibers
d. Gamma fibers
Ans. a

Ref: Cohen 10/e p50

30. According to scientists recent studies says about pattern of enamel prism demineralization true is:
a. Head is more resistant to dissolution
b. Tail is more resistant to dissolution
c. Head and tail both are more resistant to dissolution
d. Head and tail both are not resistant to dissolution
Ans. b

Ref: Sturdevant 4/e p18

31. Concavity at cervical one third with vertical fracture line or a tooth with wedge shaped defect at cervical third with vertical crack lines radiating represents:
a. Abrasion
b. Abfraction
c. Erosion
d. Attrition
Ans. b

Ref: Neville 2/e p58

32. Streptococci adhere to the oral surfaces/tooth and contribute to development as they:
a. Produce extracellular polysaccharides
b. Ferment carbohydrates
c. Penicillinase resistant
d. Produce acid during metabolism
Ans. a

Ref: Nikiforuk 1/e p176

33. Necrotic maxillary central incisor with open apex > 1 mm in IOPA, treatment will be:
a. Routine GP obturation
b. Glutaraldehyde pulpotomy
c. Formocresol pulpotomy
d. One step MTA Apexification
Ans. d

Ref: International Endodontic Journal Mar 2007 Vol 40 Issue 3 page 186

34. Dentin Bonding Agent has both hydrophilic and hydrophobic end binds with:
a. Hydroxyapatite of enamel
b. Collagen of dentin
c. Calcium of tooth
d. Composite
Ans. c

Ref: Skinner 10/e p387

35. Radiating pain from pulp transmitted by:
- a. C fiber
- b. A delta
- c. A gamma
- d. Beta

Ans. a

Ref: Cohen 10/e p52

36. All of the following helps in reducing the discoloration of amalgam restored tooth except:
- a. Greater condensation
- b. Void in restoration
- c. Use of varnish over the restoration
- d. Restoration involving root

Ans. b

Ref: Craig 13/e p24

37. Tooth with most predictable single root canal is:
- a. Mandibular centrals
- b. Maxillary canine
- c. Maxillary centrals
- d. Mandibular premolars

Ans. c

Ref: Nisha Garg Endodontics 1/e p136

38. Present caries risk status of an adult is measured by:
- a. Thickness of the plaque on same day
- b. Total number of restored tooth
- c. Pit and fissure sealed teeth
- d. Total number of teeth in the mouth

Ans. b

Ref: Dental Clinics of North America 54(2010) p 497

39. Radiotherapy associated caries is due to infection of which part most probably:
- a. Lower jaw
- b. Parotid gland
- c. Maxillary sinus
- d. Tongue

Ans. b

Ref: White and Pharaoh 6/e p25

40. In long surgical procedure the intubation method is:
- a. Nasotracheal cuffed tube
- b. LMA
- c. Endotracheal tube
- d. Nasotracheal uncuffed tube

Ans. a

Ref: Fonseca Trauma 3/e Vol 1 p 152

41. Which amount of fluoride can lead to skeletal fluorosis in child on long term use?
- a. 0.5–1 ppm
- b. 2–2.5 ppm
- c. 3–6 ppm
- d. 4–7 ppm

Ans. c

Ref: Soben Peter 4/e p281

42. Major difference between self etch primer and total etch adhesive:
a. Bond strength
b. Amount of smear layer removal
c. Time
d. No need of a wet bonding agent
Ans. b

Ref: Sturdevant 5/e p254

43. In statistics sample represents:
a. Subset of sample
b. Group of samples
c. Represent each member of populations
d. Is a representative of population
Ans. c

Ref: Soben Peter 3/e p23

44. When the sample size is small and observations are dependent of each other which test is used for significance of difference between two mean?
a. Paired t test
b. Unpaired t test
c. Z test
d. Fischer test
Ans. a

Ref: Kothari Statistics 2/e p196

45. Eradication means:
a. Treatment of all patients with disease
b. Interruption/termination of transmission of disease
c. Reduction of prevalence of disease in a predetermined area
d. Cessation of disease progress in a geographical region
Ans. b

Ref: Park 19/e p36

46. Relationship between socioeconomic status of population and incidence of caries in the year 2014 is studied under:
a. Descriptive epidemiology
b. Analytical epidemiology
c. Case control study
d. Cohort study
Ans. a

Ref: Soben Peter 4/e p56

47. Crude mortality rate is:
a. Per 10
b. Per 100
c. Per 1000
d. Per 1,00,000
Ans. c

Ref: Park 17/e p159

48. Randomized control trials are conducted in:
a. Phase I
b. Phase II
c. Phase III
d. Phase IV
Ans. c

Ref: K.d. Tripathi Pharmacology 6/e p79

49. True about Wilson curve is:
a. Determine posterior plane of occlusion
b. Posterior teeth parallel to inward pull of masseter
c. Anteroposterior curve
d. Helps in achieving compensating curve during arrangement of masseter
Ans. d

Ref: Nallaswamy 1/e p194

50. Retromolar pad does not have insertion of:
a. Temporalis
b. Medial pterygoid
c. Fibers of buccinator
d. Pterygomandibular raphe
Ans. b

Ref: Nallaswamy 1/e p57

51. Major drawback of nonrigid connector is:
a. Excessive load on ridge away from abutment
b. Force is evenly divided over the ridge
c. Excessive force on ridge near the abutment
d. There is no predictable pattern of distribution of load
Ans. a

Ref: Osborne and Lammie RPD 4/ e p 266

52. Hybrid prosthesis is:
a. Removable appliance
b. It takes support completely from the implant
c. Fixed appliance with removable component, takes support from soft tissues, hard tissues and residual ridge or anatomical structures
d. Fixed appliance with removable component, takes support from soft tissues, hard tissues or implants and residual ridge or anatomical structures
Ans. d

Ref: Misch 3/e p123

53. Magnets in orthodontics obeys:
a. Electrostatic law
b. Coulomb's law
c. Gravitational law
d. Inverse square law
Ans. d

Ref: Profitt 4/e p372

54. Maximum increase in height of children is at:
a. 1st year
b. 2nd year
c. 3rd year
d. 4th year
Ans. a

Ref: Bishara Orthodontics 1/e p39

55. Facebow mostly used to fabricate:
a. Multiple tooth restoration
b. Three unit FPD
c. Single tooth restoration
d. Short span tooth supported RPD
Ans. a

Ref: Shillingburg 3/e p25

56. Property of internal occlusal rest are all except:

a. Retention
b. Vertical stop
c. Support
d. Horizontal stabilization

Ans. a

Ref: Mc Cracken RPD 11/e p71

57. On examination of a patient who has worn new dentures for 2 months irritation is noted on the lingual side of mandibular residual ridge from canine premolar region or midline to canine unilaterally, retention of the mandibular denture is adequate.What treatment procedure should be instituted to correct the problem?

a. Relining the mandibular denture
b. Shortening the lingual flange
c. Remarking the mandibular denture
d. Remounting and equilibrating the denture

Ans. d

Ref: Winkler 2/e p324

58. Spoon shape of occlusal rest:

a. Easy to fabricate
b. It extends upto central fossa
c. Provide bulk and distribute forces in better way
d. Directs forces along long axis of the teeth

Ans. d

Ref: Mc Cracken 11/e p67

59. Crib causes all except:

a. Acts as a reminder
b. Prevent tongue thrusting
c. Distribute forces on posterior teeth
d. Provides suction and exert force on anterior palate

Ans. d

Ref: Orthodontics by Phulari 1/e p431

60. Which of the following is a self correcting anomaly in a 10 year old child?

a. Posterior cross bite
b. Anterior open bite
c. Anterior cross bite
d. Flaring of maxillary incisors

Ans. d

Ref: Profitt 4/e p101

61. A mother of 12-year-old girl complaints of large anteriors and proclination. Cephalometry is carried out which shows SNA 105 degrees IMPA 90 degrees and mandibular angle 97 degree. What would be your advice to the mother?

a. Self correcting
b. Surgery required
c. Simple appliance for 2–4 weeks
d. Jaw repositioning and long term treatment needed

Ans. b

Ref: Athanasious Cephalometry 1/e p229

62. Permissive occlusal splint, occlusion scheme used is:

a. Uniform occlusal contact in centric relation and canine guided in lateral excursion
b. Uniform occlusal contact in centric relation and group function in lateral excursion
c. Uniform occlusal contact in centric relation as well as during lateral excursion
d. Uniform occlusal contact of posterior in centric relation and canine guided in lateral excursions

Ans. d

Ref: Dawson 2/e p380

63. **Orthodontic mixed dentition space analysis for tooth size prediction with this table:**
    a. Hixon and oldfather analysis
    b. Moyers analysis
    c. Nance analysis
    d. Bolton ratio
    Ans. b

Ref: Profitt 4/e p197

64. **The angle that does not get changed by orthodontic treatment is:**
    a. SNA
    b. SNB
    c. ANB
    d. Saddle angle
    Ans. d

Ref: Gurkeerat 2/e p510

65. **Translatory tooth movement is best done by:**
    a. Interrupted force
    b. Moment of force
    c. Intermittent force
    d. Continuous force
    Ans. b

Ref: Profitt 4/e p339

66. **True about Lateral cephalometry in child is:**
    a. Keep the distance to be 60 inch
    b. Keep the distance to be 70 inches
    c. Assume head circumference to be 9 inches and keep the distance of 60 inches away from the X ray tube
    d. Assume head circumference to be 6 inches and keep the distance of 60 inches away from the X ray tube
    Ans. d

Ref: OP Kharbanda 2/e p210

67. **Relative to heterogenous population the incidence of malocclusion in a homogenous population generally is:**
    a. Lower
    b. Slightly lower
    c. Slightly more
    d. Almost the same
    Ans. a

Ref: Profitt 4/e p123

68. **Australian wire is a round austenitic wire most commonly used with Begg differential light force technique, is manufactured by:**
    a. Cold treated and heat drawn
    b. Heat treated and cold drawn
    c. Annealed and cold drawn
    d. Spring drawn and cold treated
    Ans. b

Ref: Begg and Kesling 3/e p94

69. **COGS Analysis was given by:**
    a. Burstone and Nanda
    b. Burstone and Levine
    c. Burstone and Legans
    d. Burstone and Merril
    Ans. c

Ref: Orthodontics by Phulari 1/e p287

70. Physioprint is the term used to describe:

a. Facial mask of patient taken before and after treatment
b. Physiological assessment of growth changes
c. A test to assess mental growth and correlated dental growth
d. Photographic orientation technique that permits measurement of facial contours and volume

Ans. d

Ref: O.P.Kharbanda 1/e p226

71. Ulnar sesamoid calcification starts at:

a. Birth
b. Prepubertal growth spurt
c. At the start of puberty
d. End of puberty

Ans. c

Ref: Bhalajhi 3/e p167

72. Cutting edges of the orthodontic instruments are made up of:

a. Austenite carbon steel
b. Ferritic carbon steel
c. Martensitic carbon steel
d. Cementite carbon steel

Ans. c

Ref: Philips 11/e p637

73. Pitch of Hyrax screw is:

a. 0.8 mm
b. 0.25 mm
c. 1 mm
d. 0.5 mm

Ans. a

Ref: O.P.Kharbanda 2/e p439

74. In intrusion the centre of rotation is:

a. Infinity
b. Outside tooth
c. CEJ
d. Apical one third

Ans. b

Ref: Profitt 3/e p228

75. The 37 % orthophosphoric acid typically dissolves about .... Micrometres of enamel surface and creates a zone of etched enamel rods for about 15–25 micrometres

a. 1–5 mm
b. 5–10 mm
c. 10–15 mm
d. 15–20 mm

Ans. b

Ref: Brantley 1/e p107

76. Mandibular condyles grows by which of the following mechanism:

a. Appositional growth
b. Subperiosteal surface edition
c. Endochondral bone formation
d. Endosteal bone growth

Ans. b

Ref: Profitt 2/e p37

77. Normal facial index is:
a. 75 %
b. >80 %
c. 75-80%
d. 15 %
Ans. b

Ref: Orthodontic Diagnosis by Rakosi 1/e p109

78. Which of the following cement has most anticariogenic effect while used for placing bands on molars to prevent caries:
a. Polycarboxylate
b. GIC
c. Silicate
d. Zinc phosphate
Ans. b

Ref: AJO-DO 1988 (6) p 273-289

79. According to the norms of the orthodontic study models the total height of the maxillary and mandibular casts should be close to:
a. 55 mm
b. 60 mm
c. 70 mm
d. 90 mm
Ans. c

Ref: :Gurkeerat Singh 2/e p80

80. Hardening heat treatment is commonly used for:
a. Nickel titanium wires
b. Titanium wires
c. Elgiloy wires
d. Stainless steel wires
Ans. c

Ref: Profitt 4/e p361

81. While giving an inferior alveolar nerve block, LA solution is deposited to:
a. Pterygopalatine fossa
b. Masticator space
c. Submandibular space
d. Pterygomandibular space
Ans. d

Ref: Malamed 4/e p195

82. If impacted third molar is to be extracted in patients planned for BSSO then extraction should be done:
a. At the time of surgery
b. Six months before surgery
c. One month before surgery
d. One month after surgery
Ans. b

Ref: Fonseca Trauma vol 2 p 305

83. Injection of 2% LA with adrenaline given to patient on beta blockers will lead to:
a. Hypertension and tachycardia
b. Hypotension and tachycardia
c. Hypotension and bradycardia
d. Hypertension and bradycardia
Ans. d

Ref: Carranza 11/e p546

84. The main barrier for diffusion of LA into the nerve is:
   a. Neural membrane
   b. Perineurium
   c. Endoneurium
   d. Epineurium
   Ans. b

Ref: Malamed 4/e p18

85. PSA block is used to anesthetize completely:
   a. All maxillary molars
   b. Maxillary second and third molars
   c. All mandibular molars
   d. Only first maxillary molars
   Ans. b

Ref: Malamed 4/e p164

86. The most potent topical anesthesia is:
   a. Tetracaine
   b. Benzocaine
   c. Prilocaine
   d. Mepivacaine
   Ans. a

Ref: Malamed 5/e p75

87. Maxillary tori are removed by:
   a. Bone bur and osteotome
   b. Chisel and mallet
   c. Bone rongeur
   d. Bone file
   Ans. a

Ref: Peterson principle of OMFS 2/e p170

88. Choice of intubation in bilateral TMJ ankylosis for oral surgeries is:
   a. North pole RAE tube
   b. South pole RAE tube
   c. Cricothyrotomy
   d. Tracheostomy
   Ans. a

Ref: Ajay Yadav 5/e p46

89. During maxillofacial trauma in the presence of oral bleeding the choice of intubation is:
   a. Cricothyroidotomy
   b. Tracheostomy
   c. Fiberoptic intubation
   d. Awake intubation
   Ans. a

Ref: Fonseca Trauma 4/e p56

90. Which drug is avoided in patients with TMJ ankylosis with history of OSA?
   a. NSAIDs
   b. Opioids
   c. Aminoglycosides
   d. Antihistamine
   Ans. b

Ref: Fonseca Trauma 2/e p289

91. **Jannetta procedure is:**
   a. Microvascular decompression
   b. Radiofrequency gangliolysis
   c. Radiofrequency neurolysis
   d. Percutaneous ganglion glycerolysis
   Ans. a

Ref: Fonseca 3/e vol 1 p 151

92. **During gap arthroplasty trigeminal nerve stimulation during surgery cause:**
   a. Bradycardia
   b. Tachycardia
   c. Torsades de pointes
   d. Paroxysmal atrial tachycardia
   Ans. b

Ref: Clinical Neurocardiology by Caplan 1/e p1197

93. **True about tracheostomy is:**
   a. Increase dead space
   b. Decrease dead space
   c. Increase tracheal secretion
   d. All of the above
   Ans. b

Ref: Bailey and Love 25/e p721

94. **Throat pack is used in:**
   a. After LMA
   b. Cuffed endotracheal tube
   c. Uncuffed tube
   d. In all oral surgical intubations
   Ans. d

Ref: Dolenska 1/e p110

95. **Rehrmann flap used in:**
   a. Oroantral fistula
   b. Vestibuloplasty
   c. Ridge augmentation
   d. Alveoloplasty
   Ans. a

Ref: Peterson 2/e p772

96. **A Patient came with tender fluctuating swelling with history of fever, dyspnea, odynophagia, normal oral cavity and oropharynx BP 94/60, pulse 95/min, P02 98%, Treatment will be**
   a. IV Antibiotics
   b. I and D
   c. Awake fiberoptic intubation
   d. ICU admission and CECT Neck
   Ans. b

Ref: Neelima Malik 1/e p554

97. **A 9-year-old child is having recurrent pain in lower right molar region with fever from last night only proximal caries in primary first molar way to proceed is:**
   a. IOPA first
   b. Thermal vitality test
   c. Electric pulp test
   d. Test cavity
   Ans. a

Ref: McDonalds 8/e p390

98. In a child permanent anteriors are small in size, all primary teeth are normal in size, type of hypoplasia is:
a. Focal hypoplasia
b. Hypomaturation type
c. Hypocalcification
d. Generalized developmental
Ans. d

Ref: McDonald 8/e p85

99. Children able to keep his head erect in which age group:
a. 3–4months
b. 6–7 months
c. 10–12 months
d. 20–24 months
Ans. b

Ref: O P Ghai 2/e p45

100. On eruption of deciduous first molar child shows:
a. Bowel control
b. Focus on light
c. Walk without support
d. 2–3 Word sentences formation
Ans. c

Ref: McDonald 8/e p36

101. Procedural sedation in child helps in all except:
a. Helpful in routine day care patients
b. Helps to manage misbehaving patients
c. Increase quality of dental treatment
d. Provide psychological support to the child
Ans. a

Ref: McDonald 8/e p287

102. Baby can breathe even while suckling because of:
a. Higher position of larynx
b. Short soft palate
c. Wide and short tongue
d. Small pharynx
Ans. a

Ref: Grays Anatomy 40/e p313

103. Intellectual deficiency syndrome, IQ is in the range of:
a. 75–90
b. 45–50
c. 50–75
d. 90–110
Ans. c

Ref: O.P.Ghai 1/e p339

104. In which of the following condition GA and conscious sedation not required:
a. Mental retardation
b. Controlled epileptic patient
c. Cerebral palsy
d. Emotionally unstable and apprehensive
Ans. b

Ref: McDonald 8/e p315

105. Small bone are supplied by:
a. Subperiosteal vessels
b. Epiphyseal vessels
c. Periosteal vessels
d. Nutrient artery
Ans. c

Ref: Carranza 10/e p67

106. Full thickness flap is advantageous than partial thickness in all except:
a. Better esthetics
b. Less shrinkage
c. Better color matching
d. For large defects involving wide area
Ans. d

Ref: Carranza 8/e p432

107. Which of the following hormone in pregnancy is more associated with blood vessels and increased permeability:
a. Prolactin
b. Testosterone
c. Estrogen
d. Progesterone
Ans. d

Ref: Carranza 11/e p571

108. Microorganism are able to damage immunoglobulin produced by host through:
a. Hyaluronidase
b. Catalase
c. Collagenase
d. Protease
Ans. d

Ref: Carranza 11/e p1330

109. Maximum microbes accumulation occurs in:
a. Buccal
b. Occlusal
c. Lingual
d. Interproximal
Ans. d

Ref: Carranza 11/e p328

110. Which of the following structures is not present in PDL?
a. Fibronectin
b. Mature elastic fibers
c. Myelinated nerve fibers
d. Angioblast and undifferentiated cells
Ans. b

Ref: Carranza 9/e p41

111. Method of plaque control on concavities of root is:
a. Interdental brush
b. Dental Floss
c. Toothbrush
d. Toothpick
Ans. a

Ref: Carranza 9/e p663

112. Diode laser wavelength in period is:
a. 400–800 nm
b. 450–950 nm
c. 1060–1250 nm
d. 2000–12980 nm
Ans. b

Ref: Carranza 11/e p956

113. Juvenile periodontitis causing bacteria belongs to which species:
a. Fusobacterium
b. Actinomycetes
c. Prevotella
d. Streptococci
Ans. c

Ref: Carranza 9/e p412

114. Effects of radiation therapy are directed at all except:
a. RNA
b. DNA
c. Mitochondria
d. Cell membrane
Ans. a

Ref: White andPharaoh 5/e p26

115. Low dose therapeutic radiation will cause all in less time except:
a. Mucositis
b. Teratogenesis
c. Carcinogenesis
d. Mutagenesis
Ans. a

Ref: White and Pharaoh 5/e p19

116. Which of the following features are not seen in malignant transformation of a lymph node:
a. Decreased vascularity
b. Microcalcifications
c. Loss of fatty hyaline layer
d. Hypoechogenicity
Ans. a

Ref: Grainger 2/e p337

117. A patient experiences postoperative nausea and vomiting after dental treatment is due to all of the following except:
a. Opioid
b. Ingested blood
c. Acetaminophen
d. Nitrous oxide
Ans. c

Ref: Peterson 2/e p100

118. Co prescription of Amoxicillin with clavulanic acid is an example of:
a. Synergism
b. Antagonism
c. Displacement
d. Cumulative action
Ans. a

Ref: KD Tripathi 6/e p55

119. Which of the following is the drug of choice for antibiotic associated pseudomembranous colitis?

a. Ciprofloxacin
b. Clindamycin
c. Oral vancomycin
d. Linezolid

Ans. c

Ref: Goodman and Gilman 12/e p688

120. Which of the following drugs is useful against pseudomonas?

a. Streptomycin
b. Cephalexin
c. Cefotaxime
d. Piperacillin-Tazobactam

Ans. d

Ref: KDT 7/e p724

121. Xylometazoline nasal drops given before nasotracheal intubation to:

a. Dilatation of orifices
b. Decrease secretion
c. Constriction of nasal mucosa
d. Dilatation of posterior conche

Ans. c

Ref: Goodman and Gilman 11/e p166

122. Regarding furosemide true is:

a. Used in pulmonary edema
b. Acts at PCT
c. Causes hypercalcemia
d. Given by parenteral route only

Ans. a

Ref: Goodman and Gilman 11/e p485

123. Which of the following is not a 4-Aminoquinoline

a. Mefloquine
b. Primaquine
c. Amodiaquine
d. Chloroquine

Ans. b

Ref: KDT 6/e p816

124. True about phenytoin is:

a. Not teratogenic
b. Drug of choice for absence seizures
c. Nystagmus and ataxia
d. First pass metabolism

Ans. c

Ref: KDT 7/e p414

125. What can be given to 62 years old hypertensive patient with high lipids and atherosclerosis?

a. Heparin
b. Low dose aspirin
c. Amlodipine
d. Digoxin

Ans. c

Ref: KDT 6/e p870

126. Which of the following is incorrect about NSAIDs?

a. Can be used topically
b. Decrease the antihypertensive action of diuretics
c. Used in neuropathic pain
d. Should be avoided in renal failure

Ans. d

Ref: KDT 7/e p720

127. Route of choice for analgesic in cancer patient:

a. IV
b. Oral
c. Sublingual
d. Topical

Ans. b

Ref: WHO guidelines 2015

128. Virus is usually cultured as:

a. Rogosa blood agar
b. Non-embryonated eggs
c. Embryonated eggs
d. Sabouraud's medium

Ans. c

Ref: Ananthanarayan 7/e p437

129. Sunlight has sterilizing effect because:

a. It has short wavelength
b. It has long wave length
c. Ozone is present in the environment
d. Heat is present

Ans. a

Ref: Park 19/e p109

130. Identify the disease shown in the karyotype:

a. Downs syndrome
b. Prader Willi syndrome
c. Bloom syndrome
d. Cri-du-chat syndrome

Ans. d

Ref: Robbins 6/e p445

131. Chromosome becomes unstable due to damage:

a. Autosome
b. Sex chromosome
c. Centromere
d. Telomere

Ans. d

Ref: Robbins 9/e p191

132. H5N1 avian influenza has not become an epidemic till now. What is the important reason behind this:

a. It has avian influenza genes
b. Segmented RNA genome
c. Seen only in wild birds and not in domestic poultry
d. Human to human transmission is rare

Ans. d

Ref: Robbins 8/e p715

133. Commercially available DETTOL is:
a. Halogen
b. Alcohol
c. Phenol
d. Quarternary ammonium compound
Ans. c

Ref: Ananthanarayan 7/e p30

134. Stain used in candida hyphe and yeast:
a. PAS
b. H and E
c. Carbol fuchsin
d. D acridine orange
Ans. a

Ref: Neville 2/e p195

135. Pleomorphic bacteria is:
a. Bacteria in clusters
b. Rod shaped
c. Dumbbell shaped
d. Changing shape with time
Ans. d

Ref: Jawetz 12/e p337

136. Introduction of DNA with the help of electricity is:
a. Electrolysis
b. Electrotransfer
c. Electroporation
d. Electrofusion
Ans. c

Ref: Lippincott 5/e p485

137. Disinfectant used in laboratories:
a. Soap solution
b. Sodium hypochlorite
c. Alcohol
d. Chlorhexidine
Ans. b

Ref: Jawetz Microbiology 10/e p442

138. What is injected in tuberculin mantoux test?
a. Antigen abstract
b. Live attenuated
c. Killed bacteria
d. Live bacteria in less concentration
Ans. a

Ref: Jawetz 22/e p298

139. Tissue culture is:
a. Micropropagation
b. Macropropogation
c. Chemical propagation
d. Vegetative propagation
Ans. a

Ref: Lipincott 5/e p22

140. In HIV altered ratio is:
a. Helper T cell to suppressor T cell
b. NK cells to B cells
c. B cells to T cells
d. Lymphocytes to monocytes
Ans. a

Ref: Harsh Mohan 3/e p152

141. A boy complaints of unprovoked bite by a local dog in the community. The dog was caught later by the authorities and appeared to be healthy. The most appropriate course of action would be:
a. Test the dog for rabies antibodies
b. Immediately carry out euthanasia of dog
c. Withhold vaccination and observe dog for 10 days for signs of rabies
d. Give post exposure prophylaxis with cell culture derived vaccine
Ans. c

Ref: Park 19/e p229

142. In a rural clinic a 3-year-old child is brought by her mother and is emaciated. Her Hb was 5g/dl. The girl also had odema over her knees and ankles with discrete rash on her knees, elbows and ankles. The most likely worm causing these infestations is:
a. Whipworm
b. Roundworm
c. Hookworm
d. Pinworm
Ans. c

Ref: Jawetz 22/e p972

143. False about virus:
a. They are either DNA or RNA
b. Lytic and lysogenic phases occur together
c. There is no incubation period that helps in diagnosis
d. Encapsulated ones are susceptible to environmental changes
Ans. b

Ref: Jawetz 22/e p361

144. Nutritive value of zero was found for:
a. Starch
b. Fructose
c. Maltose
d. Cellulose
Ans. a

Ref: Harpers Biochemistry 26/e p109

145. When A=B=C=D then which is true for B and C?
a. B and C are always constant as their rate of formation is equal to the rate of consumption
b. B and C are in state of equilibrium
c. A and B are increasing
d. A and B are decreasing
Ans. a

Ref: Jawetz 22/e p254

146. Increase in lactate and pyruvate is seen in deficiency of:
a. Niacin
b. Thiamine

c. Retinoic acid
d. Pyridoxine
Ans. b

Ref: Harper 26/e p489

147. Which is associated with coronary heart disease?
a. VLDL
b. HDL
c. LDL
d. Triglycerides
Ans. c

Ref: Harper 26/e p209

148. A child presents with pellagra like dermatitis and aminoaciduria. Two siblings have the same condition and it is absent in two other siblings as well as parents. Which of the following is most likely:
a. Phenylketonuria
b. Alkaptonuria
c. Hartnup's disease
d. Von Gierke disease
Ans. c

Ref: Nelson 19/e p446

149. Growth not modified by:
a. Growth hormone
b. Insulin
c. Prolactin
d. Vasopressin
Ans. d

Ref: KDT 5/e p597

150. Mydriasis is due to:
a. Relaxation of ciliary muscles
b. Contraction of ciliary muscles
c. Relaxation of radial muscles
d. Contraction of radial muscles
Ans. d

Ref: KDT 6/e p108

151. Which of the following is true for the pulmonary neuroendocrine cells?
a. Secrete catecholamines
b. Have only cholinergic nerve supply
c. Contain serotonin
d. Respond to a decrease in PO2
Ans. d

Ref: Ganong 23/e p791

152. Characteristics of blood flow in capillaries:
a. High velocity and high stress
b. High velocity and low stress
c. Low velocity and pulsatile
d. Low velocity and higher sheer stress
Ans. d

Ref: Physiology by Boron 2/e p332

153. Iron absorption occurs chiefly from:
a. Stomach
b. Small intestine
c. Esophagus
d. Small intestine and abdomen
Ans. d

Ref: Ganong 23/e p612

154. A cell membrane is damaged by insertion of microneedle, repair shall occur by:
a. Enzymatic reactions
b. Hydrophobic interactions
c. An active process involving hydrolysis of ATP
d. Lateral movement of proteins
Ans. d

Ref: Lippincott 5/e p75

155. When chemoreceptors are activated it causes:
a. Tachycardia
b. Bradycardia
c. Hypovolemia
d. Hypervolemia
Ans. a

Ref: Lippincott 5/e p334

156. In radiograph of non-accidental injury, not seen is:
a. Sternal fracture
b. Metaphysis corner fracture
c. Parietal bone fracture
d. Costochondral and rib junction fracture
Ans. c

Ref: Grainger 2/e p871

157. Minimum tumor burden needed to be detected by PET scan:
a. 2–3 ccm
b. 3–5 ccm
c. 8–12 ccm
d. 13–16 ccm
Ans. a

Ref: Grainger 2/e p133

158. Role of fixer is:
a. It takes away extra developer solution
b. It binds developer to film
c. It strengthens or fixes the silver halides on to X-ray film
d. It removes the extra silver halides which are unfixed
Ans. d

Ref: White and Pharaoh 5/e p97

159. Hutchinson triad does not include:
a. Corneal involvement
b. Peg lateral incisors
c. Sensory nerve deafness
d. Depressed nasal bridge
Ans. d

Ref: Neville 3/e p190

160. Generalized microabscess in oral mucosa histopathology shows exocytosis. Neutrophil infiltration, history of use of new toothpaste, the treatment option is:

a. Fluconazole
b. Systemic antifungal
c. Beclomethasone mouth rinse
d. Systemic antibiotic and NSAIDs

Ans. c

Ref: Neville 2/e p304

161. Oral lesion seen in Hepatitis C:

a. Leukoplakia
b. Erythroplakia
c. Gingivitis
d. Lichen Planus

Ans. d

Ref: Burket 11/e p90

162. Disease that involves the parotid glands in children but occur only once in his life is:

a. Mumps
b. Measles
c. Herpes
d. Varicella

Ans. a

Ref: Neville 3/e p321

163. Gold 750 fineness means:

a. 75 Karat
b. 75%
c. 750%
d. 750 Grams

Ans. b

Ref: Philips 11/e p575

164. Sialagogue is:

a. Reduce the flow of saliva
b. Increase the flow of saliva
c. Is a dye for sialography
d. Is a dye used for nasolacrimal system

Ans. a or b

Ref: Burket 10/e p222

165. All are true about dentigerous cyst except:

a. Unilocular
b. Always associated with mandibular erupted third molar
c. OPG is diagnostic
d. Multivariants are associated with nevoid BCC

Ans. b

Ref: Neville 1/e p78

166. Brush cytology process is:

a. Brush rotated 5–6 times over the lesion
b. To fix extracted tissue brush cytology is useful
c. Used after excision of lesion by scalpel
d. Brush is placed at the border of the lesion and passed once over the lesion

Ans. a

Ref: Marx and Sterns Pathology 3/e p229

167. Herpetic paronychia is related to:
a. No relation with herpes
b. Congenital syphilis
c. Tertiary syphilis
d. Nail and finger
Ans. d

Ref: Neville 2/e p217

168. Vitamin D deficiency causes:
a. Amelogenesis imperfecta
b. Hyperdontia
c. Accelerated eruption
d. Delayed eruption
Ans. d

Ref: Shafer 6/e p636

169. Generalized gingival inflammation profuse salivation and scalding of skin from palm and foot diagnosis is:
a. Lichen Planus
b. Psoriasis
c. Heavy metal poisoning
d. Contact dermatitis
Ans. c

Ref: Burket 11/e p126

170. Granulomatous gingivitis cause:
a. Recent dental visit
b. Recurrent gingivitis, multiple repeated episodes of vasculitis
c. History of fast food intake
d. Broad spectrum antibiotics
Ans. a

Ref: Neville 2/e p142

171. A 40-year-old woman has ameloblastoma, histopathologic picture is:
a. Peripheral palisading strand with central loose stellate reticulum
b. Peripheral palisading strand with peripheral loose stellate reticulum
c. Peripheral palisading strand with central stromal retraction artefact
d. Central loose stellate reticulum shows marked nuclear atypia and numerous mitotic figures
Ans. a

Ref: Shafer 6/e p274

172. True about involucrum in osteomyelitis is:
a. Extracted dead bone
b. New bone fill the cavity space
c. Newly formed bone surrounding necrosed bone in osteomyelitis
d. Newly formed bone separated from necrosed bone in osteomyelitis
Ans. c

Ref: Neville 2/e p126

173. Cyst involving all three germ layers is:
a. Dermoid
b. Teratoid
c. Branchial
d. Thyroglossal
Ans. b

Ref: Neville 2/e p32

174. Thickness of die spacer depends upon:
a. Type of restoration
b. Film thickness of luting cement and amount of shrinkage
c. Type of inlay wax pattern
d. Type of cement used for cementation
Ans. b

Ref: Shillingburg 3/e p312

175. Energy required to liquefy a solid is known as:
a. Sublimation
b. Vapourization
c. Latent heat of fusion
d. Condensation
Ans. c

Ref: Philips 10/e p22

176. Retarder in alginate is:
a. Sodium phosphate
b. Calcium sulphate
c. Potasium alginate
d. Diatomaceous earth
Ans. a

Ref: Skinners 10/e p240

177. Mercury and silver alloy reaction when mixed, the product is:
a. Tin reacts with Hg
b. Cu reacts with Hg
c. Dissolution of Ag in Hg
d. Precipitation of Ag with Hg
Ans. d

Ref: Philips 11/e p502

178. Ductility represents:
a. Plastic strain
b. Flexural stress
c. Percentage elongation
d. Percentage compression
Ans. c

Ref: Craig 11/e p79

179. Main drawback of Be in Ni–Cr alloys:
a. Health hazard
b. Increase flow of alloy
c. Reduce fusion temperature
d. Refine grain bending
Ans. a

Ref: Philips 11/e p197

180. Angle of wetting is zero, it reflects that attraction between the molecules is:
a. No such correlation
b. Molecules of adhesive are attracted to molecules of adherend less than they are attracted to themselves
c. Molecules of adhesive are attracted to molecules of adherend as much as or more than they are attracted to themselves
d. Molecules of adhesive are attracted to molecules of adherend exactly same as than they are attracted to themselves
Ans. c

Ref: Philips 11/e p37

181. In dental material setting time is measured by which test:

a. Vickers
b. Rockwell
c. Cold bend
d. Vicat needle

Ans. d

Ref: Craig 11/e p361

182. Tongue Epithelium is:

a. Specialized mucosa
b. Stratified Squamous
c. Keratinized stratified and specialized
d. Non keratinised stratified and specialized

Ans. c

Ref: Orban 12/e p237

183. Enamel calcification starts at:

a. From cervical area
b. From cusp tips
c. Between outer enamel epithelium and DEJ
d. Apical region

Ans. b

Ref: Tencate 7/e p169

184. Cementum is rich in which collagen fibers:

a. Type 1
b. Type 3
c. Type 4
d. Type 9

Ans. a

Ref: Carranza 11/e p33

185. First mature oral tissue:

a. Lip
b. Posterior tongue
c. Tip of tongue
d. All soft tissues mature simultaneously

Ans. a

Ref: Profitt 3/e p75

186. Tubule of serous acinar cell gland is lined by:

a. Simple cuboidal
b. Simple columnar
c. Stratified columnar
d. Stratified squamous

Ans. a

Ref: Tencates 8/e p266

187. Neonatal line is accentuation of:

a. Striae of Retzius
b. Hunter Schreger bands
c. Perikymata
d. Prominent DEJ

Ans. a

Ref: Orbans 7/e p44

188. Chlorhexidine used for hand disinfection uses concentration of:
a. 1 %
b. 0.2 %
c. 0.5 %
d. 0.12 %
Ans. a

Ref: Bailey and Love 25/e p208

189. Enamel spindles are:
a. Enamel rods formed linearly by successive apposition of enamel in discrete increments
b. Thin leaf like faults between enamel rod groups that extend from the enamel surface towards the DEJ
c. Hypomineralized structures of enamel rods that project between adjacent groups of enamel rods from the DEJ
d. Odontoblastic processes that cross the DEJ into the enamel
Ans. d

Ref: Sturdevant 4/e p19

190. What is the investigation of choice in a patient with acute head injury?
a. PET
b. NCCT
c. CECT
d. MRI
Ans. b

Ref: Grainger 2/e p172

191. Grade 1 axillary lymph node is:
a. Lateral to pectoralis major
b. Medial to pectoralis major
c. Medial to pectoralis minor
d. Lateral to pectoralis minor
Ans. d

Ref: Schwartz 11/e p227

192. Which of the following is the ideal time for repair of cleft palate:
a. 2–3 years
b. 5–6 years
c. 9–12 months
d. 18–24 months
Ans. c

Ref: O.P.Kharbanda 2/e p690

193. Doppler ultrasound all are true except:
a. Direction of blood flow
b. Degree of stenosis
c. Provide information about blood velocity
d. Monophasic tracing measure normal flow
Ans. d

Ref: Harrison 16/e p2387

194. Hypothyroidism in children:
a. Myxedema
b. Cretinism
c. Gigantism
d. Acromegaly
Ans. b

Ref: Guyton 11/e p942

195. Microbes of hospital induced infection carries in which part of health worker:
a. Skin
b. Throat
c. Hair
d. Nail
Ans. b

Ref: Jawetz 22/e p892

196. Juvenile onset diabetes is another name of:
a. Type 1
b. Type 2
c. Type 3
d. Type 4
Ans. a

Ref: Ganong 23/e p435

197. Which disease has been eradicated?
a. Chicken pox
b. Small pox
c. Cholera
d. Measles
Ans. b

Ref: Harrison 18/e p1808

198. Blood product of mother to child is advisable in:
a. Packed RBC in autoimmune thrombocytopenic purpura
b. Platelets in autoimmune thrombocytopenic purpura
c. Plasma in autoimmune thrombocytopenic purpura
d. In case to prevent any graft rejection
Ans. b

Ref: Harrison 14/e p2977

199. Inorder to manage inventory the blood banks like to release unit which is close to expiration which one of the following is close to expiration among these?
a. SAGM 35 days
b. CPDA 27 days
c. ACD 14 days
d. SAGM 25 days irradiated same day
Ans. d

Ref: Ajay Yadav 5/e p34

200. A 45-years-old female diabetic patient on insulin is brought to hospital in an unconscious state. What is the first line of treatment?
a. IV infusion of dextrose
b. IV insulin
c. Blood glucose test
d. IV dexamethasone solution
Ans. c

Ref: Harrison 18/e p3006

AIIMS Dental (May 2015)

1. **Most common cause of CSF leakage in middle cranial fossa fracture is due to:**
   a. Sphenoidal sinus
   b. Tegmen tympani
   c. Frontal sinus
   d. Cribriform plate
   Ans. b

Ref: Fonseca 4/e Trauma p 487

2. **A patient with neuromuscular incoordination reports to your clinic. Best way to do occlusal discrepancy correction is:**
   a. Take interocclusal records using carborundum paste
   b. Take interocclusal records and do occlusal correction in the articulator
   c. No need to correct occlusal discrepancy for neuromuscular patients
   d. Direct method on patient's mouth as jaw relation is difficult
   Ans. b

Ref: Bouchers 13/e p276

3. **Facial plane angle is:**
   a. N-Pog to basion sella
   b. FHP to Sn-Go
   c. Sn to N-Pog
   d. FHP to N-Pog
   Ans. d

Ref: OP Kharbanda 1/e p227

4. **90 degree activation of pendulum appliance creates how much distal force on molars:**
   a. 350 gm
   b. 250 gm
   c. 75 gm
   d. 125 gm
   Ans. b

Ref: Profitt 4/e p580

5. **Collum angle decreases in:**
   a. Class II div 1
   b. Class II div 2
   c. Class III cases
   d. Bimax cases
   Ans. b

Ref: OP Kharbanda 1/e p

6. **Density of base metal alloys compared to gold alloys is:**
   a. Double
   b. Half
   c. Similar
   d. Four times increased
   Ans. b

Ref: Craig 11/e p485

7. **Centric holding cusp is:**
   a. Mesiolingual cusp of mandibular first molar
   b. Mesiopalatal cusp of maxillary first molar
   c. Distolingual cusp of mandibular first molar
   d. Mesiobuccal cusp of maxillary first molar
   Ans. b

Ref: Shillingburg 3/e p340

8. **In edgewise appliance first order bend are:**
   a. Horizontal
   b. Vertical
   c. Bends are not given at all
   d. Is horizontal and then vertical
   Ans. a

Ref: Profitt 4/e p410

9. **Wrought metal in cast RPD is used for:**
   a. Reciprocal arm
   b. Retentive arm
   c. Shoulder
   d. Major connector
   Ans. b

Ref: Stewart 3/e p82

10. **Least modulus of elasticity is of:**
    a. Cobalt chromium
    b. Beta titanium
    c. Stainless steel
    d. NiTi
    Ans. d

Ref: Profitt 4/e p362

11. **Phosphate bonded investment should be completely carbon free otherwise:**
    a. Black casting
    b. Smooth casting
    c. Carbon makes the casting brittle
    d. Investment chips off when molten metal enters the mold space
    Ans. c

Ref: Philips 12/e p208

12. **In dentinogenesis imperfecta which gene is involved:**
    a. Chromosome 6
    b. Chromosome 8
    c. Chromosome 4
    d. Chromosome 21
    Ans. c

Ref: McDonald 8/e p96

13. **Giemsa stain of biopsy shows oral petechiae, hepatosplenomegaly with ascites enlarged macrophage with round organism, the likely diagnosis is:**
    a. Kala-azar
    b. Mucor mycosis
    c. Infectious mononucleosis
    d. Herpes Zoster
    Ans. c

Ref: Neville 2/e p225

14. In costochondral graft, chondral part is taken with:
a. Rib cutter
b. Rib shear
c. No 11 blade
d. 701 bur
Ans. c

Ref: Peterson OMFS 2/e p788

15. Preoperative CT scan shows internal maxillary artery in ankylosis,which of the following is used to cut:
a. Oscillating saw
b. Piezoelectric handpiece
c. Rotary cutting
d. Chisel mallet
Ans. b

Ref: PeterWard Booth 3/e p423

16. Distal portion of mandibular 3rd molar is covered by ascending ramus:
a. Position B
b. Distoangular
c. Level A
d. Class II
Ans. d

Ref: Neelima Malik 2/e p124

17. Le Clerc procedure is done for:
a. Disimpaction of maxilla
b. Recurrent dislocation
c. Cleft lip
d. Disk displacement
Ans. b

Ref: Peterson OMFS 2/e p1045

18. In a rheumatoid arthritis patient with TMJ ankylosis progressively exhibiting anterior open bite and decreased mouth opening,what is indicated?
a. Neocondyle distraction
b. Costochondral graft
c. Gap Arthroplasty
d. Titanium and plastic graft for TMJ Reconstruction
Ans. d

Ref: Okeson TMJ 2/e p301

19. In mandible fracture with gonial flaring plating should be best done with:
a. Lingual surface
b. Buccal surface
c. Lower surface
d. Upper surface
Ans. c

Ref: Peterson 1/e p871

20. Simplifying of fracture is done in:
a. Greenstick fracture
b. Comminuted mandibular fracture
c. Bilateral condyle and symphysis
d. Panfacial trauma /single line fracture of angle
Ans. b

Ref: Trauma Guidelines International 2/e p332

21. Which of the following is most common cause of pulmonary embolism?
a. Endarteritis
b. Lymphadenitis
c. Thrombophlebitis
d. Hemorrhage
Ans. c

Ref: NBDE Straight pick 1996 Dec Micro-Patho p 8

22. A patient complain of frequent maxillary denture fracture on evaluation on articulator no occlusal discrepancy is seen, what can be the actual cause?
a. Poor retention
b. Improper extension of maxillary denture
c. Lack of mucosal resiliency in hard palate
d. Poor denture base material flexural properties
Ans. c

Ref: Prosthodontics by Nallaswamy 1/e p255

23. A 7-year-old patient with history of trauma 2 hour back reported with Ellis Class III fracture on right central incisor, normal physiologic mobility, what will be the treatment for this?
a. Apexification
b. Apexogenesis
c. Orthodontic extrusion of tooth
d. Reimplantation and splinting with composite
Ans. b

Ref: Cohen 10/e p845

24. A patient complaints of sore throat after 24 hours of denture delivery, most likely cause is:
a. Extended maxillary denture
b. Extended maxillary denture in pterygoid notch area
c. Extended mandibular denture
d. Allergy to acrylic
Ans. c

Ref: Winkler 1/e p213

25. Low grade malignancy seen with:
a. Adenoid cystic carcinoma
b. Acinic cell carcinoma
c. Comedo ductal adenocarcinoma
d. Pleomorphic adenoma
Ans. b

Ref: Neville 2/e p423

26. Mandibular arch within the maxillary arch is called:
a. Cross bite
b. Deep bite
c. Reverse bite
d. Scissor bite
Ans. d

Ref: Graber 5/e p12

27. Diagnosis of Sjogren syndrome is confirmed by:
a. Absence of anti SS Antibody
b. Positive rheumatoid factor
c. Lip biopsy
d. Lymph node biopsy
Ans. c

Ref: Neville 2/e p401

28. **Cranial base length is:**
   a. Sella to Bolton
   b. Nasion to Sella
   c. Nasion to Bolton
   d. Nasion to Menton
   Ans. c

Ref: Gurkeerat Singh 2/e p512

29. **Hardness of stone surface is affected by:**
   a. Rubber based impression material
   b. Hydrocolloid impression material
   c. Impression wax
   d. Impression compound
   Ans. b

Ref: Bouchers 13/e p126

30. **Silver stain tissue biopsy of uncontrolled diabetic patient with sequestering alveolar segment and nasal pus discharge show large nonspecific hyphae with right angle branching the diagnosis will be:**
   a. Candidiasis
   b. Leishmaniasis
   c. Mucormycosis
   d. Aspergillosis
   Ans. c

Ref: Burket 10/e p78

31. **Casting of base metal crown is done in:**
   a. High refractory silica
   b. Phosphate bonded investment
   c. Gypsum bonded investment
   d. Silica bonded investment
   Ans. b

Ref: Shillingberg 3/e p366

32. **Most likely to collapse in blowout fracture is:**
   a. Roof of orbit
   b. Medial wall of orbit
   c. Floor of orbit
   d. Lateral wall of orbit
   Ans. c

Ref: Peterson 2/e p467

33. **ADA specification number of orthodontic wire is:**
   a. 25
   b. 29
   c. 30
   d. 32
   Ans. d

Ref: Brantley 1/e p33

34. **Stiffness is:**
   a. Degree of plastic deformation
   b. Resistance to plastic deformation
   c. Degree of elastic deformation
   d. Resistance to elastic deformation
   Ans. d

Ref: Philips 11/e p53

35. Pre carve burnishing is useful for all except:
a. Marginal adaptation
b. Increase surface hardness
c. Bring further excess mercury to surface
d. Decrease the number and size of voids
Ans. b

Ref: Sturdevant 4/e p682

36. In archial analysis facial type III:
a. Anterior cranial base does not pass through O
b. Palatal plane does not pass through O
c. Occlusal plane does not pass through O
d. Mandibular plane does not pass through O
Ans. c

Ref: OP Kharbanda 1/e p189

37. Bacteria are populated most commonly in:
a. Lingual surface
b. Buccal surface
c. Interproximal surface
d. Occlusal surface
Ans. c

Ref: Carranza 11/e p328

38. Janetta surgical procedure:
a. Microvascular decompression
b. Radiofrequency neurolysis
c. Radiofrequency gangliolysis
d. Percutaneous ganglion glycerolysis
Ans. a

Ref: Fonseca 3rd ed vol 1 p 151

39. House Brackmann scale is for which nerve?
a. Optic
b. Hypoglossal
c. Facial
d. Trigeminal
Ans. c

Ref: Peter Ward Booth 2/e p312

40. Prior to reimplantation tooth is soaked in 3% citric acid. This is done to:
a. Etch the surface
b. Remove PDL
c. Disinfect the tooth
d. Increase surface reactivity
Ans. b

Ref: Cohen 10/e p649

41. Alignment of teeth in a curve from anterior to posterior is called:
a. Monson curve
b. Bonwills curve
c. Curve of Wilson
d. Curve of Von Spee
Ans. d

Ref: Nallaswamy 1/e p194

42. **Radiations affect all three germ layers causes:**
    a. Dermoid cyst
    b. Teratoid cyst
    c. Branchial cyst
    d. Thyroglossal cyst
    Ans. b

Ref: Neville 2/e p32

43. **Recently two methods of CPAP conventional and bubble CPAP were compared in the conventional method 90 out of 160 shows extubation failure while 40 out of 160 showed extubation failure in the bubble method which test would be the best to compare the statistical significance between the rates of extubation:**
    a. Paired test
    b. Chi square test
    c. Student test
    d. ANOVA
    Ans. b

Ref: Park 20/e p755

44. **In emergency cricothyrotomy is done:**
    a. Below the cricoid
    b. Above the cricoid
    c. Below the thyroid cartilage
    d. Through the isthmus
    Ans. c

Ref: Fonseca 4/e p56

45. **In a study done for the evaluation of prevalence caries in a given population the ratio of its standard deviation to the mean of data is called as:**
    a. Standard error of mean
    b. Coefficient of variance
    c. Standard deviation
    d. Coefficient of skewness
    Ans. b

Ref: Park 20/e p754

46. **In a country the incidence of disease is high and prevalence of the disease is low then:**
    a. Diseases is fatal or can be cured easily
    b. Disease is not curable
    c. No incidence and low prevalence
    d. They are not related
    Ans. a

Ref: Park 20/e p58

47. **Metallic taste after application of stannous flouride is due to:**
    a. Stannous Trifluoro phosphate
    b. Stannic trifluorophosphate
    c. Calcium tri-flouro-stannate
    d. Tin hydroxyphosphate
    Ans. d

Ref: Marya 2/e p213

48. **In a stainless steel crown on a deciduous molar with overhanging margin, gingival pain and inflammation occurs due to:**
    a. Engaging undercut
    b. Crown margins causing irritation

c. Excess cement
d. Plaque retention
Ans. d

Ref: Aaratho Rao 5/e p225

49. Activity of plaque in proximal area remains normal for:
a. 120 min
b. 180 min
c. 60 min
d. 30 min
Ans. a

Ref: McDonald 8/e p200

50. A child suffers from trauma which causes lateral luxation of the primary central incisor. The incisor is not in occlusion and does not cause interference. What should be done?
a. Reduce the opposing tooth
b. Immediate repositioning and splinting
c. Reduce both affected and opposite tooth
d. The incisor should be allowed for passive and spontaneous reposition
Ans. d

Ref: McDonald 8/e p479

51. Powder liquid ratio in chemically activated resin:
a. 3:1 by vol, 2:1 by weight
b. 2:1 by vol, 3:1 by weight
c. 1:2 by vol, 2:1 by weight
d. 2:1 by volume 1: 3 by weight
Ans. a

Ref: Bouchers 12/e p192

52. The color of oxygen cylinder is:
a. Blue
b. Black with white shoulders
c. Grey with white shoulders
d. White with black shoulders
Ans. b

Ref: Neelima Malik 2/e p164

53. Dental arch form is ultimately determined by:
a. Facial type
b. Facial growth pattern
c. Angle's classification
d. Balance between facial and intraoral musculature
Ans. d

Ref: Tencate 5/e p123

54. Life span of RBC is:
a. 100 Days
b. 120
c. 60
d. 90
Ans. b

Ref: Guyton 11/e p426

55. **Calorific value of fat is:**
   a. 7 Kcal
   b. 9 kCal
   c. 14 Kcal
   d. 19 Kcal
   Ans. b

Ref: Satyanarayana 1/e p279

56. **Lymph from tongue not drained by:**
   a. Central
   b. Ventral
   c. Marginal
   d. Posterior
   Ans. b

Ref: BDC 6/e p268

57. **Oroantral fistula in maxillary third molar region is preferably closed by:**
   a. Palatal island
   b. Palatal mucoperiosteal
   c. Bridge
   d. Buccal mucoperiosteal
   Ans. a

Ref: Vinod Kapoor 2/e p186

58. **Infection from lower lip reaches blood stream through:**
   a. Pterygoid plexus
   b. Superior labial artery
   c. Inferior labial artery
   d. Brachiocephalic vein
   Ans. d

Ref: BDC 4/e p150

59. **Cross section of minor connector designed to closely adapt to tooth surface:**
   a. Round
   b. Flat
   c. Half round
   d. Triangular
   Ans. d

Ref: McCraken 11/e p54

60. **Calcified structures of oral cavity develops from:**
   a. Endoderm only
   b. Ectoderm and mesoderm
   c. Ectoderm and endoderm
   d. Endoderm and mesoderm
   Ans. b

Ref: Grays 37/e p137

61. **An athlete has habit of chewing gums, develop asymptomatic swelling in preauricular region, on palpation bony hard in nature also seen as radiopaque in PA view, most probable diagnosis is:**
   a. Osteosarcoma
   b. Parotitis
   c. Traumatic myositis ossificans
   d. Benign masseteric hypertrophy
   Ans. d

Ref: Marx and Stern 2/e p45

62. Which is true about Immediate denture?

a. All teeth extracted on the same day
b. No extraction
c. Anteriors extracted first and on the day of denture insertion posteriors are extracted
d. Posteriors extracted first and on the day of denture insertion anteriors are extracted

Ans. d

Ref: Bouchers 12/e p128

63. Taking consideration of the systemic factors and displacement of gingival tissue which is the best?

a. Ferric sulphate
b. Aluminium chloride
c. Adrenaline
d. Lignocaine

Ans. b

Ref: Shillingberg 3/e p362

64. Latency period for distraction osteogenesis in a 8-month-old child is

a. 0–2 days
b. 5–7 days
c. 1 week
d. 2 week

Ans. a

Ref: Peterson 2/e p1342

65. Which of the following wire can be bent for maximum times before it gets fractured?

a. NiTi
b. Co-Cr-Ni
c. Beta Titanium
d. Stainless Steel

Ans. b

Ref: Brantley 1/e p78

66. Anterior upper facial height: Lower facial height is:

a. 55:45
b. 45:55
c. 60:40
d. 40:60

Ans. b

Ref: OP Kharbanda 2/e p240

67. In Caldwell Luc procedure antrostomy is done through:

a. Middle meatus
b. Superior meatus
c. Inferior meatus
d. Inferior and middle meatus

Ans. c

Ref: Peterson 2/e p308

68. Palatine process began to fuse at:

a. 6 weeks post fertilization
b. 8 weeks post fertilization
c. 10 weeks post fertilization
d. 12 weeks post fertilization

Ans. a

Ref: OP Kharbanda 1/e p93

69. For long duration to maintain the vitality of PDL an avulsed tooth should be stored in:

a. HBSS
b. Viaspan
c. Saline
d. Milk
Ans. b

Ref: AAPD Trauma Manual

70. Acute oral bullae with ballooning degeneration, lipschutz bodies with nuclear 3–4 microns are present, the diagnosis is:

a. Oral herpes
b. Pemphigus
c. Psoriasis
d. Aphthous ulcer
Ans. a

Ref: Neville 2/e p223

71. Carbon monoxide transfusion in lung is diffusion limited as:

a. Base of lung is poorly ventilated
b. Diffusion of CO across blood gas barrier is low
c. PCO2 rises in blood immediately on exposure
d. Carboxy hemoglobin has high avidity
Ans. d

Ref: Ganong 23/e p803

72. Hyperactive mentalis activity is seen in:

a. Class II div 2
b. Class II div 1
c. Class III
d. Deepbite
Ans. b

Ref: Gurkeerat Singh 2/e p549

73. Muscle responsible for opening of mandible:

a. Temporalis
b. Medial pterygoid
c. Lateral pterygoid
d. Buccinator
Ans. c

Ref: BDC 4/e p168

74. Loop and helices in orthodontics:

a. No effect on force
b. Increase range
c. No relation
d. Increase force
Ans. b

Ref: Graber 5/e p366

75. Color of bile is due to:

a. 2 alpha mercaptopurine
b. Bilirubin
c. Copper
d. Creatinine
Ans. b

Ref: Ganong 23/e p585

76. Which of the following is not a physiological method of heat loss from the body?
a. Vasodilation
b. Posture
c. Peripheral vasoconstriction
d. Sweating
Ans. c

Ref: Guyton 11/e p895

77. In case with increased carbohydrate intake the excess carbohydrate is stored as:
a. Trypsin
b. Protein
c. Glycogen
d. Trans fatty acids
Ans. c

Ref: Lipincott 3/e p124

78. Some bacteria get encapsulated to:
a. To multiply
b. To produce spores
c. Achieve protection from phagocytosis
d. To increase penetration capacity
Ans. c

Ref: Ananthanarayan 7/e p14

79. Co-prescription of amoxicillin with clavulanic acid is an example of:
a. Synergism
b. Antagonism
c. Cumulative action
d. Displacement
Ans. a

Ref: KDT 6/e p677

80. True about Wilson curve is:
a. Posterior teeth parallel to inward pull of masseter
b. Helps in achieving compensatory curve during arrangement of posteriors
c. Determine posterior plane of occlusion
d. Anteroposterior curve
Ans. b

Ref: Nallaswamy 1/e p194

81. A silver amalgam restoration is to be done in a posterior tooth with a proximal box extension with wide faciolingual width. Which wedging technique should be used to well adapt the matrix band:
a. Double wedge
b. Wedge wedge
c. Piggy back
d. Single wedge
Ans. a

Ref: Nisha Garg 1/e p215

82. Which of the following is the property of ceramic?
a. Equal compressive and tensile strength
b. Low compressive and high tensile strength
c. High compressive and low tensile strength
d. High compressive and high compressive strength
Ans. c

Ref: O Brian 3/e p180

83. **Most common sign of airway obstruction:**
    a. Strenuous breathing
    b. Increase pulse rate
    c. Decrease pulse rate
    d. Slow pounding pulse
    Ans. a

Ref: Neelima Malik 3/e p358

84. **Which is a feature of ageing PDL:**
    a. Increase in cell size
    b. Increase in cell activity
    c. Increase in cell number
    d. Decrease in number of elastic fibers
    Ans. d

Ref: Carranza 10/e p95

85. **Transient Bell's Palsy during mandibular nerve block after injection of LA occurs due to needle piercing into:**
    a. Temporalis
    b. Maxillary artery
    c. Parotid gland
    d. Buccinator
    Ans. c

Ref: Malamed 5/e p200

86. **Serum chemistry analysis in a patient reveals PCO_2 30 mm Hg, PO_2 105 mm Hg, and pH 7.46 this indicates partially compensated:**
    a. Metabolic acidosis
    b. Respiratory acidosis
    c. Metabolic alkalosis
    d. Respiratory alkalosis
    Ans. d

Ref: Ganong 22/e p735

87. **Dermal and oral manifestation are seen most commonly in:**
    a. Myelocytic
    b. Monocytic
    c. Aleukemic
    d. Lymphocytic
    Ans. b

Ref: NBDE July 1981 Oral Radiology p 24

88. **Streptococci is important organism in causing dental caries as it is:**
    a. Penicillinase resistant
    b. Ferment carbohydrate
    c. Produce extracellular polysaccharide
    d. Produce acid during metabolism
    Ans. c

Ref: Nikiforuk 1/e p167

89. **Which of the following has little or no significance:**
    a. Mandibular canine erupting before mandibular premolar
    b. Mandibular incisor erupting before mandibular molar
    c. Mandibular second premolar erupting before mandibular molar
    d. Mandibular canine and premolar erupting before mandibular molar
    Ans. b

Ref: McDonald 8/e p178

90. **Leeway space is due to:**
    a. Difference between maxillary permanent and deciduous canines
    b. TSALD
    c. Space difference between deciduous incisors and their succedaneous permanent teeth
    d. Space difference between deciduous canine and molar and their succedaneous permanent teeth
    Ans. d

Ref: Bishara 1/e p57

Prosthodontics SR Papers (July 2015)

1. **Superior constrictor of pharynx has insertion at:**
   a. Posterior wall of pharynx, oro and nasopharynx
   b. Posterior wall of oropharynx
   c. Posterior wall of oro and laryngopharynx
   d. Pterygomandibular raphae
   Ans. c

   Ref: BD Chaurasia 4/e p 328

2. **Binder in Phosphate bonded investment is:**
   a. MgO
   b. Cristoballite
   c. Quartz
   d. Carbon
   Ans. a

   Ref: Philips 11/e p 310

3. **Paralleling tool touches the cervical third of a tooth, to establish guide plane what should be done:**
   a. Tilting and jacket crown if required
   b. Tilting enameloplasty and jacket crown
   c. Enameloplasty or jacket crown whichever required
   d. Tilting and enameloplasty if required
   Ans. a

   Ref: McCracken 11/e p 256

4. **All are false except:**
   a. Glue and gelatin form a layer over hemihydrates resulting in decrease in solubility in water
   b. Borax and NaCl aid as retarder due to insoluble hemihydrate
   c. Cooler water significantly affect the setting time
   d. Gypsum < 20 % helps in fast setting
   Ans. d

   Ref: Philips 11/e p 265

5. **Centric slide is the movement of mandible:**
   a. From the working side to centric occlusion
   b. From the first contact to centric relation
   c. From maximum intercuspation to centric relation
   d. From first contact from centric relation to maximum intercuspation
   Ans. a

   Ref: Nallaswamy 1/e p 256

6. **Wax pattern stored in refrigerator before investment procedure what should be done:**
   a. Allow the pattern to come to room temperature
   b. Margins are reheated and readapted
   c. Not allowed to return to room temperature
   d. Not stored in refrigerator
   Ans. b

   Ref: Craig 12/e p 312

7. **First step in conducting research is:**
   a. Formulating study question
   b. Formulating null hypothesis
   c. Calculation of sample size
   d. Presentation in ethical committee and to get ethical clearance
   Ans. a

Ref: Mahajan 5/e p 19

8. **Martensitic type of stainless steel is used for the fabrication of cutting edge of surgical instruments because:**
   a. Martensitic is brittle
   b. Martensitic has higher strength
   c. Martensitic has high corrosion resistance
   d. Martensitic has low corrosion resistance
   Ans. b

Ref: Philips 11/e p 638

9. **In cast gold alloys with change in gold content true is:**
   a. Mechanical properties increase with increase in gold content
   b. Mechanical properties increase with decrease in gold content
   c. Mechanical properties decrease with decrease in gold content
   d. Mechanical properties are not affected with decrease in gold content
   Ans. b

Ref: Philips 11/e p 638

10. **Regarding horizontal bone augmentation which of the following statement is not true**
    a. Distraction osteogenesis
    b. Ridge split or expansion
    c. Non Stage guided regeneration
    d. Simultaneous rudge augmentation
    Ans. c

Ref: Carl Misch 3/e p 214

11. **A cast mandibular guidance appliance as described by Robinson and Rubright is appropriate for**
    a. Cases where mandible can be manipulated into acceptable centric relation but patient lacks motor control
    b. Cases where flange guidance prosthesis can be fabricated
    c. Mandibular guidance therapy
    d. Return to guidance appliance after completion of mandibular guidance therapy
    Ans. a

Ref: Journal of Prosthetic Dentistry 1964; 14: 992–999

12. **Freedom in centric occlusal philosophy is indicated in all except:**
    a. Neuromuscular incoordination:
    b. Heavy habitual centric relation
    c. Interferences between CO and CR
    d. Not able to hold in CR
    Ans. b

Ref: Heartwell 1/e p 132

13. **All are true except:**
    a. Gum Arabic is added to reduce water consumption
    b. Alpha hemihydrate consists of prism like crystals and Beta hemihydrate has orthorhombic structure
    c. Alpha and beta hemihydrates are two phases of gypsum
    d. They have differences in consumption of water
    Ans. c

Ref: Philips 11/e p 257

14. Electrognathography allows to track:
a. Lower jaw movements three dimensionally, as the jaw traverses through space from rest to centric
b. Skull movements two dimensionally, as the skull moves during function
c. Skull movements three dimensionally, as the skull moves during function
d. Lower jaw movements two dimensionally, as the jaw traverses through space from rest to centric
Ans. a

Ref: Heartwell 3/e p 329

15. Obstructive Sleep Apnea is characterized by all except:
a. Strenous breathing
b. Unconscious awakening in night
c. Pharyngeal muscle fatigue
d. Oxygen saturation affecting cardiovascular and metabolic system
Ans. b

Ref: Maxillofacial Prosthetics by Davenport 2/e p 241

16. True about magnets is all except:
a. Hard magnets have low corrosion resistance
b. Alnico magnets were first to be used
c. Hard magnets-low coercivity
d. Soft magnets are easier to magnetize and demagnetize
Ans. c

Ref: Davenport 2/e p 712

17. About Hobo and Takayama philosophy of full mouth rehabilitation the differences between anterior and posterior guidance should not be more than .... Degrees:
a. 3
b. 5
c. 7
d. 10
Ans. b

Ref: Hobo Oral Rehabilitation 1/e p 35

18. Best cement that provides benefit of durability and ease of retrievability of an implant supported metal ceramic crown is:
a. Zinc polycarboxylate
b. Zinc phosphate
c. Zinc oxide eugenol
d. Glass Ionomer cement
Ans. b

Ref: Craig 11/e p 155

19. Dr. Bernard Giesenhyen is famous for his bone augmentation technique usually called:
a. Roll flap
b. Onlay graft
c. Pouch and tunnel
d. Bone ring
Ans. d

Ref: Babbush 2/e p 138

20. From anterior view the articular disc in TMJ is:
a. Uniform
b. Medially thick
c. Posteriorly thick
d. Thinnest in the centre
Ans. b

Ref: Okeson 5/e p 9

21. In case of cast partial denture for duplication of master cast to fabricate refractory cast, which material is not used:
a. PVS
b. Polyether
c. Agar
d. Alginate
Ans. b

Ref: Craig 11/e p 346

22. Common complication of zygoma implants are all except:
a. Post operative sinusitis
b. Subconjunctival hematoma
c. Oroantral fistula
d. Itching
Ans. d

Ref: Fonseca 3/e p 1123

23. According to ADA specification number 24 all indications of base plate wax are correct except:
a. Type I- building veneers
b. Type II-trial fitting of pattern in the mouth
c. Type III-Trial in tropical countries
d. Type IV-For fabrication of denture base plate
Ans. d

Ref: Philips 11/e p 292

24. Half life of methyl methacrylate monomer in human body is:
a. 24 hours
b. 36 hours
c. 20–40 minutes
d. Not absorbed, directly excreted from kidney
Ans. c

Ref: Philips 11/e p 754

25. Implant safe instruments for debridement of implant surface include all except:
a. Plastic
b. Gold
c. Graphite
d. Stainless steel
Ans. d

Ref: Misch 3/e p 1076

26. Best acceptable theory of setting of amalgam is:
a. Hydration
b. Colloidal
c. Phase conversion
d. Dissolution–precipitation
Ans. d

Ref: Philips 11/e p 259

27. Approach for management of severely extruded abutment tooth, loss of which will create distal extension area is:
a. Cast restoration
b. Extraction
c. Occlusal reconstruction
d. Endodontic treatment planning
Ans. d

Ref: Misch 2/e p 241

28. Adhesive cannot be given in ear prosthesis because:
a. Nerve and vessels are present
b. Facial skin is more mobile
c. Thickness of the skin
d. More sweat glands are present
Ans. b

Ref: Davenport 2/e p 286

29. Incorrect about microwave curing of denture:
a. PMMA can be cured in normal microwave
b. PMMA is activated by heat of microwave
c. Specially designed plastic flanks are used
d. Polymerisation occurs at increased rate
Ans. c

Ref: Philips 11/e p 734

30. Which of the following is incorrect?
a. Molten alloy flow from cusp to marginal area
b. Two staged burnout for plastic sprue
c. Sprue former flare more in high density alloys, while constricted in low density alloys
d. Diameter of the sprue former is greater than the thickest portion of the wax pattern
Ans. d

Ref: Philips 11/e p 323

31. A patient complaints that his cast partial denture impinge on mucosa during function. On examination dentist found denture base with no imperfections or overextensions. The reason is:
a. Improper reciprocal arm
b. Improper retentive arm
c. Occlusal contact is high
d. Improper support or rest seat
Ans. d

Ref: Heartwell 2/e p 132

32. About laterotrusive movement true is:
a. Mandible shifts to left
b. During left lateral movement contact occurs between inner incline of maxillary buccal cusp and outer incline of mandibular buccal cusp
c. Both sides of teeth move in same direction
d. Lingual to lingual laterotrusive movement occur between the inner inclines of mandibular lingual cusp and inner inclines of mandibular lingual cusp
Ans. d

Ref: Okeson 5/e p 87

33. Which of the following is correct regarding angulation of both the jaws:
a. Maxillary anterior distally, posterior mesially
b. Mandibular anteriors straightly inclined, posteriors inclined mesially
c. Mandibular anteriors mesially inclined, posteriors inclined mesially
d. Maxillary anterior teeth are inclined distally, posterior teeth inclined distally
Ans. c

Ref: Okeson 6/e p 62

34. VHN of Zirconia is:
a. 350
b. 500
c. 700
d. 1300
Ans. d

Ref: Journal of Prosthodontics, 2013 April p239

35. Pipers stage IIIa for TMJ Dislocation is:
a. Medial click
b. Lateral lock
c. Lateral click
d. Medial lock
Ans. c

Ref: Dawson 2/e p 312

Stage I	Structurally intact TMJ
Stage II	Intermittent click
Stage III a	Lateral pole click
Stage III b	Lateral pole lock
Stage IV a	Medial pole click
Stage IV b	Medial pole lock
Stage V a	Perforation with acute degenerative joint disease
Stage V b	Perforation with chronic degenerative joint disease

36. All are true about residual ridge resorption except:
a. Loss of bundle bone
b. Maxillary buccal cortical bone resorbs more than palatal or lingual bone
c. Rate of resorption of maxillary bone is 0.1 mm/year and mandibular bone is 0.4 mm/year
d. 60% reduction in vertical height, 40% reduction in width
Ans. a

Ref: Winkler 2/e p 23

37. Wrought alloy is:
a. Having granular grain structure
b. Not used in prosthodontics
c. Used in reciprocating and retentive arm of cast partial denture
d. Used in retentive arm only
Ans. b

Ref: Stewart RPD 2/e p 67

38. Main complication during implant placement for an ear prosthesis:
a. Soft tissue overlying mastoid
b. Presence of nerves and vessels
c. Air cells in mastoid sinus
d. Presence of sigmoid sinus under mastoid process
Ans. b

Ref: Peterson 2/e p 304

39. Soft lining materials are all except:
a. Silicon based
b. Polyphosphate
c. Polyurethane
d. Vinyl resin
Ans. c

Ref: Boucher 12/e p 200

40. Mandibular and maxillary cast partial dentures are to be given, frameworks have been adjusted for occlusion individually. On placement of both the frameworks the teeth are in hyperocclusion when placed together, the premature contacts are due to:
a. Teeth are in occlusion
b. Both maxillary and mandibular framework
c. Maxillary natural teeth against maxillary framework
d. Mandibular natural teeth against maxillary framework
Ans. b

Ref: Stewart 2/e p 1227

41. Which of the following is false about O-ring:
a. Hardest O-ring 80–90 Shore A
b. Softest O-ring 30–40 Shore A
c. Water based lubricants damage the O-rings
d. They are composed of nitrile, silicon, ethylene, propylene fluorocarbon
Ans. c

Ref: Misch 2/e p 768

42. Randomized control trials are based on:
a. CONSORT
b. PRISMA
c. STROBE
d. STARD
Ans. a

Ref: Community Dental Health by Jong 2/e p 122

43. True about zirconia is:
a. May create problems during MRI
b. Yield strength of zirconia is 700-800
c. It has lower modulus of elasticity
d. Radioactive isotopes may cause radioactive emission
Ans. d

Ref: Babbush 2/e p 189

44. Pre surgical nasoalveolar moulding includes all except:
a. Improvement of esthetics of nasolabial complex
b. Successful in delayed management of both unilateral and bilateral cleft anomalies
c. Positioning of deformed soft tissue and cartilage in cleft surgery
d. Columellar elongation to form nasocolumella through a non surgical approach
Ans. b

Ref: Davenport 2/e p 119

45. True about outermost surface of condyle:
a. Mesenchymal cells lining outer surface
b. Fibrous connective tissue and hyaline cartilage to bear functional load
c. Fibrous connective tissue lining to bear the functional load
d. Chondroblasts and chondrocytes line outer surface
Ans. b

Ref: Okeson 5/e p 9

46. All are true with respect to all on four concept except:
a. Eliminates the need for bone graft
b. Reduced postoperative complications
c. Cost is less
d. Good biomechanics
Ans. d

Ref: Ajay Vikram Singh 2/e p 578

47. In the chewing cycle before the initiation of crushing phase there is:
a. Mandible shifts slightly upward and then laterally
b. Food is placed on the occlusal table between the teeth
c. Lateral movements 5–6 mm from the midline
d. Simultaneous downward and, lateral movement
Ans. c

Ref: Okeson 5/e p 45

48. The minimum acceptable power of study should be:
a. 0.5
b. 0.6
c. 0.7
d. 0.8
Ans. d

Ref: Mahajan 6/e p 14

49. Errors in occlusion during processing of complete dentures are due to all except:
a. Incomplete closure of flask
b. Rapid heating of the flask
c. Warpage of the denture due to heat produced during finishing
d. Too much pressure application
Ans. b

Ref: Manappallil 2/e p 127

50. Patient complaints of looseness of RPD during function, the problem lies in:
a. Support
b. Stability
c. Retention
d. Reciprocation
Ans. c

Ref: McCracken 11/e p 92

51. TMJ is called ginglimoidal joint because:
a. Gliding and rotation
b. Hinge and gliding
c. Hinge movement
d. Hinge movement and gliding along the axes of condyle
Ans. c

Ref: Okeson 6/e p 12

52. RPD is given in:
a. Bilateral stabilization
b. Patient cannot afford the prosthesis
c. Severely resorbed ridge
d. Fixed prosthesis cannot be given
Ans. d

Ref: Nallaswamy 1/e p 268

53. Water powder ratio in Type III gypsum is:
a. 0.45–0.50
b. 0.25–0.28
c. 0.28–0.30
d. 0.35–0.40
Ans. c

Ref: Philips 11/e p 273

54. Mandibular guiding appliance should be given
a. Immediately after surgery
b. 2 weeks after surgery
c. 3 months after surgery
d. After radiation and chemotherapy
Ans. b

Ref: JPD 1964: 14: 992–99

55. A patient with bruxism is advised to wear splint for 6 months. True statement is:
a. Bruxism will heal spontaneously
b. Bruxism gets cured
c. Appliance can be discontinued
d. The appliance reduces the proprioceptive inputs to the brain
Ans. d

Ref: Okeson 6/e p 468

56. In an edentulous patient with Parkinsons disease the best treatment option is:
a. Fixed implant retained prosthesis
b. Conventional complete denture
c. Implant tissue supported overdenture
d. Implant supported overdenture
Ans. d

Ref: Babbush 1/e p 120

57. True statement regarding the role of nasal turbinates in maxillectomy defects are all except:
a. Nasal turbinates should be removed as they enlarge with time
b. In small lesions involving midline or soft palate they are not utilized
c. Removing the inferior turbinate the prosthesis can be contoured to fit into the nasal cavity
d. Undercuts along the line of palatal resection into nasal or paranasal cavity or medial wall of defect can increase retention
Ans. a

Ref: Applied Anatomy Last 5/e p 179

58. A 25-year-old female presented with defect in midfacial region maxilla and nose resected. The premaxilla was missing and a few loose abutment teeth are present. The patient is a known case of Non Hodgkin Lymphoma, has undergone surgery radiotherapy and chemotherapy 6 months ago. The best treatment modality to improve her esthetics:
a. Obturator and nasal prosthesis retained with magnets
b. Obturator and nasal prosthesis retained with adhesive
c. Implant retained obturator and nasal prosthesis
d. Obturator and spectacle retained acrylic nasal prosthesis
Ans. a

Ref: Davenport 2/e p 232

59. About evisceration true statement is:
a. The sclera and extraocular muscles are preserved
b. The sclera and extraocular muscles are sacrificed
c. All the contents of the orbit along with eyelids are removed
d. All the contents of the orbit are removed
Ans. a

Ref: Curtis 3/e p 298

60. Blatterfein survey lines:
a. Low, high, medium, diagonal
b. Near zone, far zone
c. Low, High, intermediate, perpendicular
d. Esthetic and unesthetic zone
Ans. a

Ref: Nallaswamy 1/e p 311

61. Which of the following is true about muscle spindles:
a. Stimulation of alpha nerve fibers cause contraction of intrafusal fibers
b. Spindles are arranged parallel to each other
c. Muscle spindles are supplied by two afferent nerve one larger and other smaller one
d. Intrafusal and extrafusal muscle spindle with connective tissue form muscle spindle
Ans. c

Ref: Okeson 6/e p 32

62. All of the following are true about immediate implants except:
a. The presence of microthreads leads to more bone resorption in the crestal area
b. Not recommended in the thin gingival biotypes

c. Jumping defect of 2 mm or less may heal spontaneously
d. A movement equal to 150 micrometre may lead to formation of fibrous encapsulation around the implant
Ans. a

Ref: Misch 2/e p 118

63. Regarding ring liner the false statement is:
a. The ends of the liner should be overlapped instead of a butt joint
b. The ring liner should not be squeezed as it will result in non uniform expansion
c. The length of the liner is somewhat shorter than the ring itself
d. If thickness is increased it will result in more expansion
Ans. a

Ref: Philips 11/e p 323

64. Sigma implant is:
a. Titanium
b. Subperiosteal
c. Zirconia
d. Stainless steel implant
Ans. c

Ref: Misch 3/e p 321

65. DIEM 2 concept for edentulous patients was given by:
a. Misch
b. Branemark
c. Tarnow
d. Paulo Malo
Ans. d

Ref: Babbush 3/e p 120

66. Best tool to measure the productivity and validity of publication of scientific research is determined by:
a. Impact factor
b. Visibility in pubmed
c. Citation index
d. H index
Ans. d

Ref: Park 15/e p 332

67. Surface modification of implant is done by all except:
a. Tetracycline
b. Metronidazole
c. Gentamycin
d. Simvastatin
Ans. b

Ref: Misch 2/e p 453

68. Arrangement of teeth in monoplane occlusion:
a. Maxillary buccal cusp tip lies over the crest of the mandibular ridge
b. Maxillary occlusal forces lie over the slopes of the mandible
c. Reduced horizontal overlap results in cheek biting
d. In case of orthognathic ridge relation, anterior teeth are arranged with no overjet
Ans. c

Ref: Misch 2/e p 223

69. The probing depth of healthy peri implant sulcus is:
a. 0 mm
b. 1–2 mm
c. 2.5–4 mm
d. 6–7 mm
Ans. c

Ref: Misch 3/e p 434

70. Not true about mitotic jaw reflex:
a. Jaw opening
b. Contraction
c. No relay to the cerebral cortex
d. Responsible for maintenance of tonicity of the muscle
Ans. a

Ref: Okeson 5/e p 42

71. Disadvantage of fluid resin technique:
a. Expensive
b. Technique sensitive
c. Inferior adaptation to the tissue surfaces
d. Teeth movement like processing
Ans. d

Ref: Philips 11/e p 736

72. Which of the following is correct regarding angulation of both the jaws:
a. Maxillary anterior distally, posterior mesially
b. Mandibular anterior are inclined straight, posteriors are inclined mesially
c. Mandibular anteriors are inclined mesially posteriors are inclined mesially
d. Maxillary anterior teeth are inclined distally, posterior teeth inclined distally
Ans. c

Ref: Okeson 6/e p 62

73. Cantilever fixed prosthesis comprise of all except:
a. More lateral forces on the abutment tooth
b. Midpoint between most mesial and distal abutment is defined as mechanical advantage
c. Non axial forces are applied on the periodontium of the abutment teeth
d. Type II lever mechanism
Ans. d

Ref: J Prosthetic Dentistry 1992; 67 484–7

74. Lateral pole disc derangement is due to all except:
a. Muscle innervations
b. Distalising after intercuspal interference
c. Distalising of non working condyle
d. Trauma
Ans. c

Ref: Dawson 3/e p 281

75. Nonrigid connector is indicated in:
a. To provide less force in prosthesis
b. To provide less forces in the anterior segment
c. In long span fixed dental prosthesis
d. Excessive reduction of tooth for contouring is required
Ans. d

Ref: Shillingburg 3/e p 97

76. Pankey Mann Schyuler and Takayama and Hobo occlusal philosophies differ mainly in:
a. Plane of occlusion
b. Number of contacts during lateral movements
c. Number of interocclusal records made
d. Type of articulator used
Ans. c

Ref: Davenport 2/e p 321

77. Which of the following is not true:
a. Thickness of Ce-TZP coping can be a minimum of 0.3 mm
b. Ce-TZP is stronger than Y-TZP
c. Ce-TZP/alumina nanocomposites is the toughest ceramic available
d. Ce-TZP/ Alumina nanocomposites show LTAD (Low temperature ageing degradation)
Ans. b

Ref: JPD 57 (2013) 236–261

78. A patient needs mandibular and maxillary implants and has to undergo radiotherapy. At what time implant should be placed:
a. Placement before the radiation therapy
b. 6 months after the radiation therapy
c. Immediately after radiotherapy
d. After surgery immediately before chemo and radiotherapy
Ans. d

Ref: Misch 3/e p 460

79. To evaluate the path of insertion of RPD, what should be checked:
a. Guideplanes, retentive undercuts, interferences, esthetics
b. Guideplanes, retentive undercuts, interferences, edentulous areas
c. Guideplanes, retentive undercuts, occlusion, esthetics
d. Guideplanes, retentice undercuts, remaining teeth, esthetics
Ans. b

Ref: McCrackens 11/e p 72

80. When a person looks forward the contraction of cervical muscle occurs, to balance this contraction which muscles are activated:
a. Suprahyoid, splenius capitis, sternocleidomastoid, trapezius
b. Suprahyoid, infrahyoid, splenius capitis, sternocleidomastoid
c. Masseter, Suprahyoids and infrahyoids
d. Suprahyoid, Infrahyoid, splenius capitis, masseter, trapezius
Ans. c

Ref: Okeson 5/e p 32

Oral Surgery SR Papers (July 2015)

1. **Burning mouth syndrome is called:**
   a. Glossopyrosis
   b. Glossoptosis
   c. Glossitis
   d. Glossophagia
   Ans. a

Ref: Shafer 7/e p 856

Burning mouth syndrome (BMS) is an idiopathic condition characterized by a continuous burning sensation of the mucosa of the mouth (Glossodynia) typically involving the tongue, with or without extension to the lips and oral mucosa. Classically, burning mouth syndrome (BMS) is accompanied by gustatory disturbances (dysgeusia, parageusia) and subjective xerostomia. By definition, no macroscopic alterations in oral mucosa are apparent. Burning mouth syndrome (BMS) occurs most frequently, but not exclusively, in perimenopausal and postmenopausal women.

2. **A patient of head injury shows pinpoint radiodensities on NCCT head with loss of sulci and gyri Definition is:**
   a. EDH
   b. SDH
   c. DAI
   d. SAH
   Ans. c

Ref: 1. Fonseca Vol 1 3/e p 226

2. Sanders MJ and McKenna K. 2001. Mosby's Paramedic Textbook, 2/e, Ch 22, 'Head and Facial Trauma'. Mosby.

Diffuse axonal injury (DAI) is a brain injury in which damage in the form of extensive lesions in white matter tracts occurs over a widespread area. DAI is one of the most common and devastating types of traumatic brain injury, and is a major cause of unconsciousness and persistent vegetative state after head trauma. It occurs in about half of all cases of severe head trauma.

The outcome is frequently coma, with over 90% of patients with severe DAI never regaining consciousness. Those who do wake up often remain significantly impaired.

DAI can occur in every degree of severity from very mild or moderate to very severe. Concussion may be a milder type of diffuse axonal injury.

Diagnosis

DAI is difficult to detect since it does not show up well on CT scans or with other macroscopic imaging techniques, though it shows up microscopically. However, there are characteristics typical of DAI that may or may not show up on a CT scan. Diffuse injury has more microscopic injury than macroscopic injury and is difficult to detect with CT and MRI, but its presence can be inferred when small bleeds are visible in the corpus callosum or the cerebral cortex. MRI is more useful than CT for detecting characteristics of diffuse axonal injury in the subacute and chronic timeframes. Newer studies such as Diffusion Tensor Imaging are able to demonstrate the degree of white matter fiber tract injury even when the standard MRI is negative. Since axonal damage in DAI is largely a result of secondary biochemical cascades, it has a delayed onset so a person with DAI who initially appears well may deteriorate later. Thus; injury is frequently more severe than is realized, and medical professionals should suspect DAI in any patients whose CT scans appear normal but who have symptoms like unconsciousness.

MRI is more sensitive than CT scans, but MRI may also miss DAI, because it identifies the injury using signs of edema, which may not be present. There may be some pinpoint hyperdense lesions too often.

DAI is classified into grades based on severity of the injury. In Grade I, widespread axonal damage is present but no focal abnormalities are seen. In Grade II, damage found in Grade I is present in addition to focal abnormalities, especially in the corpus callosum. Grade III damage encompasses both Grades I and II plus rostral brainstem injury and often tears in the tissue.

3. **Gene involved in cherubism is:**
   a. SH4BP2
   b. SH4BP5
   c. SH3BP1
   d. SH3BP2

   Ans. d

Ref: Neville 2/e p 187

Mutations in the SH3BP2 gene have been identified in about 80 percent of people with cherubism. In most of the remaining cases, the genetic cause of the condition is unknown.

The SH3BP2 gene provides instructions for making a protein whose exact function is unclear. The protein plays a role in transmitting chemical signals within cells, particularly cells involved in the replacement of old bone tissue with new bone (bone remodeling) and certain immune system cells.

Mutations in the SH3BP2 gene lead to the production of an overly active version of this protein. The effects of SH3BP2 mutations are still under study, but researchers believe that the abnormal protein disrupts critical signaling pathways in cells associated with the maintenance of bone tissue and in some immune system cells. The overactive protein likely causes inflammation in the jaw bones and triggers the production of osteoclasts, which are cells that break down bone tissue during bone remodeling. An excess of these bone-eating cells contributes to the destruction of bone in the upper and lower jaws. A combination of bone loss and inflammation likely underlies the cyst-like growths characteristic of cherubism.

4. **In alloplastic reconstruction of TMJ, head of the condyle should be placed at:**
   a. Posteriormost position on the fossa
   b. Superiormost position on the fossa
   c. Anteriormost position on the fossa
   d. 1 mm below the fossa to create the joint space

   Ans. a

Ref: Okeson 2/e p 232

5. **The position of the lingual nerve is:**
   a. 2 mm inferior and 0.5 mm lingual to lingual alveolar crest
   b. 2 mm inferior and 2 mm lingual to lingual alveolar crest
   c. 5 mm inferior and 5 mm lingual to lingual alveolar crest
   d. 5 mm inferior and 2 mm lingual to lingual alveolar crest

   Ans. a

Ref: Chamberlain and Kiesselbach et al in AJOMFS 1988, (4) vol 3 p 211–24

The mean horizontal distance of the nerve from the lingual plate is having been reported to range from 0.58 mm to 3.45 mm. The nerve has been shown to contact the lingual plate directly from 22% to 62% of the time. The mean vertical distance of the lingual nerve below the alveolar crest has similarly been demonstrated to be from 2.28 mm to 8.32 mm. Additionally, the nerve can be found above the lingual crest in 4.6% to 17.6% of cases and lie within the retromolar tissues in 0-15%.

Kiesselbach and Chamberlain were the first to present quantitative data on the position of the lingual nerve in the mandibular third molar area. The position of the lingual nerve was measured in 34 cadaver dissections and 256 cases of third molar extraction cases. The average horizontal distance of the nerve from the lingual plate was 0.58 ± 0.90 mm and the nerve contacted the lingual plate of the third molar in 62% of the cases. The average vertical distance of the lingual nerve was 2.28 ± 1.96 mm below the alveolar crest. In 17.6% of the dissections, however, the nerve was found at the level of the alveolar crest or higher and even in the retromolar tissues. Of the 256 extraction cases, the nerve was visualized above the lingual plate of the third molar region in 4.6% of the cases. Furthermore, 8.8% of the dissections showed 0.5 mm. thick flat nerves, thus demonstrating that a 25 gauge needle also 0.5 mm thick—could seriously damage the lingual nerve during anesthetic injections.

6. **Most preferred transport media is:**
   a. Viaspan
   b. HBSS
   c. Saliva
   d. Normal saline
   Ans. a

Ref: AIIMS Protocol, JOE 2014 (5) p 123–45*

7. **Polyglycolic sutures are:**
   a. Absorbable natural
   b. Nonabsorbable natural
   c. Absorbable synthetic
   d. Nonabsorbable synthetic
   Ans. c

Ref: Vinod Kapoor 2/e p 20

Needles

Eyed or reusable needles are needles with holes or eyes which are supplied separate from their suture thread. The suture must be threaded on site, as is done when sewing at home. The advantage of this is that any thread and needle combination is possible to suit the job at hand. Swaged, or atraumatic, needles with sutures comprise a pre-packed eyeless needle attached to a specific length of suture thread. The suture manufacturer swages the suture thread to the eyeless atraumatic needle at the factory. The chief advantage of this is that the doctor or the nurse does not have to spend time threading the suture on the needle, which may be difficult for very fine needles and sutures. Also, the suture end of a swaged needle is narrower than the needle body, eliminating drag from the thread attachment site. In eyed needles, the thread protrudes from the needle body on both sides, and at best causes drag. When passing through friable tissues, the eye needle and suture combination may thus traumatise tissues more than a swaged needle, hence the designation of the latter as 'atraumatic'.

There are several shapes of surgical needles. These include:

- Straight
- 1/4 circle
- 3/8 circle
- 1/2 circle. Subtypes of this needle shape include, from larger to smaller size, CT, CT-1, CT-2 and CT-3.
- 5/8 circle
- Compound curve
- Half-curved (also known as ski)
- Half-curved at both ends of a straight segment (also known as canoe)

The ski and canoe needle design allows curved needles to be straight enough to be used in laparoscopic surgery, where instruments are inserted into the abdominal cavity through narrow cannulas.

Needles may also be classified by their point geometry; examples include:

- Taper (needle body is round and tapers smoothly to a point)
- Cutting (needle body is triangular and has a sharpened cutting edge on the inside curve)
- Reverse cutting (cutting edge on the outside)
- Trocar point or tapercut (needle body is round and tapered, but ends in a small triangular cutting point)
- Blunt points for sewing friable tissues
- Side-cutting or spatula points (flat on top and bottom with a cutting edge along the front to one side) for eye surgery
- Finally, atraumatic needles may be permanently swaged to the suture or may be designed to come off the suture with a sharp straight tug. These 'pop-offs' are commonly used for interrupted sutures, where each suture is only passed once and then tied.

8. **A 70-year-old male patient has undergone resection and reconstruction of mandible. On 7th postoperative day, he presents with 98.8 degrees F fever and TLC count 10,000. The treatment is:**

a. IV fluids
b. Local infection control at the surgical site
c. Check ESR
d. Check for immunodeficiency

Ans. b

Ref: Peterson 1/e p 77

9. Noninvasive way to measure saturation of the patient:

a. Capnography
b. End tidal CO_2
c. Polysomnography
d. Pulse oximetry

Ans. d

Ref: Fonseca 3/e p 332

10. Not a reversible COX inhibitor:

a. Aspirin
b. Tenoxicam
c. Nabumetone
d. Naproxen

Ans. a

Ref: Katzung 9/e p 764

11. Which of the following indices is not used to evaluate the difficulty of extraction:

a. Parent scale
b. Pell-Gregory index
c. Peterson index
d. Pederson scale

Ans. c

Ref: Howe 2/e p 21

12. Which of the following bones transmits the cranial nerve carrying the sensation of smell:

a. Cribriform plate of ethmoid
b. Lacrimal bone
c. Lesser wing of sphenoid
d. Greater wing of sphenoid

Ans. a

Ref: Last Applied Anatomy 5/e p 219

13. The opening of frontal sinus is:

a. Anterolateral
b. Anteromedial
c. Posteromedial
d. Posterolateral

Ans. b

Ref: Chaurasia 3/e p 198

14. Circumzygomatic suspension is used in:

a. Lefort I
b. Lefort II
c. ZMC
d. NOE

Ans. a

Ref: Fonseca 3/e p 129

15. In a patient with Lefort III fracture, protocol for management of meningitis should be:
 a. Started if CSF leak is present
 b. Used immediately along 'with or without' waiting for any symptom
 c. Not necessary
 d. Is mandatory always
 Ans. a

Ref: Harrison 18/e p 2217

16. In a patient, forced duction test is positive and there is muscle entrapment:
 a. Muscle repair surgery is needed
 b. Facelift is often done
 c. Orbital floor reconstruction should be done
 d. Give steroids and other medicines and defer surgery for a week
 Ans. c

Ref: Fonseca 3/e vol 2 p 671

17. In the management of angle fracture, maximum complications occur with:
 a. Reconstruction plates
 b. 2 miniplates
 c. Closed reduction and IMF
 d. 2 AO plates
 Ans. d

18. Early secondary alveolar grafting, TRUE is:
 a. At 2–4 years
 b. After the eruption of lateral incisor, but before the eruption of canine
 c. After rhinoplasty or palatal or lip repair
 d. At 7–12 years
 Ans. a

Ref: Ward Booth 2/e p 871

19. Crouzon syndrome is:
 a. Craniofacial dysostosis
 b. Cleidocranial dysplasia
 c. Syndactly
 d. Apertognathia
 Ans. a

Ref: Ward Booth 2/e p 1123

Crouzon syndrome is an autosomal dominant genetic disorder known as a branchial arch syndrome. Specifically, this syndrome affects the first branchial (or pharyngeal) arch, which is the precursor of the maxilla and mandible. Since the branchial arches are important developmental features in a growing embryo, disturbances in their development create lasting and widespread effects.

This syndrome is named after Octave Crouzon, a French physician, who first described this disorder. He noted the affected patients were a mother and her daughter, implying a genetic basis. First called 'craniofacial dysostosis', the disorder was characterized by a number of clinical features. This syndrome is caused by a mutation in the fibroblast growth factor receptor II, located on chromosome 10.

Breaking down the name, 'craniofacial' refers to the skull and face, and 'dysostosis' refers to malformation of bone.

Now known as Crouzon syndrome, the disease can be described by the rudimentary meanings of its former name. What occurs in the disease is that an infant's skull and facial bones, while in development, fuse early or are unable to expand. Thus, normal bone growth cannot occur. Fusion of different sutures leads to different patterns of growth of the skull. Examples include: trigonocephaly (fusion of the metopic suture), brachycephaly (fusion of the coronal suture), dolichocephaly (fusion of the sagittal suture), plagiocephaly (unilateral premature closure of lambdoid and coronal sutures), oxycephaly (fusion of coronal and lambdoidal sutures), Kleeblattschäedel (premature closure of all sutures).

Treatment

A child with Crouzon syndrome wearing a corrective cranial band.

Surgery is typically used to prevent the closure of sutures of the skull from damaging the brain's development. Without surgery, blindness and mental retardation are typical outcomes. Craniofacial surgery is a discipline of both plastic surgery and oral and maxillofacial surgery (OMS) . To move the orbits forward, craniofacial surgeons expose the skull and orbits and reshape the bone. To treat the midface deficiency, craniofacial surgeons can move the lower orbit and midface bones forward. For jaw surgery, either plastic surgeons or oral and maxillofacial (OMFS) surgeons can perform these operations. Crouzon patients tend to have multiple sutures involved, most specifically bilateral coronal craniosynostoses, and either open vault surgery or strip craniectomy (if child is under 6 months) can be performed. In the later scenario, a helmet is worn for several months following surgery.

Once treated for the cranial vault symptoms, Crouzon patients generally go on to live a normal lifespan.

Dental Significance

For dentists, this disorder is important to understand since many of the physical abnormalities are present in the head, and particularly the oral cavity. Common features are a narrow/high-arched palate, posterior bilateral crossbite, hypodontia (missing some teeth), and crowding of teeth. Due to maxillary hypoplasia, Crouzon patients generally have a considerable permanent underbite and subsequently cannot chew using their incisors. For this reason, people with Crouzon syndrome sometimes eat in an unusual way—eating chicken drumsticks with a fork, for example, or breaking off pieces of a sandwich rather than taking a bite into it.

20. All are visible in Pierre Robin syndrome except:
  a. Ankyloglossia
  b. Macroglossia
  c. Cleft palate
  d. Short mandible

  Ans. a

Ref: Shafers 7/e p 721

Pierre Robin syndrome (abbreviated to PRS, and also known as Pierre Robin malformation, Pierre Robin anomaly or Pierre Robin anomalad) is a congenital condition of facial abnormalities in humans. PRS is a sequence, i.e. a chain of certain developmental malformations, one entailing the next. The 3 main features are cleft palate, retrognathia (abnormal positioning of the jaw or maxilla) and glossoptosis (airway obstruction caused by backward displacement of the tongue base). A genetic cause to PRS was recently identified. Pierre Robin sequence may be caused by genetic anomalies at chromosomes.

Signs and Symptoms

PRS is characterized by an unusually small mandible (micrognathia), posterior displacement or retraction of the tongue (glossoptosis), and upper airway obstruction. Incomplete closure of the roof of the mouth (cleft palate) is present in the majority of patients, and is commonly U-shaped.

Causes and Associated Conditions

It is not known how this abnormality occurs in infants, but one theory is that, at some time during the stage of the formation of the bones of the fetus, the tip of the jaw (mandible) becomes 'stuck' in the point where each of the collar bones (clavicle) meet (the sternum), effectively preventing the jaw bones from growing. It is thought that, at about 12 to 14 weeks gestation, when the fetus begins to move, the movement of the head causes the jaw to 'pop out' of the collar bones. From this time on, the jaw of the fetus grows as it would normally, with the result that, when born, the jaw of the baby is much smaller (micrognathia) than it would have been with normal development, although it does continue to grow at a normal rate until the child reaches maturity.

However, association with gene loci 2q24.1-33.3, 4q32-qter, 11q21-23.1, and 17q21-24.3 has been found. Recent studies have indicated that genetic dysregulation of SOX9 gene prevents the SOX9 protein from properly controlling the development of facial structures, which leads to isolated PRS. Similarly, KCNJ2 gene also has a role to play. Overlap with certain other genetic syndromes like Patau syndrome has also been found.

PRS may occur in isolation, but it is often part of an underlying disorder or syndrome. The most common is Stickler syndrome. Other disorders causing PRS, according to Dr. Robert J. Sphrintzen Ph.D of the Center for Craniofacial Disorders, Montefiore Medical Center, are velocardiofacial syndrome, fetal alcohol syndrome and Treacher Collins syndrome. For more disorders associated with PRS, see Dr Shprintzen's article entitled. 'The Implications of the Diagnosis of Robin Sequence'.

Diagnosis

The syndrome is generally diagnosed clinically shortly after birth. The infant usually has respiratory difficulty, especially when supine. The cleft palate is often U-shaped and wider than in cleft palate that is not associated with this syndrome.

Management

The goals of treatment in infants with Robin sequence focus upon breathing and feeding, and optimizing growth and nutrition despite the predisposition for breathing difficulties. If there is evidence of airway obstruction (snorty breathing, apnea, difficulty taking a breath, or drops in oxygen), then the infant should be placed in the sidelying or prone position, which helps bring the tongue base forward in many children. One study of 60 infants with PRS found that 63% of infants responded to prone positioning (Smith and Senders, 2006, Int J Pediatr Oto). 53% of the infants in this study required some form of feeding assistance, either nasogastric tube or gastrostomy tube feedings (feeding directly into the stomach). In a separate study of 115 children with the clinical diagnosis of PRS managed at 2 different hospitals in Boston (Evans et al., 2006, Int J Pediatr Oto), respiratory distress was managed successfully in 56% without an operation (either by prone positioning, short-term intubation, or placement of a nasopharyngeal airway). In this study, gastrostomy tube feedings were placed in 42% of these infants due to feeding difficulties.

Gastroesophageal Reflux (GER) seems to be more prevalent in children with Robin sequence (Dudkiewicz, March 2000, CPCJ). Because reflux of acidic contents in the posterior pharynx and upper airway can intensify the symptoms of Robin sequence, specifically by worsening airway obstruction, it is important to maximize treatment for GER in children with PRS and Reflux symptoms. Treatment may include upright positioning on a wedge (a tucker sling may be needed if the baby is in the prone position), small and frequent feedings (to minimize vomiting), and/or pharmacotherapy (such as proton pump inhibitors).

21. During surgery in an 8-year-old child:

a. Parent's legal guardian cannot give consent
b. Consent from parent's/legal guardian only
c. Consent from parent's/legal guardian with assent to the child
d. Consent can be taken from children below 12 years of age

Ans. c

Ref: Reddy 19/e p 112

22. Sellick's maneuver is done for:

a. Pressure over cricoid to prevent aspiration
b. Pressure on hyoid bone to prevent bleeding from branches of carotid artery
c. Pressure on bilateral angles of mandible to reduce a parasymphyseal fracture
d. BURP (Backward, Upward, Rightward pressure) over larynx to assist intubation

Ans. a

Ref: Fonseca 3/e p 149

Sellick's maneuver, the application of pressure to a patient's cricoid cartilage during endotracheal intubation, is supposed to prevent aspiration. The procedure was named after British anesthetist Brian A. Sellick, following an article in the prestigious British medical journal 'The Lancet' (Sellick). In a series of cadaver experiments, the cadavers' stomachs were filled with water and cricoid pressure was applied. Then the cadavers were placed into a steep Trendelenburg position.

Sellick found that cricoid pressure, when applied, did not cause regurgitation of fluid into the pharynx. Thus, we in the medical community assumed it worked. In fact, during residency in the late 1980s, I was taught that it would stop regurgitation pressures up to 100 cm/H_2O. It became an integral part of rapid sequence induction (RSI)—especially when dealing with a trauma patient who invariably had just ingested a pepperoni pizza and several liters of beer.

Several researchers have subsequently looked at Sellick's maneuver and have come to the conclusion that it probably does little good and, in fact, can sometimes obscure the view of the operator. In 1983, in a study to determine how much pressure is routinely applied during Sellick's maneuver, researchers found that while over 78 percent of anesthetists surveyed routinely used the maneuver, 70 percent had experienced a problem with its application. Interestingly, the average force applied was 44.6 N while 47 percent of anesthetists failed to reach a force of 44 N. This indicated that the applied pressure varied greatly. (Howells)

KG Allman found that application of cricoid pressure, even by experienced anesthetists, caused some degree of airway obstruction and, in some cases, caused complete airway obstruction. (Allman) Other researchers reported a case of cricoid cartilage fracture following cricoid pressure during RSI for status asthmaticus. (Heath) British researchers, in 2005 performed a systematic review of the literature regarding cricoid pressure/Sellick's maneuver and wrote, "There is little evidence to support the widely held belief that the application of cricoid pressure reduces the incidence of aspiration during a rapid sequence intubation." (Butler) Australian researchers completed a detailed review of the procedure in the last month's issue of Annals of Emergency Medicine. They concluded:

"Cricoid pressure entered medical practice on a limited evidence base but with common sense supporting its use. Given that the risks of cricoid pressure worsening laryngeal view and reducing airway patency have been well described, we recommend that the removal of cricoid pressure be an immediate consideration if there is any difficulty either in intubating or ventilating the ED patient." (Ellis)

In summary, the scientific literature is telling us that we need educated paramedics, who can apply critical thinking to problems encountered. Sellick's maneuver (cricoid pressure) is possibly helpful in some patients and not so in others. Likewise, it may be harmful in some patients and not so in others. It is simply another tool in your airway armamentarium. If it helps, use it. If not, don't. Forcing students to use cricoid pressure as part of some skills test will emphasize that the procedure should be used every time. Like many things in EMS, Sellick's maneuver is not the panacea we once thought. It is simply another possible tool to use — nothing more, nothing less.

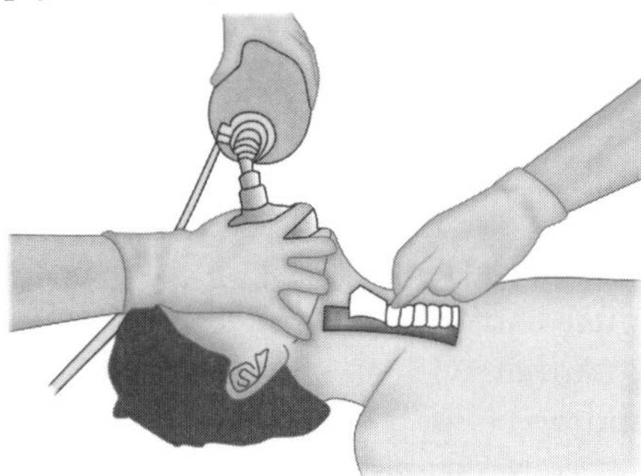

23. Due to TMJ ankylosis, there is obstructive sleep apnea in a 2-year-old child:

a. Bilateral costochondral graft
b. Bilateral sternoclavicular graft
c. Gap arthroplasty and secondary distraction osteogenesis
d. Wait till the development of ramus condylar unit

Ans. c

Ref: CCD Jan 2012 Vol 3 Issue 1/p 69–74

24. For the growth in the ramal-condylar unit, cartilage part in costochondral graft should be:

a. 4–7 mm
b. 2–4 mm
c. 7–10 mm
d. 10–12 mm

Ans. b

Ref: Ward Booth 2/e p 871

Costochondral grafts in the treatment of temporomandibular joint ankylosis.

The main causes of TMJ ankylosis are trauma and infection. Estimates of a traumatic origin range from 26% to 75% and of infection from 44% to 68%.

Also, the children were too young at the time the TMJ ankylosis set in, to have experienced trauma, for it to be the main cause. Use of the autogenous costochondral interpositional graft is an effective procedure for the prevention of reankylosis following the surgical release of TMJ ankylosis. Replacement of the condyle with a costochondral graft restores the altered biomechanics after condylectomy or gap-arthroplasty procedures. In case of a growing child, the interpositional material should not only fill the gap but should also reduce the facial deformity and induce normal growth potential of the mandible. Various growth center transplants have been used but costochondral junction graft has been found to be the material of choice as an interposition in ankylosis in growing children. The rib cartilage has capabilities similar to that of the condylar cartilage and when a costochondral graft is used to replace

TMJ apparatus and subjected to functional movements, it can function as a replacement for the mandibular condyle both histologically and physiologically. The cartilaginous portions of such grafts adapt well to the function of the reconstructed temporomandibular joint and to the ramus vertical dimension by reproducing condylar morphology. According to Macintosh, the advantages of this graft are its biological compatibility, workability and functional adaptability. The growth potential of the costochondral graft makes it the ideal choice in children. This graft has also the advantage of a predictable behavior.

The 7-step protocol in the treatment of temporomandibular joint ankylosis consists of:

(a) Aggressive excision of the fibrous and/or bony ankylotic mass
(b) Coronoidectomy on the affected side
(c) Coronoidectomy on the contralateral side, if steps a and b do not result in a maximal incisal opening greater than 35 mm or to the point of dislocation of the unaffected TMJ
(d) Lining of the TMJ with a temporalis myofascial flap or the native disc, if it can be salvaged
(e) Reconstruction of the ramus condyle unit with either distraction osteogenesis or costochondral graft and rigid fixation
(f) Early mobilization of the jaw. If distraction osteogenesis is used to reconstruct the ramus condyle unit, mobilization begins the day of the operation. In patients who undergo costochondral graft reconstruction, mobilization begins after 10 days of maxillomandibular fixation.
(g) Aggressive physiotherapy.

A mandibular opening of 30 mm is sufficient to leave patients with little or no functional deficit following reconstruction.

25. **Which nerve is damaged most frequently while taking graft from the anterior iliac crest:**
   a. Medial femoral cutaneous nerve
   b. Lateral femoral cutaneous nerve
   c. Saphenous nerve
   d. Ilioinguinal nerve

   Ans. a

Ref: Peterson 2/e p 791

26. **Calcitonin is used in the management of:**
   a. Lichen planus
   b. CGCG
   c. Ameloblastoma
   d. Pindborg tumour

   Ans. b

Ref: Thomas Oral Patho 3/e p 133

Central giant cell granulomas (CGCGs) of the jaws are rare benign intraosseous lesions that can quickly recur as indolent lesions in mandible, where they are more commonly found than in the maxilla. Conventional treatment is local curettage, which is associated with a high success rate and low recurrence rate. Recurrences have nonetheless been noted and studies suggest recurrence rates up to 20% with local curettage. A more aggressive curettage or enucleation has been recommended, possibly coupled with adjunctive treatment, such as liquid nitrogen cryotherapy. To minimize risk of poor esthetic or functional outcome, many clinicians treat aggressive CGCLs with intralesional triamcinolone, intranasal calcitonin or subcutaneous interferon alpha-2a. Radiation therapy and other chemotherapeutic agents, such as methotrexate, doxorubicin, and cyclophosphamide have been employed. Other alternative treatments include intralesional steroid injections at weekly intervals for six weeks. A number of alternative nonsurgical therapies have been advocated for the management of CGCG. Calcitonin antagonizes osteoclastic bone resorption and acts directly on other cell types in this lesion, and calcitonin receptors have been identified on giant cells of the lesion. Lim and Gibbins reported that immunohistochemistry suggests that stromal cells or fibroblasts are the etiologic basis of CGCG and that the giant cells themselves may be secondary or reactive.

27. **Massive osteolysis is also called:**
   a. Jennings syndrome
   b. Kasabach Merritt syndrome

c. Gorham's disease
d. Lobstein disease

Ans. c

Gorham's disease (pronounced GOR-amz), also known as **Gorham vanishing bone disease** and **phantom bone disease**, is a very rare skeletal condition of unknown cause, characterized by the uncontrolled proliferation of distended, thin-walled vascular or lymphatic channels within bone, which leads to resorption and replacement of bone with angiomas and/or fibrosis. Current treatments are experimental only.

The symptoms of Gorham's disease vary depending on the bones involved. It may affect any part of the skeleton, but the most common sites of disease are the shoulder, skull, pelvic girdle, jaw, ribs, and spine.

Causes

Bone mass and strength are obtained and maintained through a process of bone destruction and replacement that occurs at the cellular level throughout a person's life. Cells called osteoclasts secrete enzymes that dissolve old bone, allowing another type of cells called osteoblasts to form new bone. Except in growing bone, the rate of breakdown equals the rate of building up, thereby maintaining bone mass. In Gorham's disease that process is disrupted.

Gorham and Stout found that vascular anomalies always occupied space that normally would be filled with new bone and speculated that the presence of angiomatosis may lead to chemical changes in the bone. Gorham and others speculated that such a change in the bone chemistry might cause an imbalance in the rate of osteoclast activity to osteoblast activity such that more bone is dissolved than is replaced. Beginning in the 1990s, there were reports of elevated levels of a protein called interleukin-6 (IL-6) being detected in patients with the disease, leading some to suggest that increased levels of IL-6 and vascular endothelial growth factor (VEGF) may contribute to the chemical changes Gorham and others believed were the cause of this type of osteolysis.

In 1999 Möller and colleagues concluded, "The Gorham-Stout syndrome may be, essentially, a monocentric bone disease with a focally increased bone resorption due to an increased number of paracrine- or autocrine- stimulated hyperactive osteoclasts. The resorbed bone is replaced by a markedly vascularized fibrous tissue. The apparent contradiction concerning the presence or absence or the number of osteoclasts, may be explained by the different phases of the syndrome." They further stated that their histopathological study provided good evidence that osteolytic changes seen in Gorham's disease are the result of hyperactive osteoclastic bone. However, others have concluded that lymphangiomatosis and Gorham's disease should be considered as a spectrum of disease rather than separate diseases.

Diagnosis

In 1983, Heffez and colleagues published a case report in which they suggested eight criteria for a definitive diagnosis of Gorham's disease:

i. Positive biopsy with the presence of angiomatous tissue
ii. Absence of cellular atypia
iii. Minimal or no osteoblastic response or dystrophic calcifications
iv. Evidence of local bone progressive osseous resorption
v. Nonexpansile, nonulcerative lesions
vi. No involvement of viscera
vii. Osteolytic radiographic pattern
viii. Negative hereditary, metabolic, neoplastic, immunologic, or infectious etiology.

Management

Treatment of Gorham's disease is for the most part palliative and limited to symptom management.

Sometimes, the bone destruction spontaneously ceases and no treatment is required. But when the disease is progressive, aggressive intervention may be necessary. Duffy and colleagues reported that around 17% of patients with Gorham's disease in the ribs, shoulder, or upper spine experience extension of the disease into the chest, leading to tochylothorax with its serious consequences, and that the mortality rate in this group can reach as high as 64% without surgical intervention.

28. **Suspecting malignant ameloblastoma with expansile osteolytic lesions:**
    a. Palisaded centrally placed cells and along the outer side, there is reversal of polarity
    b. Parathyroid-related hormone

c. Age > 50 years
d. Rounded cells in follicle along the outer side of the elevated calcium levels

Ans. a

Ref: Thoma 3/e p 113

29. Mandibular fracture most frequently occurs with:

a. Completely impacted distoangular third molar
b. Completely impacted horizontal third molar
c. Completely impacted vertical third molar
d. Partially impacted mesioangular third molar

Ans. d

Ref: Howe 2/e p 55

30. A patient shows small well-defined noncorticated, well-defined radiolucent lesions on lateral skull X-ray with raised ESR with periapical lesion in relation with upper first molar showing sheets of plasma cells:

a. Multiple myeloma
b. Plasmacytoma
c. Paget's disease
d. Acute osteomyelitis of maxilla

Ans. a

Ref: Thoma 3/e p 188

31. Mechanism of fracture in Jefferson fracture is:

a. Hyperextension
b. Hyperflexion
c. Axial loading
d. Countercoup mechanism

Ans. c

Ref: Fonseca 3/e p 227

Jefferson fracture is the eponymous name given to a burst fracture of C1. It was originally described as a four-part fracture with double fractures through the anterior and posterior arches, but three-part and two-part fractures have also been described.

Pathology

Mechanism

A typical mechanism of injury is diving head first into shallow water. Axial loading along the axis of the cervical spine results in the occipital condyles being driven into the lateral masses of C1. Jefferson fracture is not normally associated with neurological deficiet although spinal cord injury may occur if there is a retropulsed fragment.

Associations

- 50% are associated with other C-spine injuries
- 33% are associated with a C2 fracture
- 25–50% of young children have concurrent head injury
- Vertebral artery injury
- Extra-cranial cranial nerve injury

Radiographic features

Plain film

Radiographs will show asymmetry in the odontoid view with displacement of the lateral mass(es) away from the odontoid peg. A distance of greater than 6 mm suggests ligamentous injury.

CT

CT demonstrates the fracture line which usually involves both the anterior and posterior arches. If there is injury to the transverse atlantal ligament, the atlantodens interval (ADI) increases. The normal ADI in the adult population is less than 3 mm; in pediatric populations, the normal distance is less than 5 mm.

MRI

The fracture will not be seen as well as with CT. However, localized soft-tissue injury will be apparent. Prevertebral hemorrhage or edema will identify injury at the level of C1/2. Ligamentous injury will also be demonstrated.
A fat-sat T2 sequence is useful in the trauma setting to help distinguish abnormal soft-tissue injury from normal fat.

Treatment and prognosis

Jefferson fractures are typically treated conservatively (hard-collar immobilization) provided the transverse atlantal ligament is considered intact (no widening of the atlanto-dens interval or intact ligament visualized on MRI).
In cases where the ligament is thought to be disrupted, the injury is considered unstable and more aggressive management is usually required. This includes halo immobilization, posterior C1-C2 lateral mass internal fixation or transoral internal fixation.

History and etymology

Named by **Sir Geoffrey Jefferson** (1886-1961), neurosurgeon from the UK

32. **Most commonly occurred single fracture of the mandible is:**
    a. Condyle
    b. Body
    c. Symphysis
    d. Angle
    Ans. d

Ref: Rowe and Williams 2/e p 112

33. **In EDCP the angulation of sliding holes is:**
    a. 45
    b. 25
    c. 85
    d. 125
    Ans. a

Ref: Killey 2/e p 19

34. **All are advantages of hexagonal screw except:**
    a. Lateral force is not required
    b. Axial force is not required
    c. Both forces are not required
    d. None of the above
    Ans. b

Ref: Ward Booth 2/e p 761

35. **All of the following are correct about EDCP except:**
    a. Converts downward force to compress alveolar gap
    b. Screws along fractured line move bone by around 0.8 cm each side
    c. Follows sliding principle
    d. Static screws are placed first along the fractured line followed by compression screws
    Ans. d

Ref: Fonseca 3/e p 1141

36. **Dautery's technique is used in:**
    a. Recurrent dislocation
    b. TMJ ankylosis
    c. Recurrent pericoronitis
    d. Parotid duct closure
    Ans. a

Ref: Neelima Malik 1/e p 200

37. Mechanism of action of povidone iodine is:
- a. Disruption of cell membrane
- b. Precipitates bacterial cell proteins
- c. Lysis of membrane and oxidizes cellular contents
- d. Damages cell wall

Ans. d

Ref: Katzung 10/e p 782

38. In mandibular canal:
- a. Vein lies inferior to nerve and artery lies buccal and superior to nerve
- b. Vein lies inferior to nerve and artery lies buccal and inferior to nerve
- c. Vein lies superior to nerve and artery lies lingual and superior to nerve
- d. Vein lies superior to nerve and artery lies lingual and inferior to nerve

Ans. c

Ref: Fonseca 3/e p 445

39. Bowlder Henry technique is related to:
- a. Cyst enucleation
- b. Tumour excision
- c. Oroantral fistula management
- d. Third molar lateral trephination

Ans. d

Ref: Enucleation of developing mandibular third molar by lateral trephination: a new approach. C.B. Henry Proc R Soc Medv.62(8); 1969 Aug

Bowdler Henry's Lateral trephination (1969): for germectomy, partially formed and unerrupted third molar (9-18 years age)

- The operation is performed as follows:
- Extended S-shaped incision is made from the retromolar fossa, across the external oblique ridge to the first molar.
- The soft tissues are readily elevated from the surface and retracted from the surface of bone and held away with Bowdler Henry retractor.

A round bur is used to trephine the position of the crypt of a third molar. When the anterior-posterior length of the crypt has been determined, the bur is used to make a vertical cut through the external plate at its anterior margin. A second cut through the outer cortex is made at the posterior end of the crypt at an angle of 450. A chisel applied in a vertical direction is used to out fracture the buccal plate, which is then delivered with a curved hemostat, thus exposing the crown of the third molar lying in its crypt.

A Warwick James' elevator is applied to the occlusal surface of the tooth and used to deliver it. Any follicular remnants are removed. The wound is irrigated and is sutured

40. According to AHA guidelines, infective endocarditis prophylaxis is needed for all except:
- a. PDA
- b. Cardial transplant recipient with valvular heart disease
- c. CHD with palliative shunt
- d. Completely repaired CHD with prosthesis during the first 6 months of the procedure

Ans. a

Ref: Carranza 10/e p 655

41. All are considered as accepted treatment protocols for OKC except:
- a. Enucleation and chemical application
- b. Cyst enucleation followed by 5% phenol application
- c. Complete marsupialization of cyst
- d. Initial marsupialization followed by late complete removal of cyst

Ans. c

Ref: Regezzi 3/e p 432

Odontogenic keratocysts (OKCs) are developmental odontogenic cysts of epithelial origin, first identified and described in 1876 and further characterized by Phillipsen in 1956.Pindborg and Hansen suggested the histologic criteria necessary to diagnose OKC in 1962. The initial terminology for an odontogenic keratocyst (OKC) was 'primordial cyst,' as the origin of the lesion was thought to be the tooth primordium. In 1992, the World Health Organization (WHO) histologic typing of odontogenic tumors listed 'odontogenic keratocyst' (OKC) as the preferred terminology for such cysts with a keratinized lining.

The odontogenic keratocyst (OKC) is known for its high recurrence rate, aggressive behavior, and its occasional association with the nevoid basal cell carcinoma syndrome (NBCCS). Three histologic variants were recognized initially: a parakeratinized variant, an orthokeratinized variant, and combination of the two. The less aggressive clinical behavior and recurrence pattern of the orthokeratinized variant ultimately warranted the designation of the orthokeratinized variant as a separate entity, 'orthokeratinized odontogenic cyst' (OOC).

NBCCS, also referred to as Gorlin-Goltz syndrome, is associated with a gene level disturbance of chromosome 9 and is transmitted as an autosomal dominant trait with high penetrance. This syndrome was established as an entity by Gorlin and Goltz in 1960 and has a low incidence of 1 in 56,000 people.

NBCCS is an ectomesodermal polydysplasia with numerous manifestations, characterized most often by cutaneous abnormalities, including multiple basal cell carcinomas, benign dermal cysts, palmar-plantar pits; craniodentofacial anomalies, such as odontogenic keratocyst (OKC), malocclusion, broad nasal bridge, and increased head circumference; skeletal anomalies, including frontal and parietal bossing and mandibular prognathism, as well as costal anomalies involving the rib and vertebrae; ophthalmologic abnormalities, including hypertelorism, congenital blindness, and strabismus; and neurologic anomalies, including calcifications of the falx cerebri, bony bridging of the sella turcica, and medulloblastoma.

The components of NBCCS can be divided into 2 groups, as suggested by Evan et al and Kimonis et al: with so-called major and minor criteria. The final diagnosis of the syndrome is achieved upon finding any 2 of the major criteria, or 1 major criterion plus 2 minor criteria.

Multiple odontogenic keratocysts (OKCs) are a well-recognized feature of NBCCS (see the image below).Usually, odontogenic keratocyst (OKC) development, which comprises one of the major criterions, occurs before the observation of other clinical findings in NBCCS, enhancing early diagnosis of the disease. Odontogenic keratocysts (OKCs) associated with this syndrome have a familial tendency, and early family detection and genetic counseling are critical. These cysts arise earlier in patients with NBCSS than in those who are unaffected by the syndrome.

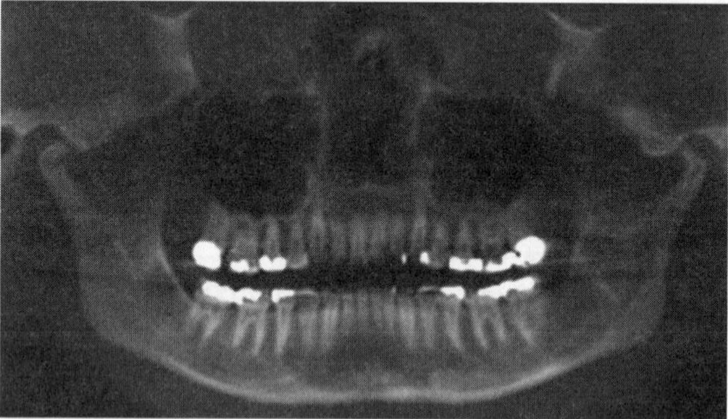

Figure: Panoramic film demonstrating mandibular odontogenic keratocysts in nevoid basal cell carcinoma syndrome.

Odontogenic keratocysts (OKCs) associated with NBCCS have occasionally been reported to transform into aggressive neoplasms such as ameloblastomas and squamous cell carcinoma. The cyst lining seen in the NBCSS-related odontogenic keratocyst (OKC) is classically parakeratinized and does not appear to be associated with the orthokeratinized variant of the OKC.

Clinically, odontogenic keratocysts (OKCs) generally present as a swelling, with or without pain. The cyst classically grows within the medullary spaces of the bone in an anteroposterior direction, causing expansion that is at first minimal. Buccal expansion is noted in approximately 30% of maxillary and 50% of mandibular lesions. It has been demonstrated that the collagenase activity in the cysts' epithelium with its resorbative properties appears to regulate the ability of the lesion to grow expansively in bone.

Radiographically, odontogenic keratocysts (OKCs) present as a well-defined radiolucent lesion that is either unilocular or multilocular, with smooth and usually corticated margins, unless they have been secondarily infected (see the images below). In 25–40% of cases, there is an unerupted tooth involved with the lesion; adjacent teeth may be displaced, but root resorption is rarely seen. Maxillary lesions tend to be smaller than mandibular lesions; however, more extensive involvement can be appreciated in the maxilla because of the cancellous nature of the bone. Larger lesions can cause bony expansion with or without perforation of the cortical plates.

42. Pedicle of pectoralis myocutaneous flap is:
   a. Dorsalis pedis artery
   b. Acromian perforator
   c. Thoracoacromial artery
   d. Perforator branch of internal mammary artery

   Ans. c

Ref: Peterson 2/e p 777

43. Meningocele is:
   a. Radiodense spaces without adjacent gliosis seen after trauma
   b. Collection of malignant cells at pia arachnoid junctions
   c. Malignant tumors within brain parenchyma
   d. Thinning of dura and arachnoid and coming out of meningeal tissues into nose sinuses and orbit

   Ans. a

Ref: Sabiston 12/e p 139

44. A patient comes to an emergency with panfacial trauma and bleeding. Bleeding from which vessel is not controlled even by ligature of external carotid artery:
   a. Ethmoid artery
   b. Sphenopalatine artery
   c. Tonsillar artery
   d. Occipital artery

   Ans. a

Ref: Chaurasia 4/e p 128

45. In which of the following conditions tooth not removed from the fracture line:
   a. Infected tooth
   b. Causing hindrance in achieving anatomic reduction
   c. Periapical infection
   d. Apical one-third of root is fractured

   Ans. d

Ref: Killey 2/e p 43

46. Vascularity is minimally damaged by which maxillary osteotomy?
   a. Cupar
   b. Wunderer
   c. Wassmund
   d. Flap design has no effect on blood vascularity

   Ans. c

Ref: Fonseca 3/e p 251

47. The process by which a material induces the osteoprogenitor cells to differentiate into osteoblasts which will form the new bone is called:
   a. Osteoconduction
   b. Osteopromotion
   c. Osteoinduction
   d. Osseointegration

   Ans. c

Ref: Babbush 2/e p 623

48. In LeFort I osteotomy to prevent septal bucking, all are done except:
   a. Anterior nasal spine reduction
   b. Reduction of nasal septum and middle turbinates
   c. Reduction of inferior turbinates
   d. Reduction of nasal septum and inferior turbinates
   Ans. a

Ref: Fonseca 2/e p 238

49. In Seddon's classification, temporary interruption of conduction without loss of axonal continuity comes under:
   a. Class I
   b. Class II
   c. Class III
   d. Class IV
   Ans. a

In 1943, Seddon described three basic types of peripheral nerve injury that include:

Neurapraxia (Class I)

It is a temporary interruption of conduction without loss of axonal continuity. In neurapraxia, there is a physiologic block of nerve conduction in the affected axons.

Other characteristics:

- It is the mildest type of peripheral nerve injury.
- There are sensory-motor problems distal to the site of injury.
- The endoneurium, perineurium, and the epineurium are intact.
- There is no Wallerian degeneration.
- Conduction is intact in the distal segment and proximal segment, but no conduction occurs across the area of injury.
- Recovery of nerve conduction deficit is full and requires days to weeks.
- EMG shows lack of fibrillation potentials (FP) and positive sharp waves.

Axonotmesis (Class II)

It involves loss of the relative continuity of the axon and its covering of myelin, but preservation of the connective tissue framework of the nerve (the encapsulating tissue, the epineurium and perineurium, are preserved).

Other characteristics:

- Wallerian degeneration occurs distal to the site of injury.
- There are sensory and motor deficits distal to the site of lesion.
- There is no nerve conduction distal to the site of injury (3 to 4 days after injury).
- EMG shows fibrillation potentials (FP), and positive sharp waves (2 to 3 weeks postinjury).
- Axonal regeneration occurs and recovery is possible without surgical treatment. Sometimes surgical intervention because of scar tissue formation is required.

Neurotmesis (Class III)

It is a total severance or disruption of the entire nerve fiber. A peripheral nerve fiber contains an axon (or long dendrite), myelin sheath (if existence), their Schwann cells, and the endoneurium. Neurotmesis may be partial or complete.

Other characteristics:

- Wallerian degeneration occurs distal to the site of injury.
- There is connective tissue lesion that may be partial or complete.
- Sensory-motor problems and autonomic function defect are severe.
- There is no nerve conduction distal to the site of injury (3 to 4 days after lesion).

- EMG and NCV findings are as axonotmesis.
- Because of lack of nerve repair, surgical intervention is necessary.

Sunderland's classification

In 1951, Sunderland expanded Seddon's classification to five degrees of peripheral nerve injury as follows:

First-degree (Class I)

Seddon's neurapraxia and first-degree are the same.

Second-degree (Class II)

Seddon's axonotmesis and second-degree are the same.

Third-degree (Class II)

Sunderland's third-degree is a nerve fiber interruption. In third-degree injury, there is a lesion of the endoneurium, but the epineurium and perineurium remain intact. Recovery from a third-degree injury is possible, but surgical intervention may be required.

Fourth-degree (Class II)

In fourth-degree injury, only the epineurium remain intact. In this case, surgical repair is required.

Fifth-degree (Class III)

Fifth-degree lesion is a complete transection of the nerve. Recovery is not possible without an appropriate surgical treatment.

Summary

Seddon-Sunderland classification

Nerve injury

Grade 1: Neuropraxia

- Conduction disruption with intact axon and preserved supportive structures.
- *Prognosis:* normally full recovery in days-weeks without surgical intervention

Grade 2: Axonotmesis

- Disrupted axon with intact endoneurium; Wallerian degeneration takes place after 1-2 weeks
- *Prognosis:* variable recovery, worse prognosis for proximal injuries and injuries who do not successfully re-implant in the muscle within 18 months

Grade 3: Neurotmesis with preservation of perineurium

Neurotmesis Refers to disruption of supporting structures

- Endoneurium is disrupted
- *Prognosis:* 60–80% recovery

Grade 4: Neurotmesis with preservation of epineurium

- *Prognosis:* nerve grafting is required

Grade 5: Neurotmesis with complete transection of nerve trunk

- *Prognosis:* bypass/jump grafting is required

Reference

- Otto D. Payton and Richard P. Di Fabio et al. Manual of physical therapy. Churchill Livingstone Inc. ISBN 0-443-08499-8 'Electrodiagnostic studies of the hand'.

50. Mazabraud's syndrome is a rare syndrome comprising of:

a. Fibroma + Fibrous dysplasia
b. Myxoma+ Fibrous dysplasia
c. Lipoma + Fibrous dysplasia
d. Myoma + Fibrous dysplasia

Ans. b

Ref: Neelima Malik 1/e p 466

- Fibrous dysplasia: usually polyostotic
- Multiple soft tissue myxomas (intramuscular myxomas): typically in large muscle groups

It is most frequently seen in women (~70%) and usually present in middle age (mean age 46; range 17–82) There is an increased risk of osseous malignant transformation.

51. In Bijaw surgery for open bite correction, maxillary impaction is decided by:
a. COGS analysis
b. Cephalometry
c. Bone scan
d. Clinical incisal show
Ans. d

Ref: Epker 2/e p 232

52. A patient who has undergone anterior maxillary subapical osteotomy feels the loss of sensations over upper anterior teeth 15 days after the surgery. This is because:
a. It occurs commonly with this procedure
b. Local infection should be suspected
c. Root trauma should be suspected
d. Avascular necrosis developing in the segment and maxillary disimpaction should be done
Ans. d

Ref: Peterson 2/e p 1233

53. In right condylar hyperplasia, bone scan shows no active growth treatment will be:
a. Bilateral IVRO
b. Bilateral BSSO
c. Distraction osteogenesis
d. IVRO on right side and right side sagittal split osteotomy
Ans. b

Ref: Chakravarty 2/e p 598

54. How to differentiate between radiolucencies present due to osteoradionecrosis or secondary to malignancies:
a. MRI
b. Contrast-enhanced CT
c. Noncontrast-enhanced CT
d. SPECT/CT
Ans. d

Ref: Grainger 2/e p 767

55. In LeFort I osteotomy, which artery is at greatest risk of hemorrhage:
a. Inferior alveolar
b. Ascending pharyngeal
c. Sphenopalatine
d. Descending palatine
Ans. d

Ref: Fonseca 3/e p 239

56. 2 cms above the Frontozygomatic suture, the layers from the skull to the skin are:
a. Subgaleal fascia, temporoparietal fascia, skin
b. Subgaleal fascia, temporoparietal fascia, temporalis fascia, SMAS, skin
c. Subgaleal fascia, temporalis fascia, temporoparietal fascia, SMAS, skin
d. Subgaleal fascia, temporoparietal fascia, SMAS, skin
Ans. c

Ref: Ellis 1/e p 80

57. Dacrocystoplasty is:

a. Orbital floor repair
b. Lacrimal duct repair
c. Parotid fistula repair
d. Repair of telecanthus with NOE fracture

Ans. b

Ref: Fonseca 3/e p 715

Ans. a

Transcutaneous lower-eyelid approaches

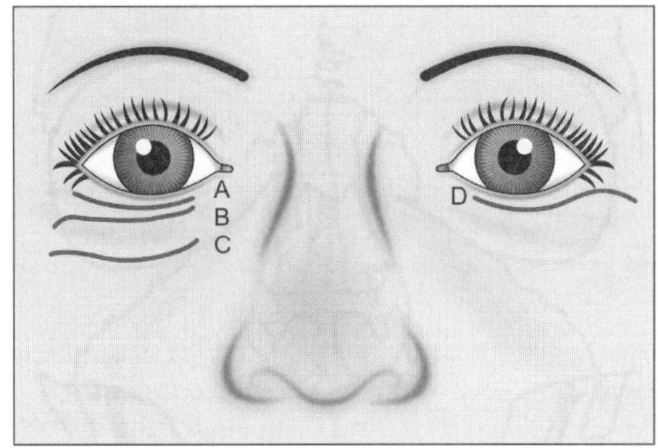

Principles

There are three basic approaches through the external skin of the lower eyelid to give access to the inferior, lower medial, and lateral aspects of the orbital cavity:

- Subciliary (A, synonym: lower blepharoplasty)
- Subtarsal (B, synonym: lower or mideyelid)
- Infraorbital (C, synonym: inferior orbital rim)

The subciliary approach can be extended laterally to gain access to the lateral orbital rim (D).
The course of the incisions is aligned to the slope of the natural skin creases which become more apparent with age.
The skin of the eyelid is the thinnest in the human body. It has little or no dermis and almost no subdermal fat.
Hypertrophic scarring and keloid formation is very uncommon following lower lid skin incisions. In general, the scars become inconspicuous with time.

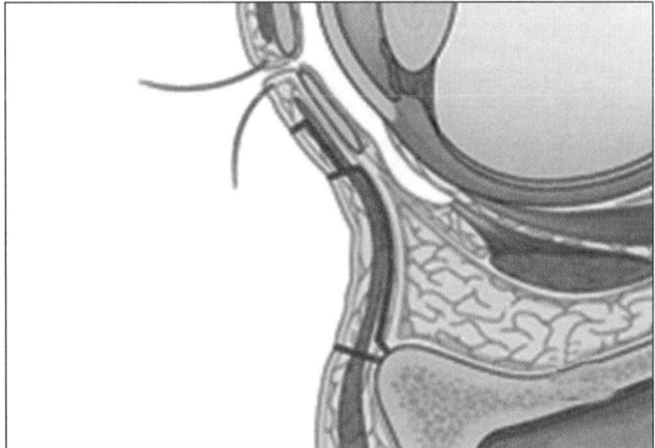

The approaches differ in the vertical position of the cutaneous incision lines. Because of this, the path and length of dissection through the layers of the lower lid vary.
Infraorbital incisions lie at the transition between the thin eyelid skin and the thicker cheek skin. They are, therefore predisposed to edema and increased visibility of the scars, even when the incision runs curvilinear within the resting skin tension lines.

That is why, the infraorbital approach has lost its former popularity. The infraorbital approach will not be detailed here.

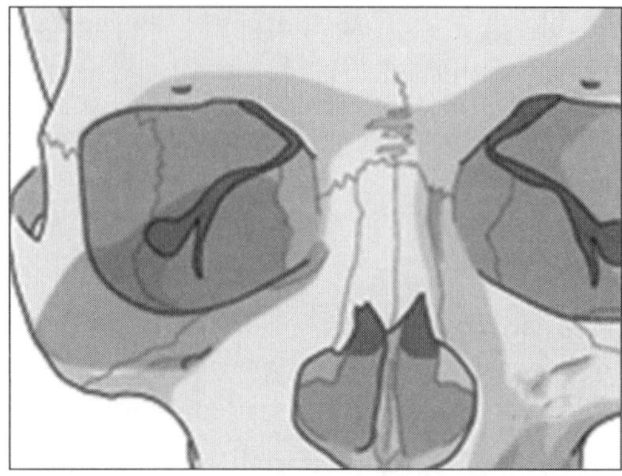

Access Areas

Transcutaneous lower-eyelid approaches yield pathways to the lower circumference of the orbital cavity and/or for the subperiosteal elevation of the upper midface and release of the cheek area.

The exposure of the infraorbital rim serves as the starting platform for the dissection of the periorbita.

The illustration outlines the approximate extent of the orbital bony surfaces which can be exposed via the subciliary, the subtarsal, and the infraorbital approach. There is little difference in the access areas along the floor, the medial and lateral rim, and the neighboring wall portions of the orbit.

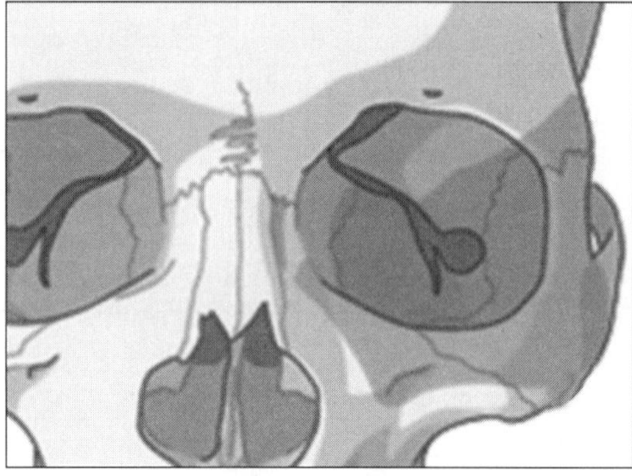

With a lateral extension of the subciliary incision, however, the entire lateral rim, with heavy traction even beyond the level of the zygomaticofrontal suture, as well the lateral orbital wall back to the zygomaticosphenoid suture become accessible.

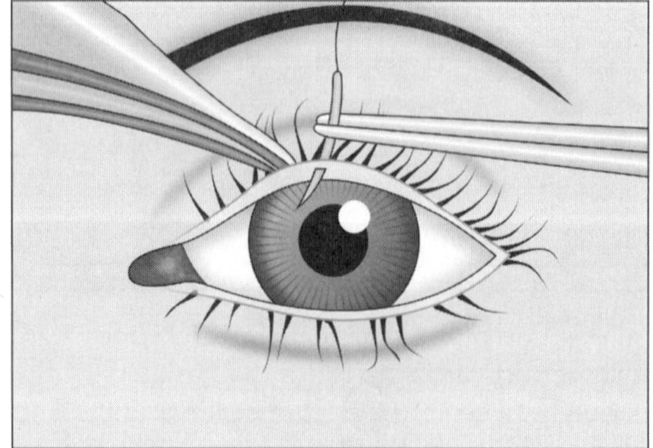

Exposure of midfacial skeleton

This illustration shows the field of bone exposure inferomedial of the infraorbital rim and across the eminence of the zygoma that can be reached after release of the retaining ligaments and muscle attachments during periosteal undermining in a downward direction.

A connection with the surgical cavity created through the upper maxillary vestibular approach allows the dismantling of the whole lower-and middle-third of the midfacial skeleton.

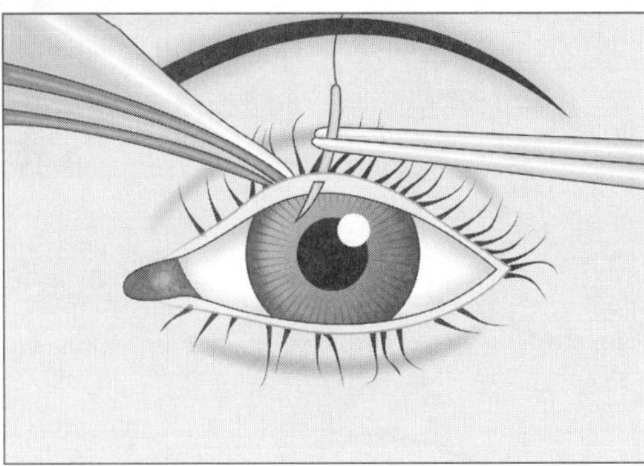

Preparation – Corneal protection

For all three kinds of transcutaneous lower-eyelid incisions, a temporary tarsorrhaphy is recommended to help protect the cornea. This is done by employing a mattress suture.

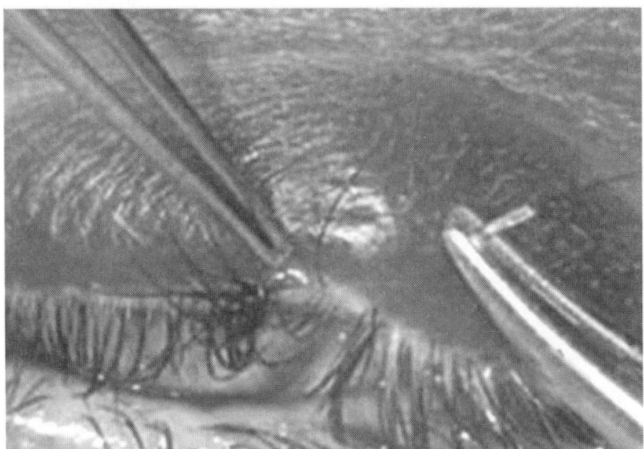

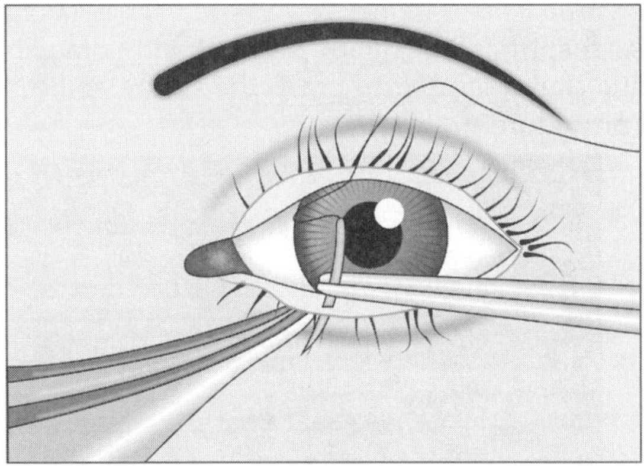

A 6.0 suture is passed through the skin of the upper eyelid and exits through the gray line of the upper lid margin. In the lower eyelid, the needle is passed from the gray line into the skin where it exits.

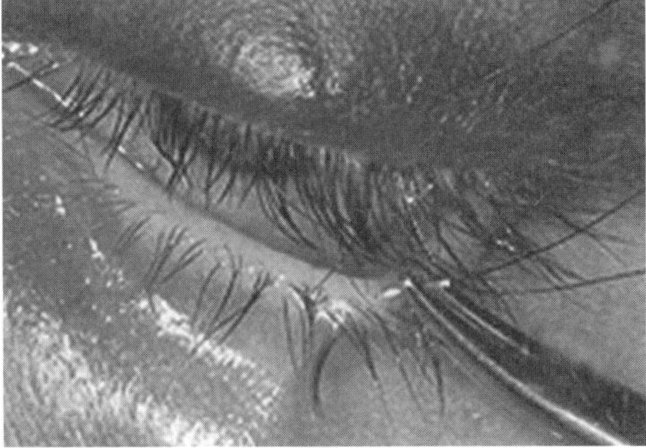

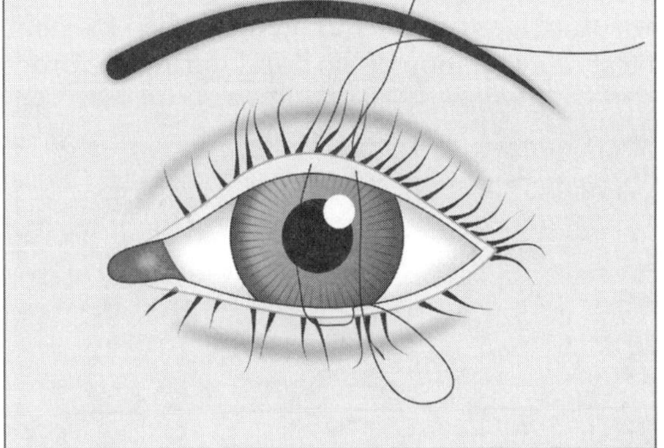

The suture is guided back picking up the same soft-tissue portions in the lower and upper eyelids to complete the mattress loop.

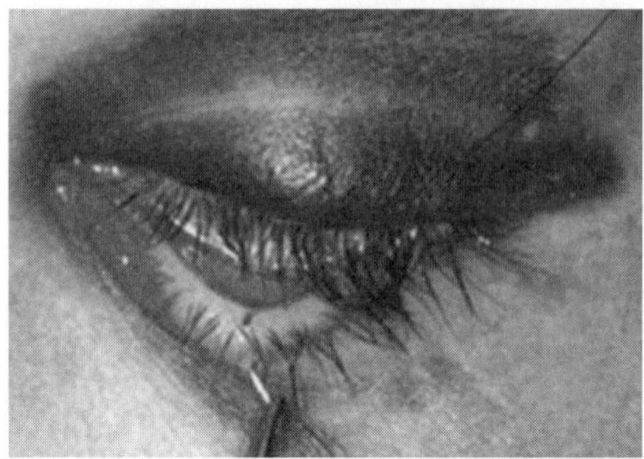

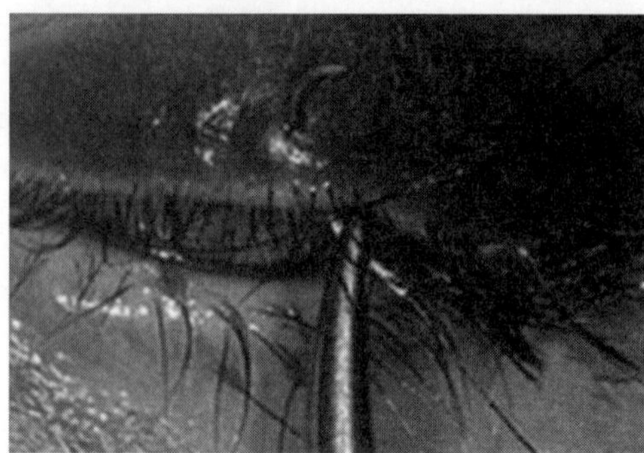

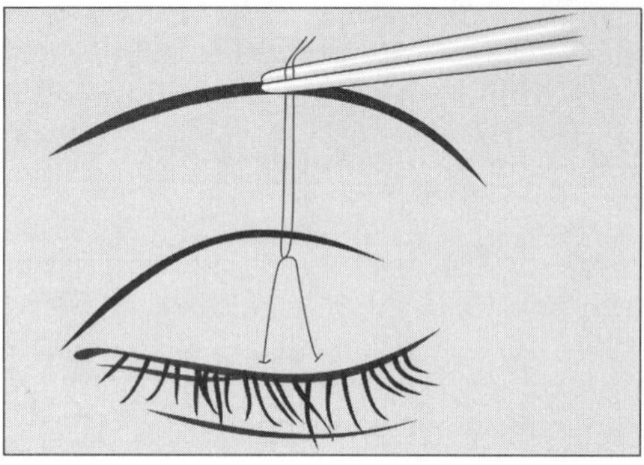

The tarsorrhaphy is not tightly secured and some space is left between the knot and the upper-eyelid skin. A hemostatic clamp is used to grasp the suture and apply traction to lower lid for full eyelid closure during the surgical procedure.

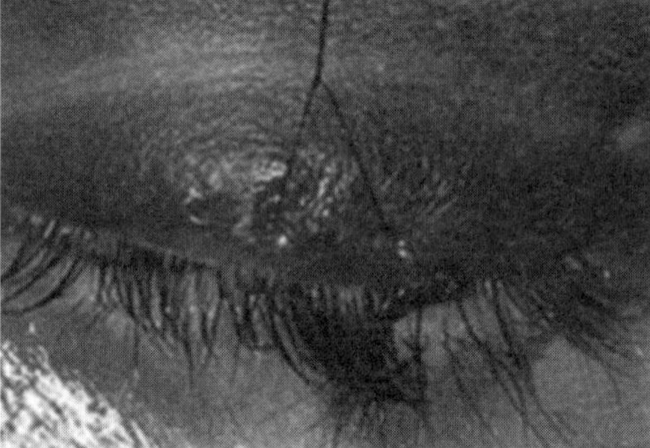

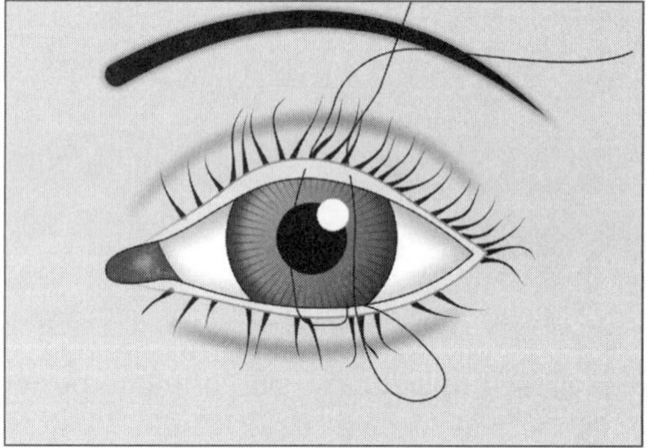

Since the suture was not fully tightened, when the hemostatic clamp is released, the lid may be opened for a forced duction test or evaluation of the pupil during the procedure.

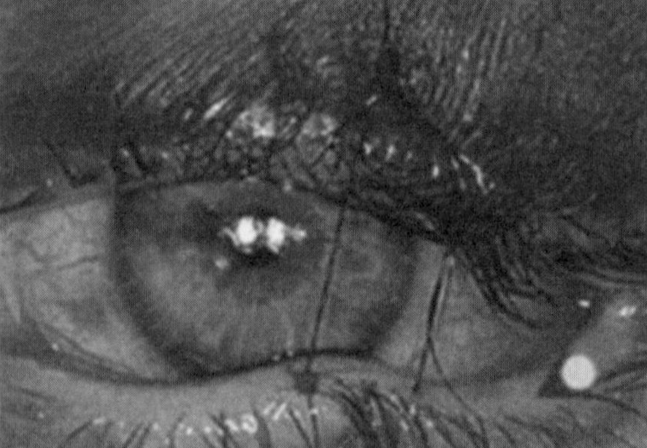

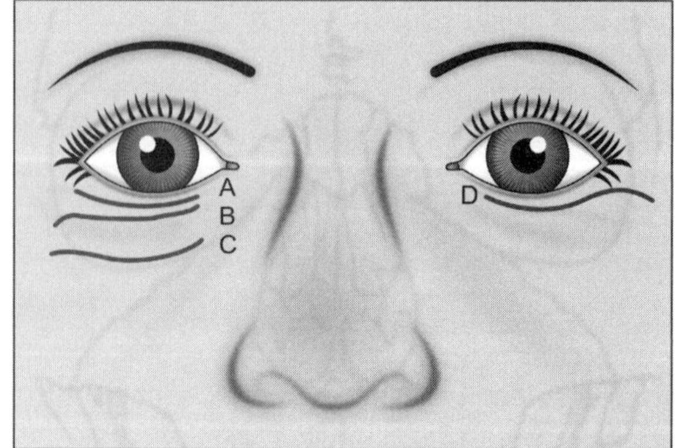

58. In edentulous mandible with less than 10 mm bone height, plating should be done with screws:
   a. In body region
   b. In angle and symphyseal region
   c. In angle region
   d. In symphyseal region
   Ans. d

Ref: Fonseca 3/e p 1012

59. In Type II NOE fracture, main central dislodged segment is stabilized by Canthopexy in which the wire is passed?
   a. Posteriorly and superiorly to lacrimal crest
   b. Anteriorly and superiorly to lacrimal crest
   c. Posteriorly and inferiorly to lacrimal crest
   d. Anteriorly and inferiorly to lacrimal crest
   Ans. a

Ref: Fonseca 3/e p 748

Periorbital zones
Zone I upper eyelid
Zone II lower eyelid
Zone III medial canthal region
Zone IV lateral canthal region

Tumor Control

Eyelid skin is prone to skin cancer, and because it is so thin, most basal cell and squamous cell carcinomas invade the underlying orbicularis muscle.

Surgical management of malignant tumors aim at disease eradication coupled with preservation of adjacent normal tissue. In the periorbital region, functional and cosmetic sequelae of removal of excessive normal tissue may have far-reaching consequences.

The tumor ablative surgeon who is unfamiliar with the periorbital anatomy and reconstructive options, may compromise margins of resection because of the unwillingness to sacrifice vital structures in the area

Mohs micrographic surgery offers highest cure rates (< 98%) while preserving maximum amount of normal tissue in an area where excess tissue for reconstruction is scarce. Orbital invasion of basal cell carcinoma is rare but calls for extensive preoperative evaluation and multidisciplinary team management.

Reconstruction Principles and Guidelines

Most resections and reconstructions are performed under local anesthesia, sometimes supplemented with i.v. dissociative anesthesia for enhanced patient comfort. Local anesthetic BMX® drops are used in the conjunctival sac, while lidocaine 2% with adrenaline 1 : 100.000 is injected with a 30 G needle. For longer operations 0.5% bupivacaine with epinephrine 1 : 200.000 is added to the mixture.

Periorbital defects are generally categorized according to location (zone I-IV), depth and size. In anterior lamellar defects, part of the eyelid thickness remains. In full thickness defects, both the anterior and posterior lamella must be reconstituted. The larger the percentage of the full thickness eyelid which is missing (0-25%/25-50%/> 50%), the more complex the reconstruction.

The ideal goal of reconstruction is to provide global protection and normal aesthetics.

Prerequisites to attain this goal may be the following:

- Lining maintaining lubrication while avoiding corneal irritation
- Lid rigidity while allowing direct global apposition
- Lid stability and orientation with proper medial and lateral canthal support
- Opening and closing ability facilitated by adequate muscle power and tone, allowed by subtle skin covering. To attain these goals, reconstruction should ideally replace the delicate, thin, pliable, well-vascularized and innervated tissues of the eyelids with kind. In general, adjacent eyelid structures may act as reservoirs for tissue harvesting and flap or graft transfer.

Distraction forces, such as gravity, edema and wound retraction may lead to complications, such as eyelid malposition (ectropion) and corneal exposure.

60. **In superior orbital fissure syndrome there is loss of direct light Ref:lex with intact consensual light Reflex is due to:**
    a. Intact afferent and efferent arc
    b. Intact afferent and damaged efferent arc
    c. Damaged afferent and efferent arc
    d. Intact efferent and damaged afferent arc
    Ans. b

Ref: Duane Ophthalmology 2/e p 916

Superior orbital fissure syndrome, also known as Rochon-Duvigneaud's syndrome, is a neurological disorder that results if the superior orbital fissure is fractured. Involvement of the cranial nerves that pass through the superior orbital fissure may lead to diplopia, paralysis of extraocular motions, exophthalmos, and ptosis. Blindness or loss of vision indicates involvement of the orbital apex, which is more serious, requiring urgent surgical intervention. Typically, if blindness is present with superior orbital syndrome, it is called orbital apex syndrome.

61. **In an 80-year-old diabetic patient mandibular fracture is managed with least complications by:**
    a. Extraoral opening and supra periosteal plating
    b. IMF
    c. Reconstruction plate
    d. External pin fixation
    Ans. b

Ref: Fonseca 3/e p 1013

62. **In panfacial trauma:**
    a. Panfacial fractures are converted to LeFort I fractures
    b. Mandibular fractures are treated first
    c. Palatal fracture is fixed first to maintain maxillary width
    d. Condyle is fixed first to maintain mandibular height
    Ans. c

Ref: Peterson 2/e p 556

63. **All are the advantages of locking reconstruction plates except:**
    a. Plate adaptation becomes easier
    b. Loosening of screws and plate occurs less
    c. Plate adaptation is not required
    d. Plate has more stability than conventional plates
    Ans. c

Ref: Peterson 2/e p 379

64. **An 80-year-old chronic alcoholic patient is admitted in endocrinology with uncontrolled diabetes and develops dusky purple discoloration and small vesicles on the lateral surface of the neck within a few hours, two days before this he complains of pain in right lower first molar. He is having:**
    a. Ludwig's angina
    b. Actinomycosis
    c. Necrotizing fasciitis
    d. Herpes
    Ans. c

Ref: Topazian 2/e p 422

65. **In mandibular symphyseal fracture while doing ORIF:**
    a. Incision is given 7–8 mm towards the attached gingiva from the junction of attached gingiva and labial mucosa
    b. Incision is given 12–15 mm towards the attached gingiva from the junction of attached gingiva and labial mucosa
    c. Incision is given 3–4 mm labially to the junction of attached gingiva and labial mucosa
    d. Incision is given 7—8 mm to the junction of attached gingiva and labial mucosa
    Ans. c

Ref: Ellis 2/e p 114

66. In orbital floor fracture, best reconstruction is done by:

a. Titanium mesh
b. Calvarial graft
c. Medpore
d. Reconstruction plate

Ans. a

Ref: Fonseca 3/e p 546

General consideration

The unique and complex anatomy of the orbit, unless prebent plates are used, requires significant contouring of the implants to restore the proper anatomy. The majority of cases require reconstruction of the orbital floor to support the globe position and restore the shape of the orbit. The reason for this is that the bony walls are comminuted and/or bone fragments are missing. Therefore, one is reconstructing missing bone rather than reducing bone fragments. This can be accomplished using various materials. There is hardly any anatomic region in the human body that is so controversial in terms of appropriate material used for fracture repair:

- Nonresorbable versus resorbable
- Autogenous/allogenous/xenogenous versus alloplastic material
- Nonprebent versus preformed (anatomical) plates
- Standard versus custom-made plates
- Nonporous versus porous material
- Noncoated versus coated plates

Many surgeons recommend using materials that allow bending to an anatomical shape, that are radiopaque (to allow for intra- or postoperative radiologic confirmation of placement), and stable over time.

Reconstruction of the dislocated orbital walls is demanding. Secondary changes to this contour are undesirable. This is why critical consideration of the use of resorbable materials is necessary.

There are different preferences of implant material depending on regional differences, variations in schools of teaching, and socio-economic factors. There is a paucity of evidence to support the ideal choice for an orbital implant. Modern imaging analysis offers a unique chance to quantitatively assess the surgical result and stability over time. This can provide valuable information for future recommendation.

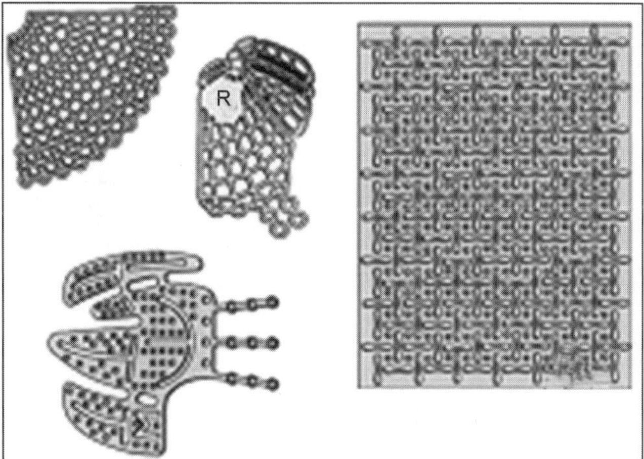

Titanium Meshes

Advantages:

- Availability
- Stability
- Contouring (eased by the artificial sterile skull)
- Adequate in large three-wall fractures (the prebent plate is limited to medial wall and orbital wall fractures only).
- Radiopacity

- Spaces within the mesh to allow dissipation of fluids
- No donor site needed
- Tissue incorporation may occur

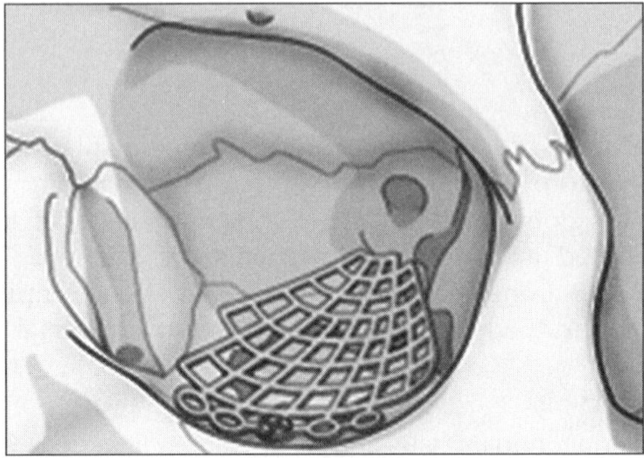

Disadvantages:

- Costs
- Possible sharp edges if not properly trimmed
- **Note:** We do not have long- term experience in a large series regarding the use of metallic mesh in young children. In several pediatric cases above the age of four it has proved to be safe.

Note: The extensive use of mesh for orbital reconstruction in traumatized orbits has been shown to be safe, with few problems due to infections and no problems with secondary displacement due to additional trauma, on condition of proper handling, contouring, and fixation of the mesh.

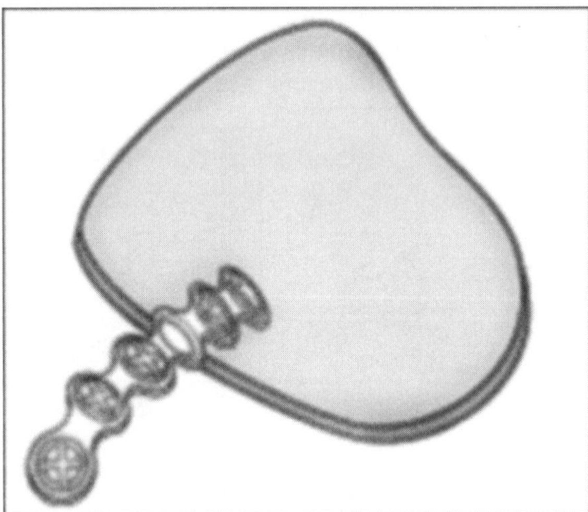

Bone graft

Illustration shows individual calvarial bone graft.

Advantages:

- Low material costs
- Smooth surface
- Variability in thickness
- Radiopacity
- Maximal biocompatibility

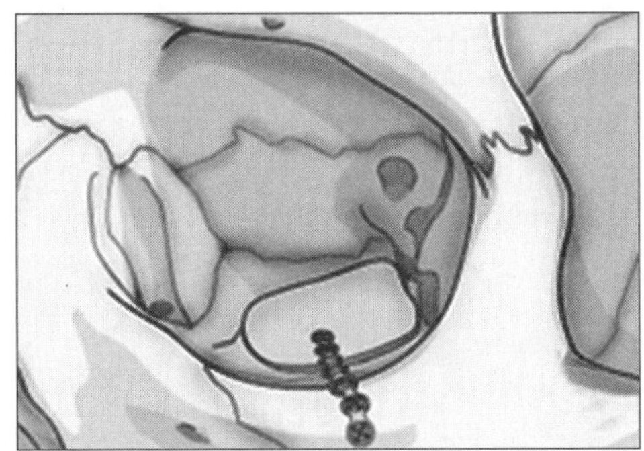

- Periorbital readily dissects off of the bone in secondary reconstruction

Disadvantages:

- Additional donor site needed (necessitating additional surgery time for harvest, pain, scar, and possible surgical complications)
- Possible contour and dimensional changes due to remodeling
- Difficult to shape according to patients anatomy
- Less drainage from the orbit than with titanium mesh

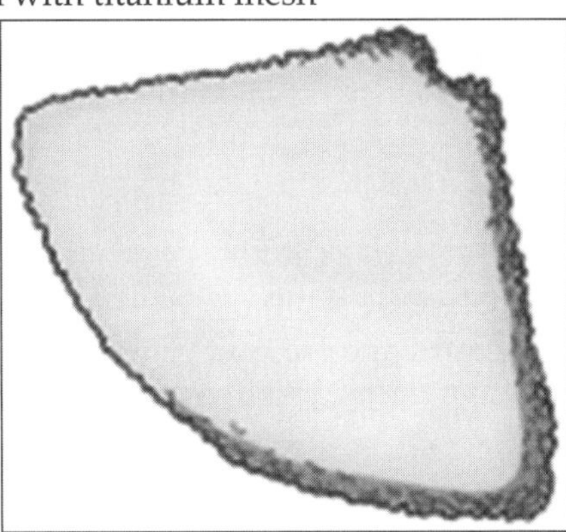

Porous polyethylene sheets (PPE)

Advantages:

- Availability
- Contouring (eased by the artificial sterile skull)
- Smooth edges
- Allows tissue ingrowth

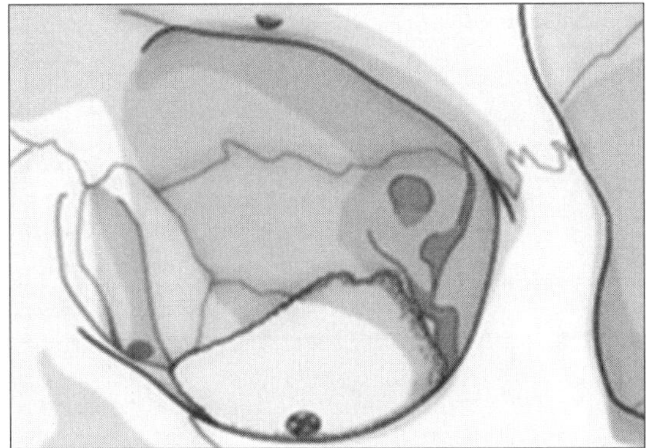

Disadvantages:

- Not radiopaque (not visible on postoperative images)
- Lack of rigidity when a very thin wafer of PPE is used, When a thicker rigid wafer is used there is a risk of causing a dystopia.
- Less drainage from the orbit than with titanium mesh

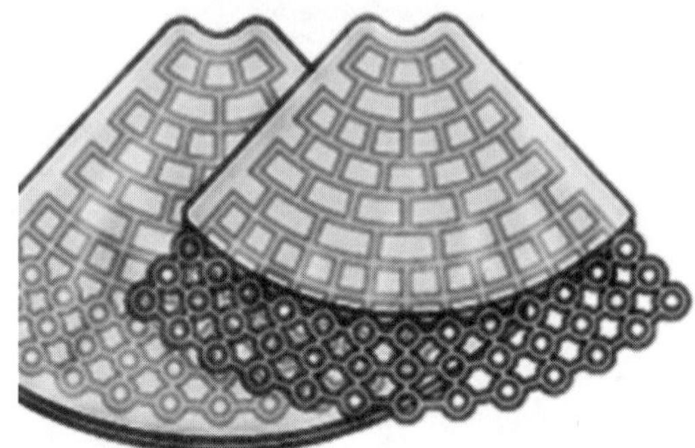

Composite of porous polyethylene and titanium mesh

By combining titanium mesh with porous polyethylene, the material becomes radiopaque, and more rigid than porous polyethylene of a similar thickness. Some surgeons also believe that there is less risk of having retained sharp barbs, which can lead to an entrapment of soft tissues during placement.

Advantages:

- Availability
- Stability
- Contouring (eased by the artificial sterile skull)
- Adequate in large three-wall fractures (the pre-bent plate is limited to medial wall and orbital wall fractures only)
- Radiopacity
- No donor site needed
- Tissue incorporation may occur

Disadvantages:

- Less drainage from the orbit than with titanium mesh.

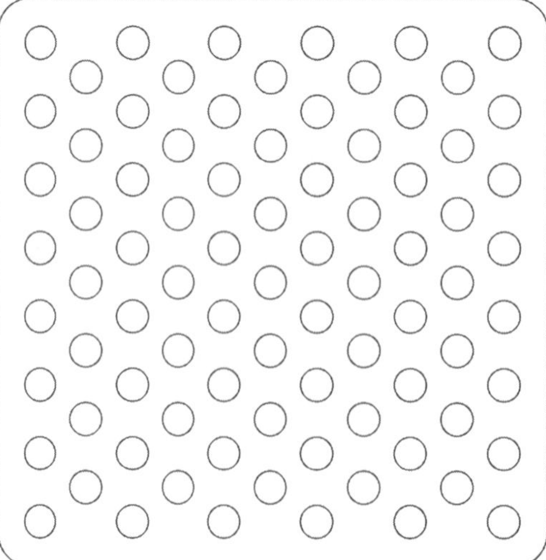

Resorbable materials

Thermoplastic and non-thermoplastic materials

Advantages:

- Availability
- Handling/contourability (only for thermoplastics)
- Smooth surface and smooth edges

Disadvantages:

- No radiopacity
- Degradation of material with possible contour loss
- Sterile infection/inflammatory response
- Difficult to shape according to patient anatomy (only for nonthermoplastics)
- Less drainage from the orbit than with uncovered titanium mesh (in case when nonperforated material is used)

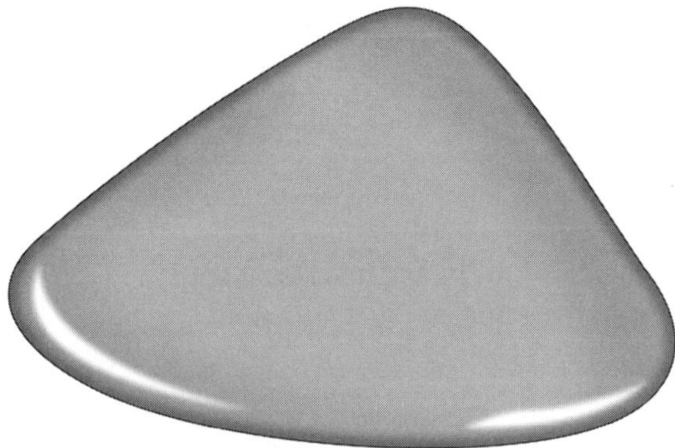

Illustration showing a nonthermoplastic PDS sheet.

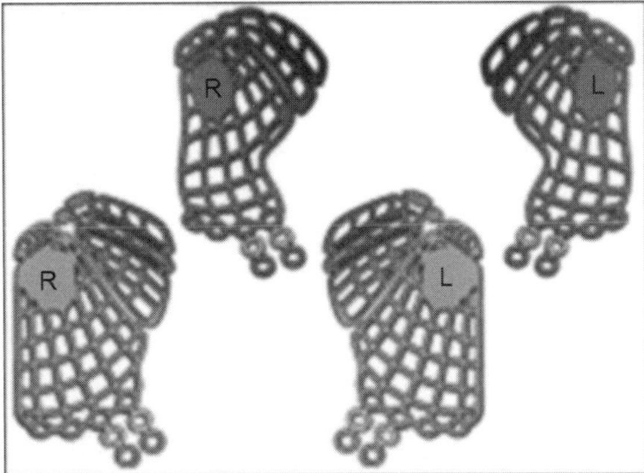

Preformed orbital implant

Advantages:

- Radiopacity
- Smooth surface
- Minimal or no contouring necessary

Disadvantages:

- Cost

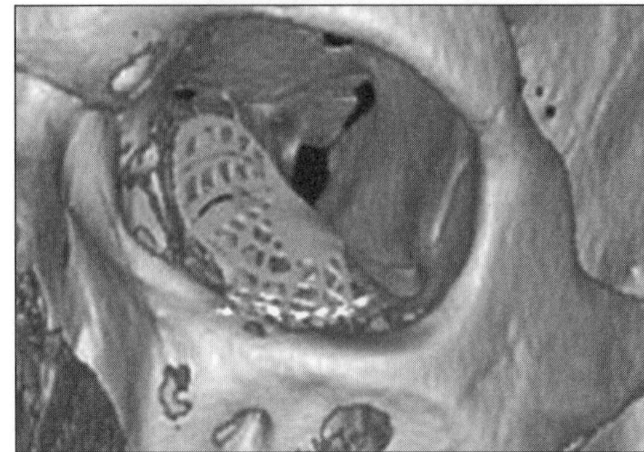

Multiplanar and 3-D view showing a preformed mesh plate placed prior to surgery into patient CT dataset.

Implant fixation

Fixation of orbital reconstruction material varies with the type and nature of the fracture.

Fixation of most materials in the orbital floor is achieved by the use of one or more screws. The diameter depends on anatomical requirements but will normally vary between 1.0, 1.3, or 1.5 mm. Alternatively, Matrix Midface screws can be used.

67. Medial wall of orbit is formed by:

a. Nasal bone, maxilla, lacrimal bone, lesser wing of sphenoid
b. Lacrimal bone, ethmoid, frontal and maxillary bone
c. Nasal bone, maxilla, lacrimal bone and greater wing of sphenoid
d. Nasal bone, maxilla, lacrimal bone and body of sphenoid

Ans. b

Ref: Chaurasia 3/e p 23

68. In orbital blowout fractures:

a. Simple reduction needed
b. Orbital repair should be done around 2 mm overcontoured
c. Steroids to be given and surgery to be deferred for initial 7 days
d. Orbital thickness is tripled

Ans. c

Ref: Fonseca 3/e p 674

69. Nerve to medial pterygoid supplies:

a. Anterior belly of digastric
b. Mylohyoid
c. Palatoglossus
d. Tensor tympani

Ans. d

Ref: Chaurasia 4/e p 155

70. Long buccal nerve is a branch of:

a. Facial
b. Anterior mandibular
c. Inferior alveolar
d. Posterior mandibular

Ans. a

Ref: Chaurasia 4/e p 151

71. Inferior oblique muscle is supplied by:

a. Occulomotor
b. Trochlear
c. Optic
d. Abducent

Ans. a

Ref: Chaurasia 4/e p 98

72. The nerve mostly affected in cavernous sinus thrombosis is:
a. Abducent
b. Trochlear
c. Occulomotor
d. Optic
Ans. a

Ref: Chaurasia 2/e p 135

73. Leave or holiday of medicines is required in patient taking bisphosphonates as:
a. Orally from last year
b. IV from last month
c. Orally from last 3 years
d. Orally from last two years with steroids
Ans. c

Ref: Katzung 10/e p 871

74. Initial sign which occurs first of all in cavernous sinus thrombosis is:
a. Congestion of retinal veins
b. Parasthesia and itching in infraorbital region
c. Headache
d. Periorbital edema
Ans. d

Ref: Гonseca 3/e p 1332

75. In costochondral graft, the chondral part is taken with:
a. Rib shear
b. Rib cutter
c. No. 11 blade
d. 701 bur
Ans. c

Ref: Peterson 2/e p 788

Sources of autogenous bone grafts for craniofacial reconstruction

Free Nonvascularized Bone Grafts

Iliac Crest

The iliac crest is one of the most common donor sites for bone grafts, both vascularized and nonvascularized. Large segments of cortical, corticocancellous, or cancellous bone can be quickly obtained for different-sized defects. Furthermore, the location of the ilium allows harvesting by a separate surgical team to save operation time. A full-thickness iliac crest graft would have two thick cortices with ample amount of trabecular bone in between and can very closely resemble the thickness and height of mandibular bone. The graft shows reasonable long-term survival, and rehabilitation with osseointegrated dental implants is possible. Mandibular defects could be filled using nonvascularized iliac bone with a 70% success rate. The graft could be implanted as corticocancellous blocks or particulate cancellous bone carried within either a titanium mesh tray or a crib of alloplastic rib bone. However, the rate of successful union drops sharply when the defect is longer than 6 cm.

Posterior iliac crest graft can also be used for craniofacial reconstruction. However, the patient has to be tilted to the prone position, which eliminates the advantage of a simultaneous two-team approach. Donor site morbidity rate for anterior iliac crest grafts is around 23%, and much less for posterior iliac crest. Complications include postoperative pain, iliac or acetabular fractures or instability, persistent hematoma, herniation of abdominal contents, vascular injury, lateral femoral cutaneous nerve injury, and unsightly contour defects along the iliac crest.

Calvarial Graft

This is one of the most popular cortical bone grafts in craniofacial reconstruction, mainly for its mechanical properties and very slow resorption rate. This makes it ideal for facial augmentation, orbital roof and floor reconstruction, and covering cranial defects. Typically, only the outer cortex is used, although a full-thickness graft could be taken and split into two grafts (Typically, the skull continues to grow until the age of 8, continues to thicken until the age of 20, and is thickest at the parietal region. This area can provide 8×10 cm of bone and is considered the safest to harvest).

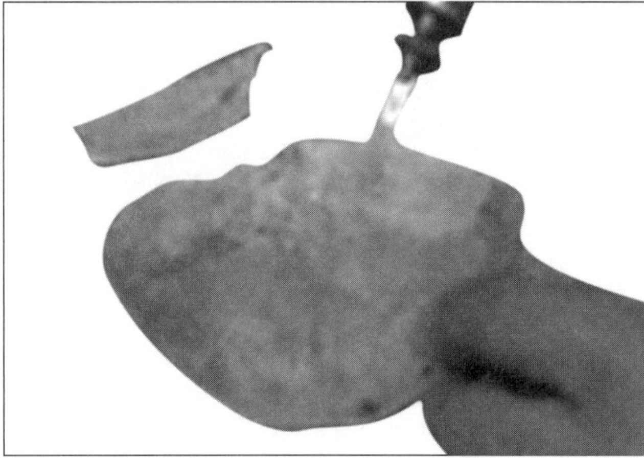

Figure: Technique of splitting cranial bone using a reciprocating saw

However, there are several key anatomic facts to consider before harvesting a calvarial bone graft:

1. Thickness of the calvarium is highly variable to the point of being unpredictable, even within the parietal region. Preoperative radiographic measurement of bone thickness should give an idea of the area of bone that can safely be harvested.
2. The dura is tightly adherent to the inner cortex and can easily be injured if the inner cortex is to be harvested with the graft.
3. Various important vascular structures exist immediately beneath the bone at various sites, including the superior sagittal sinus in the midline.
4. The two cortices fuse together and the bone can become quite thin laterally and inferiorly to the temporal line, the attachment of the temporalis muscle, and at suture sites.
5. Other anatomic variables, including transcortical emissary veins, subcortical vessels, and aberrant arachnoid plexuses (within the cortical calvarium), should also be considered.

The temporoparietal region provides more curved bone, which would be more suitable for orbital or malar reconstruction. However, straight grafts can be harvested more posteriorly (i.e., from the occipitoparietal region). In any case, the bone is typically harvested as narrow strips '5 to 6 cm long and 1.5 to 2 cm wide' to avoid graft fracture during harvest. Then, several strips can be fixed together and used as one graft.

Calvarial bone can be harvested at three levels: partial-thickness outer cortex, full-thickness outer cortex, and bicortical. Partial-thickness outer cortex can be harvested using a very sharp osteotome to curl off a sheet of cortical bone from the outer cortical plate. This technique can be used in children between the ages of 4 and 8 years and can yield enough bone to fill a small defect.

In adults, full-thickness outer cortex can safely be harvested and is, therefore the most commonly used calvarial graft. If a craniotomy has already been performed, the inner cortex can be harvested from the bone flap and used in reconstruction, leaving the outer cortex to be placed back in its original position. This technique maintains the contour of the calvarium. If large quantities of bone are needed, bicortical grafts may be harvested, followed by splitting of the two cortices to double the surface of the graft. It is obvious that harvesting a bicortical calvarial graft would have the most hazardous complications.

Complications of calvarial grafts include surface deformity at the donor and/or recipient site and graft fracture during harvest. Less commonly, dural exposure or tear can occur. If the dura is injured, the tear should be totally exposed, by expanding the bone defect with a rongeur, and patched with a temporalis fascia or, more recently, a synthetic graft. Intracranial hemorrhage after calvarial bone harvesting has been reported but is extremely rare.

Chin Graft

Up to 3 cm of cortical and corticocancellous bone can be shaved off the chin bone through an intraoral approach. This can be sufficient for small defects, such as cleft palate and orthognathic osteotomy defects. Because of its slow resorption, it can be used as an onlay graft for facial augmentation.

Retromolar Graft

A small block of cortical or corticocancellous bone can be chiseled off the area behind the third molar. This graft has the same indications as chin grafts; however, the amount of available bone is much smaller.

Tibial Graft

The anterior surface of the tibial plateau can be a good source of cortical or corticocancellous bone grafts. Mechanical stiffness of the tibial cortex can be useful in augmentation of atrophic alveolar ridge for implant placement, facial bone augmentation, or bridging an osteotomy defect.

Rib Graft

Nonvascularized rib was the first autogenous bone graft used for reconstruction of mandibular segmental defects. Osseous or osseochondral segments can be harvested from ribs 5 to 7 and can either be used in full or split thickness Costochondral grafts remain very popular in the treatment of ascending mandibular ramus and condylar defects. Side effects and complications include postoperative chest wall pain, pleural injury leading to pleuritis or pneumothorax, and facial asymmetry due to overgrowth of the graft.

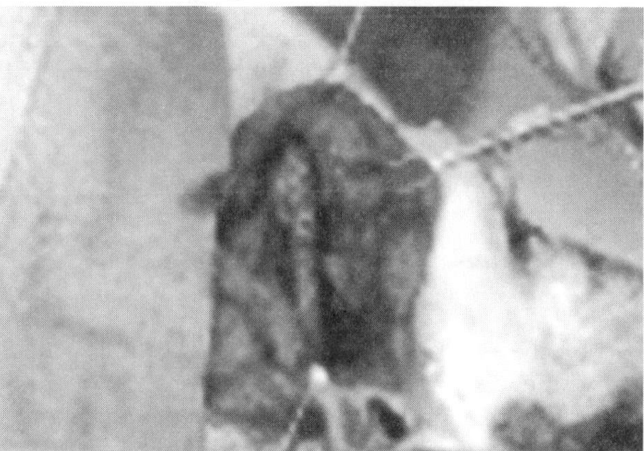

Figure: Mandibular reconstruction with an osseocartilaginous rib graft

Although they were frequently used for facial bone augmentation, bridging osteotomy defects, and orbital floor reconstruction, osseous rib grafts are now rarely used in craniofacial reconstruction. In addition to the problems mentioned previously, the amount and quality of bone obtained are inadequate for most reconstruction procedures. The availability of other sources of bone graft with better quality and quantity, as well as with safer approaches and synthetic bone substitute materials, has rendered rib grafting less popular.

Reimplantation of resected bone segments

Limited studies have tested the possibility of 'recycling' native bone segments that were removed as a part of tumor excision. Intuitively, if tumor cells were successfully eradicated from the excised segments, they would be ideal for reconstructing the remaining defects. Resected mandibular segments could be reimplanted intact or hollowed out to remove trabecular bone, with the use of the cortical bone shell as a tray for autogenous cancellous grafts. Larger long-term studies are needed to validate the safety and efficacy of this technique.

Regional Pedicled Bone Grafts

Pedicled Rib

In 1980, Cuono and Ariyan reported their successful use of the pectoralis major—attached rib as an osteomyocutaneous flap for oromandibular reconstruction. However, subsequent reports showed flap necrosis rates ranging from 21 to 75%. The rib graft can also be carried along the latissimus dorsi or serratus anterior flaps. In all the above-mentioned flaps, the pedicle only allows to rib graft to reach the lower third of the face, limiting its use to mandibular defects. As mentioned earlier, rib grafts are not suitable for such defects. Thus, these flaps are used only for soft tissue, and not bone, reconstruction

Pedicled Clavicle

Sternocleidomastoid muscle (SCM) flaps have been extensively studied but not widely used. Several reports suggested the possibility of transferring clavicular periosteum and bone segments of the clavicle itself. The bone segment can either be partial or full thickness and can be utilized in the reconstruction of small mandibular bone defects.

The technique preserves the neurovascular supply of the SCM muscle, thus allowing for its use in dynamic facial reconstruction. This is particularly advantageous in cases where restoration of facial muscles, lower lip competence, mastication, or tongue movements is attempted. However, preserving the SCM muscle raises some concern in oncology cases due to the possibility of cervical lymph node involvement. In addition, the unsightly contour defect at the donor site and in the lower neck is another disadvantage of this flap.

Pedicled Temporal Bone

The temporalis flap is one of the earliest described muscle flaps. Over the years, it became one of the main techniques for reconstructing paralyzed facial muscles and midfacial full-thickness defects. More relevant to our review, partial or full-thickness temporal bone can be raised with the muscle flap. It can be used to reconstruct maxillary, palatal, orbital rim, orbital floor, or ascending mandibular ramus defects. It can also be used as an onlay graft for facial augmentation.

However, significant donor site morbidity has been reported when calvarial bone is carried with the flap. These include limitation of mouth opening, which can be permanent, in addition to the mentioned complications of calvarial grafts.

76. Herination of brain content into orbit is called:

a. Omphalocele
b. Meningocele
c. Encephalocele
d. Hydrocele

Ans. c

Encephalocele, sometimes known by the Latin name 'cranium bifidum', is a neural tube defect characterized by sac-like protrusions of the brain and the membranes that cover it through openings in the skull. These defects are caused by failure of the neural tube to close completely during fetal development.

Diagnosis

Usually encephaloceles are noticeable deformities and are diagnosed immediately after birth, but a small encephalocele in the nasal or forehead region can go undetected. Various physical and mental developmental delays can indicate the presence of encephaloceles.

Classification

Encephaloceles of the face are generally classified as nasofrontal, nasoethmoidal, or naso-orbital. However, there can be some overlap in the type of encephalocele. They can also appear along any part of the cranial vault as they result from abnormal closure of cranial bones. The most common location for enncephaloceles is the occipital region. If the bulging portion contains only cerebrospinal fluid and the overlaying membrane, it may be called meningocele. If brain tissue is present, it may be referred to as meningoencephalocele.

Prevention

It is recommended that women who may become pregnant take 400 micrograms of folic acid daily.

Treatment

Currently, the only effective treatment for encephaloceles is reparative surgery, generally performed. during infancy. The extent to which it can be corrected depends on the location and size of the encephaloceles. However, large protrusions can be removed without causing major disability. Surgery repositions the bulging area back into the skull, removes the protrusions, and corrects the deformities, typically relieving pressure that can delay normal brain development. Occasionally, shunts are placed to drain excess cerebrospinal fluid from the brain.

The goals of treatment include:

- Closure of open skin defects to prevent infection and desiccation of brain tissue
- Removal of nonfunctional extracranial cerebral tissue with water-tight closure of the dura
- Total craniofacial reconstruction with particular emphasis on avoiding the long-nose deformity (nasal elongation that results from depression of the cribriform plate and nasal placode). Without proper management, the long-nose deformity can be more obvious after repair.

References

- Holmes, Anthony D.; Meara, John G.; Kolker, Adam R.; Rosenfeld, Jeffrey V.; Klug, Geoffrey L. (2001). 'Frontoethmoidal Encephaloceles: Reconstruction and Refinements'. The Journal of Craniofacial Surgery 12 (1): 6–18. PMID 11314190.
- 'Conditions + Treatments | Boston Children's Hospital'. Childrens hospital.org. Retrieved 2015-06-26

77. **Facial buttresses are related to:**
    a. Horizontal midface fractures
    b. Mandibular fractures
    c. Condylar fractures
    d. Rib fractures
    Ans. a

The anatomic region between the maxillary teeth and the infraorbital margin is referred to as the midface. Midface fractures typically affect certain areas. Le Fort was the first to classify the characteristics of these fractures.

Fracture classification by Le Fort (1901)

Le Fort's fracture classification is based on experimental examinations of dried skull bones and comprises three levels of fracture along the commonly occurring lines. Transverse fractures of the maxilla (outside the line of teeth) with typical lines of fracture:

LeFort I: Disarticulation of tooth-bearing part of the maxilla at the level of the floor of nose and maxillary sinuses (low-level fracture of the maxilla). The fracture line passes above the teeth roots, traversing the piriform aperture through the maxillary sinus and the pterygoid process. *Fracture line:* Piriform aperture, lateral antral wall, pterygoid process of the sphenoid bone.

LeFort II: Disarticulation of the maxilla and the nasal skeleton. The fracture line passes bilaterally from and through the nasal root caudal to the fronto nasal suture via the lacrimal bone and the orbital plate of the ethmoidal bone to the anterior and middle parts of the orbital floor, the middle part of the infraorbital margin, from there proceeding to the posterior antral wall via the lateral antral wall in an arch around the zygomatico alveolar crest, thus completely separating the pterygoid processes in the middle third, with additional fractures of the bony part of the nasal septum, the vomer and perpendicular plates of the ethmoidal bone. *Fracture line:* Above or inside the nasal bones, medial orbital wall, inferior orbital fissure, infraorbital foramen, supero-lateral antral wall, pterygoid process.

LeFort III: Disarticulation of the maxilla, the zygomatic bone and the nasal skeleton (high-level fracture of the midface) the fracture line passes medially-caudally to the fronto nasal and fronto maxillary suture via the lacrimal bone, the medial orbital wall, the orbital floor up to the inferior orbital fissure. From there, it extends caudally through the pterygopalatine fossa to the base of the pterygoid processes as well as from the anterior end of the inferior orbital fissure along the lateral orbital wall to the frontozygomatic fissure. The fracture of the midface is completed by the fracture of the zygomatic arch and the cranial bony part of the nasal septum. Le Fort III complex fractures of maxilla, zygomatic bone and nasal skeleton are relatively rare.

Possible combined fractures of the midface are:

Le Fort II fracture with fracture of the zygomatic bone
Le Fort I fracture with additional sagittal fracture
Unilateral or bilateral Le Fort II fractures combined with a unilateral fracture of the zygomatic bone

Wassmund classification of fractures (1927)

Wassmund type I fracture: Pyramidal fracture (Le Fort II) without involvement of the nasal skeleton.
Wassmund type II fracture: Equivalent to Le Fort II.

Wassmund type III fracture: Fracture of maxilla and zygomatic bones (Le Fort III) without involvement of the nasal skeleton Wassmund type IV fracture: Equivalent to Le Fort III.

Classification of midface fractures

In modern clinical practice, easily classifiable fractures of maxilla and mandible along anatomically weak points (Le Fort) rarely occur. Most injuries are complex fractures, often associated with comminuted fractures and major defects/bone loss. Therefore, the necessity of a more treatment-related classification has been recognized. Midface fractures are therefore classified according to their general position.

Lateral fractures (e.g. fractures of the zygomatic bone), centrolateral fractures (e.g. Le Fort III), and central midface fractures (e.g. Le Fort I and II, nasal bone and sagittal maxillary fractures) are differentiated. Additional classification system according to the affected region of the midface is also used:

- zygomatico-orbital complex (zygomatic bone, orbital floor),
- nasomaxillary complex (region around the piriform aperture),
- naso (orbito)-ethmoidal complex (ethmoid bone region),
- dento-alveolar complex.

Le Fort's classification, however, is still useful as a general and additional description of midface fractures as well as in orthognathic surgery.

Classification as central, centro lateral, and lateral midface fractures

Fractures of the central midface

- Le Fort I fractures
- Le Fort II fractures
- Fractures of the nasomaxillary complex:
  - Sagittal fracture of the maxilla
  - Fractures of the nasal skeleton
- Fractures of the nasoethmoidal complex
- Fractures of the dentoalveolar complex (alveolar process fractures)
- Irregular fractures
- Partial fractures and fractures where there has been bone loss

Fractures of the lateral midface

- Fractures of the zygomatico-orbital complex (fractures of the zygomatic bone and arch, isolated fracture of the lateral antral wall)
- Orbital fractures

Fractures of the centrolateral midface

- Naso-orbitoethmoidal fractures

Le Fort III fracture

Le Fort III fractures are also referred to as centrolateral fractures. The fracture line passes through the zygomatic arches, the lateral orbital wall and the frontal skull base. Combinations with other fracture lines and multiple fractures are possible. Craniofacial disarticulation (basal, pyramidal or at the level of the skull base) can be differentiated from unclassifiable fractures (comminuted fractures, fractures where there has been bone loss).

Buttress system of midface

Introduction:

The buttress system of midface is formed by strong frontal, maxillary, zygomatic and sphenoid bones and their attachments to one another. The central midface contains many fragile bones that could easily crumble when subjected to strong forces. These fragile bones are surrounded by thicker bones of the facial buttress system lending it some strength and stability.

Components of buttress system:

For better understanding the components of the facial buttress system have been divided into:

- Vertical buttresses
- Horizontal buttresses

Vertical buttress: These buttresses are very well developed. They include:

- Nasomaxillary
- Zygomaticomaxillay
  - Pterygomaxillay
  - Vertical mandible

Majority of the forces absorbed by midface are masticatory in nature. Hence the vertical buttresses are well developed in humans.

Horizontal buttresses: These buttresses interconnect and provide support for the vertical buttresses. They include:

- Frontal bar
- Infraorbital rim and nasal bones
- Hard palate and maxillary alveolus

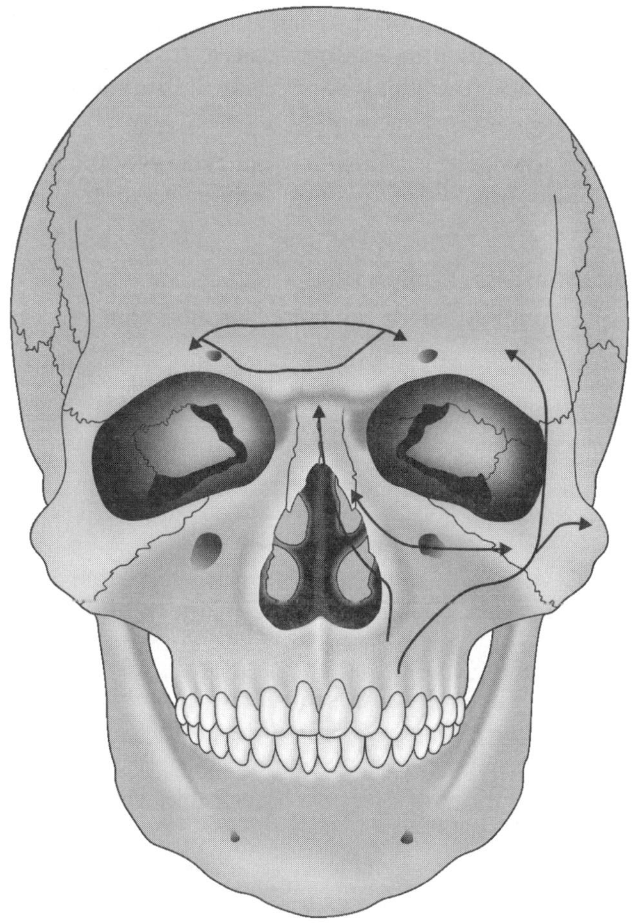

78. **The new concept in etiology of TMJ ankylosis is:**
    a. Hypercoagulabilty of blood
    b. Middle ear infection
    c. Neural theory
    d. Viral infection

Ans. a

The true traumatic microenvironment leading to TMJ ankylosis has not been identified. Although animal models and clinical observations have provided new evidence about the pathogenesis of traumatic TMJ bony ankylosis, the biological events and molecular mechanisms are far from being comprehensively understood. The hypotheses of hypertrophic nonunion and its supplement seem to grasp the nature of bony ankylosis and explain the development of the disease. A series of recent clinical and experimental studies have preliminarily verified the hypotheses at the cellular and molecular levels. Current data suggest that targeting pathways such as BMPs and Wnt signalling is likely to convert bony ankylosis into fibrous ankylosis. Alternatively, promoting MSCs of the radiolucent zone into adipocyte differentiation using FGF21 may be a promising strategy to prohibit the onset of bony ankylosis, and even avoid the occurrence of fibrous ankylosis.

79. A surgical procedure to restore the flow of tears into the nose from the lacrimal sac when the nasolacrimal duct does not function is called:

a. Dacrocystectomy
b. Dacrocystorhinostomy
c. Dacrocystotomy
d. Dacrodectomy

Ans. b

Toti first described the external approach in 1904. West described the endonasal approach in 1911. The latter approach fell out of favor because of difficult visualization and endonasal access to the lacrimal sac. However, with the newer, rigid telescopes, these difficulties have been overcome, resulting in a resurgence of the endoscopic technique. The occurrence of symptoms may be related to congenital or acquired causes.

Acquired causes include recurrent dacryocystitis and canaliculitis; dacryolithiasis; lacrimal system tumors; nasal pathology obstructing drainage; and trauma, which may be iatrogenic. An unidentifiable cause contributes to an idiopathic etiology.

Indications for dacryocystorhinostomy are as follows:

- Socially unacceptable epiphora caused by anatomic or functional lacrimal sac or nasolacrimal duct obstruction
- Chronic dacryocystitis with purulent drainage from the canaliculi
- Inflammation of the skin overlying the lacrimal sac in the region of the medial canthus
- Dacryolith formation
- Benign lacrimal sac mass

Contraindications

Relative ophthalmologic contraindications include the dry eye syndromes. Other contraindications include bleeding dyscrasias and other systemic deficiencies that would jeopardize surgery.

References

- Marcet MM, Kuk AK, Phelps PO. Evidence-based review of surgical practices in endoscopic endonasal dacryocystorhinostomy for primary acquired nasolacrimal duct obstruction and other new indications. Curr Opin Ophthalmol. 2014 Sep. 25(5):443-8.
- Sprekelsen MB, Barberan MT. Endoscopic dacryocystorhinostomy: surgical technique and results. Laryngoscope. 1996 Feb. 106 (2 Pt 1):187-9.
- Anari S, Ainsworth G, Robson AK. Cost-efficiency of endoscopic and external dacryocystorhinostomy. *J Laryngol Otol. 2007* Jul 19. 1-4.

80. Best approach for subcondylar fracture is:

a. Transparotid
b. Retromandibular
c. Trans-sphenoidal
d. Preauricular

Ans. a

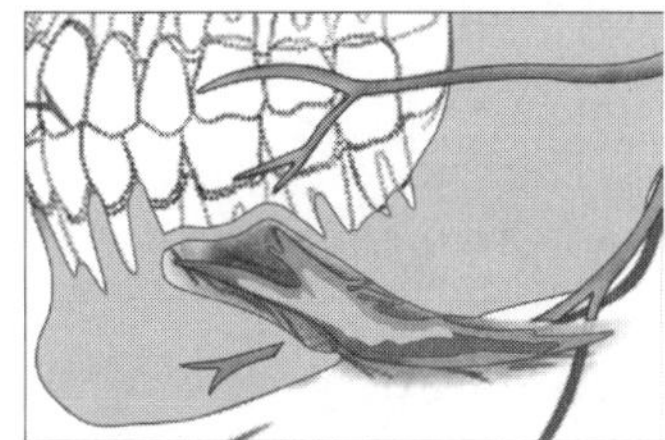

Use of existing lacerations

Frequently, patients with facial fractures also have lacerations. Very often, these existing soft-tissue injuries can be used to directly access the facial bones for management of the fractures.

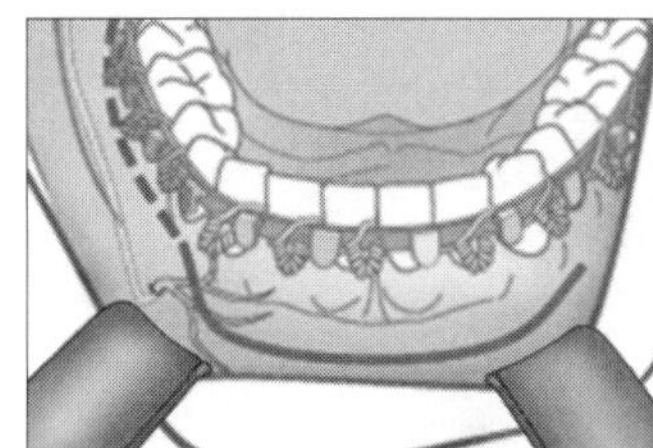

Intraoral approach to symphysis

The intraoral approach is the usual access for simple fractures of the body, symphysis, and angular regions.

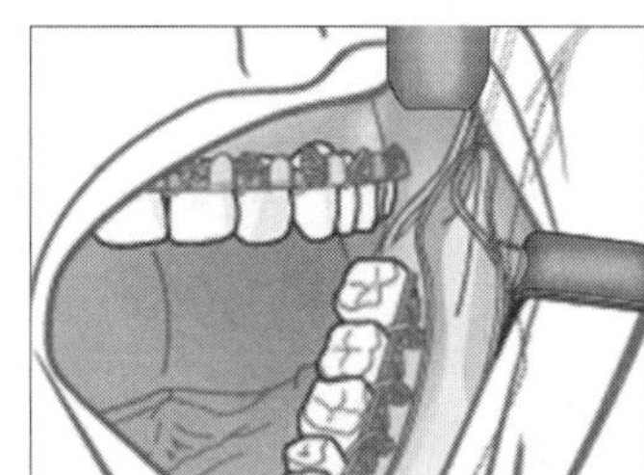

Intraoral approach to the angle

The intraoral approach is used for the majority of simple angle fractures.

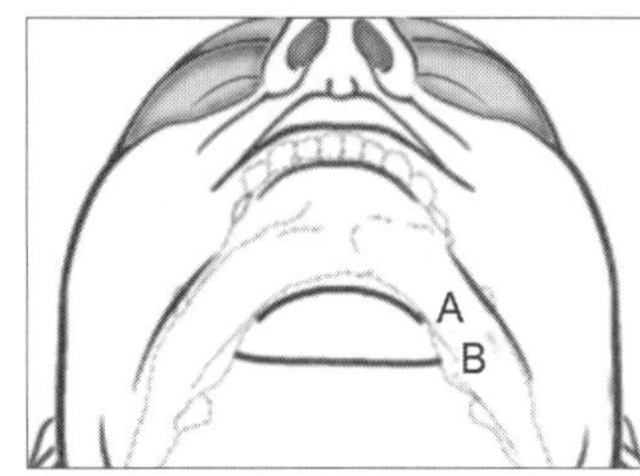

Submental approach

The submental approach is used to treat fractures of the anterior mandibular body and symphysis.

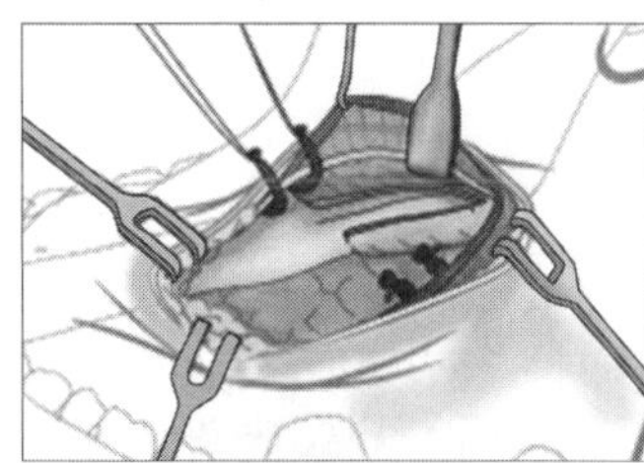

Submandibular approach

This approach is selected for fractures of the mandibular body and angle regions unsuitable for intraoral treatment.

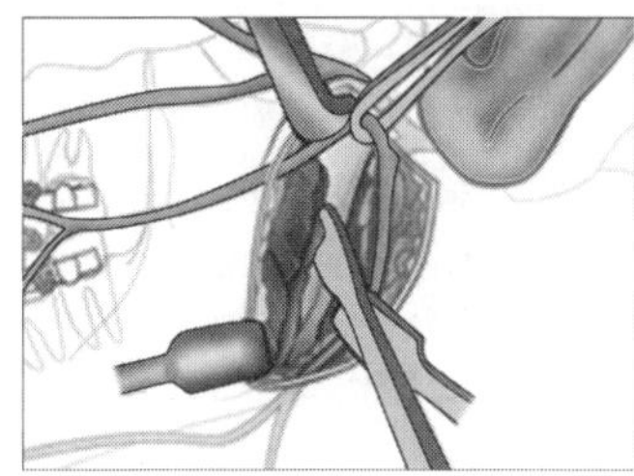

Retromandibular approaches

The retromandibular approaches expose the entire ramus from behind the posterior border. They therefore may be useful for procedures involving the area on or near the condylar process/head, or the ramus itself.

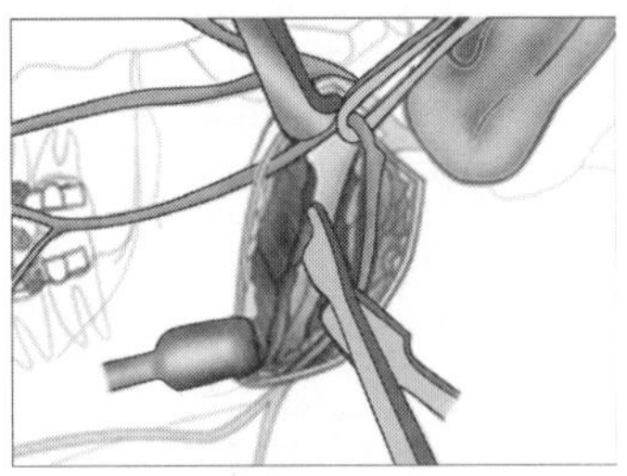

Facelift (rhytidectomy) approach

The facelift approach provides the same exposure as the retromandibular and preauricular accesses combined. The only difference is that the skin incision is placed in a more cosmetically acceptable location.

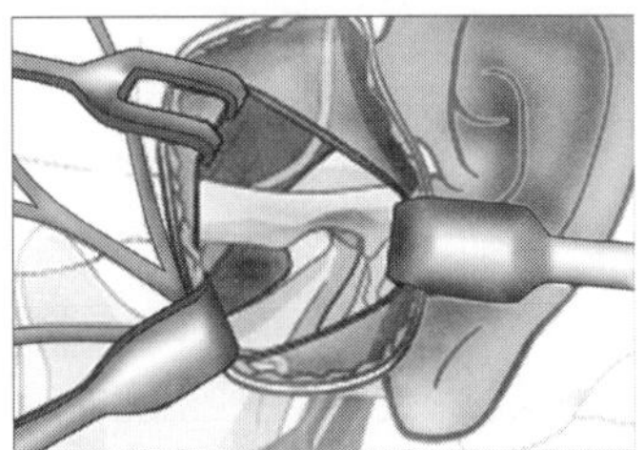

Preauricular approach

The preauricular approach can be used to access and treat fractures in the mandibular condylar head and neck region.

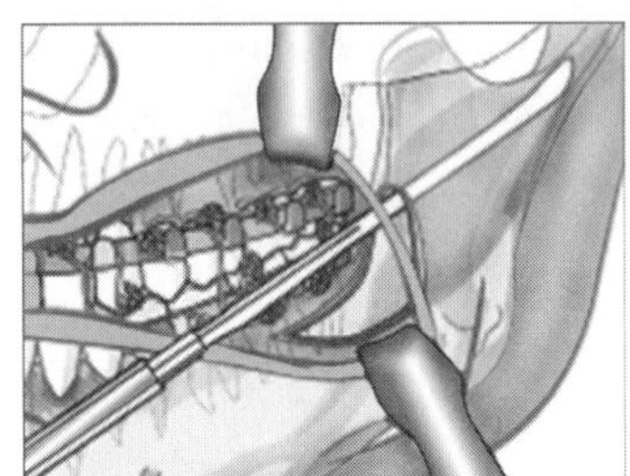

Intraoral approach to condyle

The ramus and condyle region can be exposed via an intraoral approach by extending the standard vestibular incision in a superior direction up the ascending ramus.

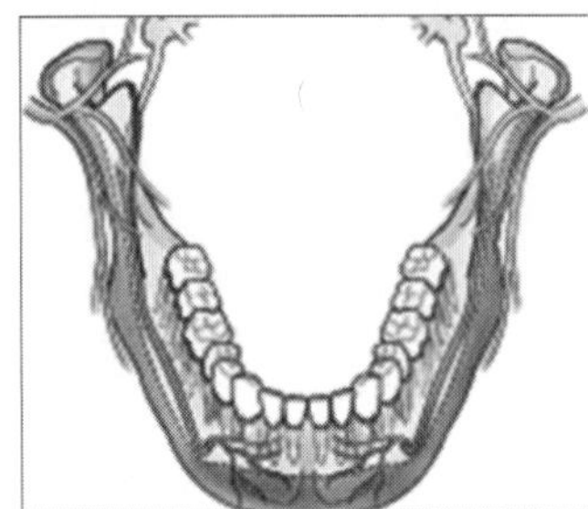

Safe zones

The safe zones for pin placement are located circumferentially around the whole continuity of the mandible along the lower and posterior borders and the condylar process.

Surgical Approaches to Subcondylar Fractures

During the application of surgical approaches, it is important to ensure that the surgeon is able to conduct anatomic reduction under direct vision of the completely exposed fractured end. To treat subcondylar fractures, several surgical approaches have been reported and each approach has its own set of advantages and disadvantages. Therefore, the choice of surgical approach depends on the need to create an optimal view of the whole subcondyle without injury to the facial nerve or to the vascularization to the condylar head during surgery.

Mini-retromandibular approach to low subcondylar fractures

The retromandibular incision was first proposed by Hinds and Girotti in 1967. It is favored by surgeons because it provides good visualization of the lower subcondyle and the entire ramus from the posterior border. Compared with the submandibular incision, this incision is closer to the subcondyle; therefore, it provides direct access to the fractured line of the subcondyle and it enables straightforward fracture management, thus facilitating the reduction of the subcondyle. Furthermore, it allows the surgeon to work perpendicularly to the fracture so that excessive retraction can be avoided and use of a transfacial trocar is not necessary. It can also avoid direct contact with the facial nerve and preserves the integrity of the parotid gland as well as its capsule and leaves a barely noticeable scar in a relatively hidden region. The skin incision of this approach is located just posterior to the mandibular ramus and the most proximal point of the incision is just below the ear lobe, runs parallel down to the posterior border of the mandible, and is limited to 25 mm in length (Figure). After the skin incision, the subcutaneous dissection allows for the extension of the surgical wound to the level of the fracture. After exposing the superficial musculoaponeurotic system (SMAS), a vertical incision is made through the SMAS behind the parotid gland. Blunt dissection is made through the parotid gland and masseteric fascia towards the posterior border of the mandible. This permits preservation of the facial nerve fibers, which are easily identified when they pass superficially to the masseter muscle and can be protected with a retractor . After reaching the mandibular angle, the pterygomasseteric sling is thinned out until the bone surface becomes visible. A sharp cut is made through the periosteum at the posterior border of the ascending ramus, opening access to the whole ramus, which is dissected subperiosteally. The periosteum at the posterior border of the ramus is then incised, and subperiosteal dissection is continued to the condylar area until the fracture line and the displaced or dislocated proximal fragment are identified. The fragment is then repositioned under direct visualization of the fracture line. Anatomical adjustment can be facilitated by pulling the mandible downwards. After aligning the fragment, stable plate or screw osteosynthesis is carried out. The posterior border of the ramus and the mandibular notch serve as reference lines for correct three dimensional repositioning.

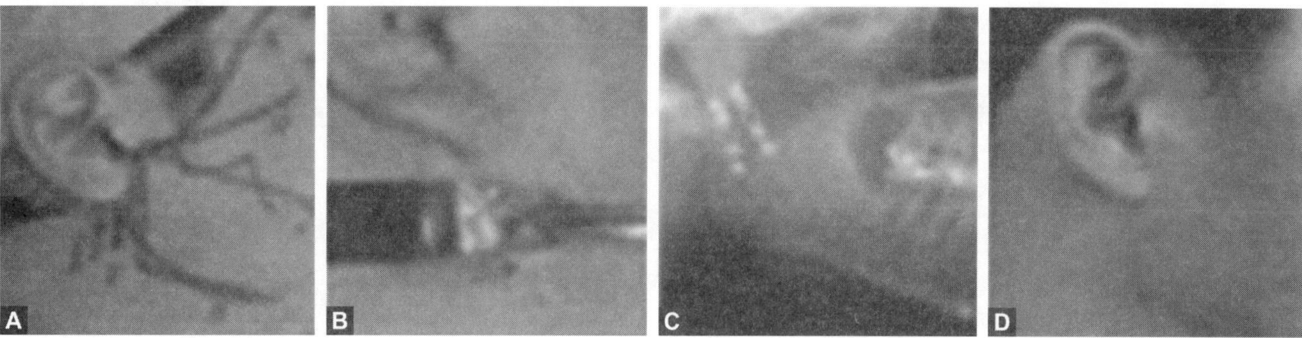

Figure: Mini-retromandibular approach to low subcondylar fractures

Wound closure is performed in layers after checking mandibular mobility and dental occlusion. A silastic drain is inserted close to the fracture line, with the exit location at the lower border of the incision line. The first step is refixation of the pterygomasseteric sling, followed by closure of the subcutaneous and cutaneous layers. The skin sutures are removed one week later. After the wound has fully healed, the scar is hardly visible.

Modified retromandibular approach to high subcondylar fractures

There are some limitations with regard to retromandibular approaches, in that, if the subcondylar fractures are located in the high subcondyle and close to the condylar head, the space that can be exposed with this approach is restricted; therefore, we modify the retromandibular incision. The modified retromandibular approach provides the same exposure as the retromandibular and preauricular accesses combined, and it may be useful for procedures involving the high subcondylar region . This approach provides a direct approach to the high subcondylar region and the distance from the skin incision to that region is reduced, compared to that of the routine retromandibular approach. The skin incision runs from the intertragal notch through the use of a gently curved incision around the ear lobule and uses the upper part of the retromandibular incision (Figure). After transection of the skin, the skin flap is elevated, taking care not to injure the great auricular nerve, which lies over the sternocleidomastoid muscle, and the subcutaneous dissection is extended to the level of the fracture. After exposing the SMAS, a vertical incision is made through the SMAS onto the parotid gland extending from the earlobe towards the gonial angle. As soon as the globular parotid tissue appears from the fascial incision, blunt dissection with a mosquito is used. When the trunk of the facial nerve or the temporofacial and cervicofacial division is exposed, the branches are retracted either superiorly or inferiorly depending on the location of the condylar fracture. Once the posterior border of the mandible is reached, an incision is made through the pterygomasseteric sling. A periosteal elevator is used in order to strip the masseter muscle from the ramus and dissect superiorly to expose the fractured end along the posterior border of the condylar process. After fracture reduction and plating, the pterygomasseteric sling is reapproximated with sutures. The wound is also reapproximated in layers, and the SMAS is resuspended. Any violation of the parotid gland capsule must be closed tightly to prevent salivary fistula. A small drain placed into the subcutaneous space may be necessary to prevent a hematoma. The skin and subcutaneous tissue are then closed.

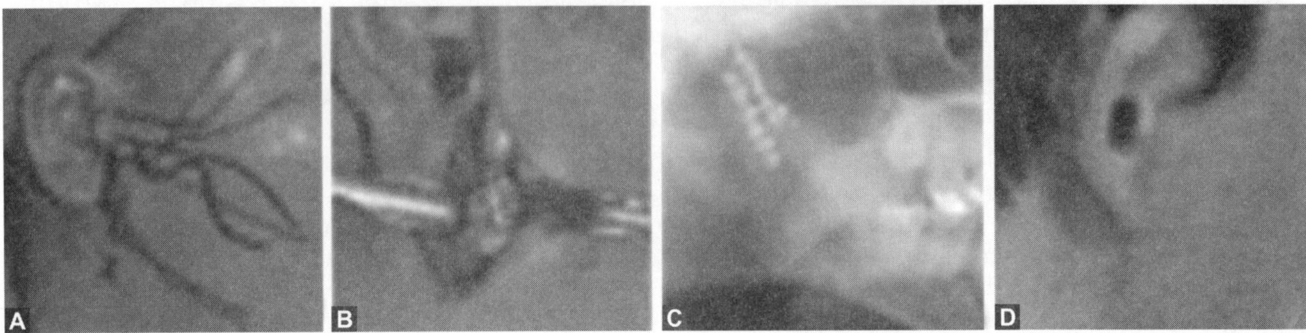

Figure: Modified retromandibular approach to high subcondylar fractures